Nursing for Public Health:

Promotion, Principles, and Practice

Edited by

Paul Linsley   Roslyn Kane   Sara Owen

University of Lincoln

OXFORD
UNIVERSITY PRESS

OXFORD
UNIVERSITY PRESS

Great Clarendon Street, Oxford OX2 6DP

Oxford University Press is a department of the University of Oxford.
It furthers the University's objective of excellence in research, scholarship,
and education by publishing worldwide in

Oxford New York

Athens Auckland Bangkok Bogotá Buenos Aires Calcutta
Cape Town Chennai Dar es Salaam Delhi Florence Hong Kong Istanbul

Karachi Kuala Lumpur Madrid Melbourne Mexico City Mumbai

Nairobi Paris São Paulo Singapore Taipei Tokyo Toronto Warsaw

With associated companies in Berlin Ibadan
Oxford is a registered trade mark of Oxford University Press
in the UK and in certain other countries

Published in the United States
by Oxford University Press Inc., New York

British Library Cataloguing in Publication Data

Data available

Library of Congress Cataloguing in Publication Data

Data available

ISBN 978-0-19-9561087

10 9 8 7 6 5 4 3 2 1

Typeset in Calibri
by Glyph International, Bangalore, India
Printed in Italy
on acid-free paper by
L.E.G.O. S.p.A. – Lavis TN

Foreword

Tony Butterworth

At the time of writing this foreword, the global financial situation is parlous, and as a consequence of this, funding for health care and the provision of nursing care is more difficult to predict than ever before. What is certain is that such resources as are available will have to be used to the very best effect. I am therefore delighted to write a foreword to this most timely publication. My pleasure is prompted by several recurrent themes that the reader will find in the chapters of this book. The themes are based on a practical understanding and delivery of nursing care that is embraced by a model of public health that uses limited resources to best advantage.

Old divisions of labour between care in hospital, care in the community or the home and services that encourage the development of healthy development and healthy adult living are redundant and nurses will need to work together with the population and its 'health career' as never before. Continuity of care and pathways of care are the rediscovered cornerstones of emerging health policies in many countries. However, realising these policies will require nurses who can understand and apply the principles of public health and its practical application. This book offers insight into those important principles and their practice.

At its most simple, understanding public health is not complicated. The mantra of public health and its three interwoven elements - primary prevention (stop it happening), secondary prevention (catch it early) and tertiary prevention (treat it effectively and promptly) offers a purposeful and pragmatic model of health care delivery that has as much value today as it has ever had.

Those necessarily simple formulations of prevention and health were started by the public health reformers of the Victorian age and were enthusiastically pursued after the second war and then once more during the baby boomer generation of the 1960's. It is clear that public health is now being re-visited by policy planners and service providers in the first decades of this Century. Just as the 'old' public health offered a revolution through great public works affecting water supply, sanitation and food, the 'new' public health can build on these fundamentals by embracing new scientific discoveries produced by the 'post-genomic' research revolution, information technology and adventurous organisational design.

Interestingly, the publication of the first edition of this book coincides with the centenary celebration of the work of Florence Nightingale our professional founder. We can see that since her inspiring and intelligent work laid the foundations for the profession, nurses have reacted to the demands of public health in noble and innovative ways. We have specialists who have responded to each of the three elements of preventive public health. Midwives and health visitors are our most visible manifestation in the contribution to primary prevention. Nurses based in primary care services (practice nurses, primary care nurse practitioners and district nurses) are in the vanguard of secondary prevention and the greater workforce of hospital based nurses offer the key to effective treatment that can be supported by outreach nurses, district nurses and nurses specialising in the care of chronic and long term conditions such as Admiral nurses working in dementia care and MacMillan nurses in cancer care. In these ways the profession makes a spectacular contribution to the population's health and well being.

Like all health care professionals we have been guilty of a creeping reductionism whereby hospital nursing retains its glamorous and exciting image of 'where it's all at' and the less publicised but fundamentally important other elements of prevention and recovery and the contribution of nurses and midwives remain less well articulated. It is important to redress this view such that continuity of care through public health is better recognized. This book allows us to do that.

Our nurse workforce is often viewed in terms of sufficient numbers and the signature tune of 'enough people in the right place at the right time' has been heard repeatedly. This focus on capacity is important but one-dimensional. Less well heard is capability, in other words the necessary education, skills and competencies that nurses must have to undertake their work effectively. This book offers insights and practical advice that consider this necessary intelligence and information. It describes interventions that span the public health model and attempts to re-balance our understanding of the patient journey. In doing so it focuses on more than the requirements for safe and effective hospital care, although these episodes are significant and important. What brings people into hospital care and what happens to them after it are of equal importance and nurses must be able to understand and work within this more complete frame of reference.

In revisiting the principles to be found in this book it may well be possible to re-examine the way in which the profession has crafted its career structures. In the United Kingdom as elsewhere Government and the profession has tried to look again at the way in which nurses work and how they are educated and deployed. One of our most recent reviews (DH 2010) has led to twenty recommendations which are both important and sensible in their focus. The trick of course lies in realising them. It can be argued that this book offers a timely contribution to the work of reviews such as that. A nursing profession that can work comfortably in a model of public health (an ambition of this book) will go some way towards realising the ambitions of modern nursing.

Finally, in writing this foreword I am struck by several underpinning messages that the profession and indeed health care services must take on board

- The fashion to dismiss ideas as 'out of date' must not be applied to well found models of nursing and public health. Good science builds and refines good ideas, it does not reject them out of hand because they may be showing their age. Public health is as relevant today as ever. The refinements and relevance of public health nursing are clearly demonstrated in this book.
- The profession has wasted both resources and time in 'retraining' nurses to work in the community setting. The particular specialities that are now demanded by hospital care are likely to be those that require further specialist training. If public health is understood and embraced during professional preparation then fitness to practice in the community becomes the norm not the unusual. Affordable health care will require this norm be firmly established.
- The profession has a duty to help the population at large understand how public health works. Connections between smoking, diet, exercise and stressful lifestyles are better understood than ever before. Nurse work must reflect this such that the promotion of healthy childhood, early behavioural interventions, screening for disease and models of prompt intervention are reflected in the way that nurses work and offer their services.
- In celebrating the work of Florence Nightingale one hundred years on, can we re-shape our profession so that we can embrace the foundations of public health, adopt new findings from science and take advantage of a clearer understanding of interventions and their outcomes?

I think these final observations and questions can and should be answered by nurses. This book sets a new tone while resting on known good practices. I welcome its publication and I am sure its readers will find it offers them support and thoughtful insights.

Tony Butterworth
Emeritus Professor of Health Care Workforce Innovation
August 2010, Manchester.

Preface and acknowledgements

Nursing for Public Health: Promotion, Principles, and Practice is an essential resource for all nursing students, nurses undertaking further study and mentors. It reflects the growing need for all nurses to become involved in the promotion of health and well-being of both their patients and of the wider population. The book seeks to provide a clear, academic and practical account of the increasing importance of public health knowledge for all nursing practice. It explores and critiques core theories, policies and models before demonstrating the essential public health skills required for all nurses practicing in the twenty-first century.

Until very recently, public health has been taught mainly at the postgraduate level, either as part of a professional qualification or degree. However, contemporary health care and nursing practice now requires that public health matters are taught increasingly at the pre-qualification stage and constitute an integral part of the future development and learning of the nurse. This book is designed to unpack the public health knowledge and skills required at the point of registration and in everyday practice respectively. Thus the text provides a comprehensive overview of contemporary nursing practice, set within the context of integrated services, collaborative practice and partnership working, identifying key challenges and some solutions for today's nurse.

All the contributors have first hand experience of working within the public health arena and are specialists within their field of practice. This not only ensures the content is mapped to key international policy and evidence, but also grounds the content of the book in reality, and provides pragmatic application.

This book has been written specifically with the purpose of informing and empowering nursing students and staff who, as the future nursing workforce, have a crucial role to play in supporting and promoting health.

We would like to acknowledge and thank all those who have contributed to this book.

Thank you to each of the authors for their enthusiasm and support and the many people who have assisted the contributors with their development of ideas for individual chapters.

Thanks also to the many people involved in the peer review process, including academics, practitioners and current undergraduate students, whose expertise, comments and constructive criticisms have helped shape the book.

We are especially grateful to two former University of Lincoln nursing students — Daniel Gray and Kati Lucas — for permitting us to include copies of their personal reflections from clinical practice in Chapter 6.

We would also like to thank the staff at Oxford University Press for supporting the publication of this book. In particular, Geraldine Jeffers the Commissioning Editor for managing the whole process so efficiently, Holly Edmundson the Commissioning Assistant for her help with the art work and Joanna Hardern the production editor for producing the final book.

We offer our special thanks to Lucinda Gazzard at the University of Lincoln, for all her hard work in managing the administration and co-ordination of the book.

Paul Linsley, Roslyn Kane, Sara Owen
University of Lincoln

Contents

Detailed table of contents

Detailed table of contents

List of figure acknowledgements

Fig.3.1 J. Kuhl, & J. Beckman (Eds.), *Action-control: From cognition to behavior* (pp. 11-39). Heidelberg, Germany: Springer.

Fig. 3.2 Prochaska, J. O. and C. C. DiClemente (1983). 'Stages and processes of self-change of smoking: Toward an integrative model of change'. *Journal of Consulting and Clinical al Psychology* 51(3): 390-395.

Fig. 3.3 Bandura, A. (1977). *Social Learning Theory*. New York: General Learning Press.

Fig. 6.2 Arnstein, S. R. (1969). 'A Ladder of Citizen Participation', *JAIP* 35(4): 216-224.

Fig. 7.2 © 2010 InTouch Technologies, Inc.

Fig. 10.1 Ewles, L. & Simnett's, I. (2003). *Planning Model: Promoting health, a practical guide* (5th edn.) Edinburgh: Bailliere Tindall. Copyright Elsevier.

Fig. 10.2 Green, L.W., & Kreuter, M.W. (4th edn. in press). Health Promotion Planning: An Educational and Environmental Approach, Palo Alto: Mayfield Publishing Co.

Fig. 12.4, Fig. 12.5 Siriwardena A.N. (2009). Using quality improvement methods for evaluating health care. *Quality Primary Care* 17: 155-159. Reproduced with permission of Radcliffe Publishing.

Fig. 12.7, Fig. 12.8 Siriwardena A.N., Shaw, D., Donohoe, R., Black, S., Stephenson, J. (2010). Development and pilot of clinical performance indicators for English ambulance services. *Emergency Medical Journal* 27: 327-331.

Fig. 12.9 Siriwardena, A.N. (2006). Releasing the potential of health services: translating clinical leadership into healthcare quality improvement. *Quality in Primary Care* 14: 128. Reproduced with permission of Radcliffe Publishing.

Fig. 12.10 Siriwardena, A.N., Apekey, T., Tilling, M., Ørner, R.J., Qureshi, M.Z., Dyas, J., & Middleton, H. (2008). Developing a psychosocial intervention for sleep problems presenting to primary care (REST: Resources for Effective Sleep Treatment). In: *'The future of primary care'*. Southampton University 15-17 September 2008'.

Fig. 13.1 © Bettmann/CORBIS.

Fig. 13.2 European Health for All database, WHO 2010 http://data.euro.who.int/hfadb/.

Fig. 13.3 Fletcher, C., Peto, R. (1977). The natural history of chronic airflow obstruction, *British Medical Journal* 1:1645-1648. Reproduced with permission from BMJ Publishing Group Ltd.

Fig. 14.1 D Dahlgren, G. and Whitehead, M.,(1998). Health Inequalities, London: HMSO.

Fig. 14.2 Cartoon by George Whitelaw, Daily Herald, 1942. Obtained with help from the British Cartoon Archive, University of Kent, www.cartoons.ac.uk. © Mirrorpix.

Fig. 15.1 © Crown copyright.

Fig. 15.2, Fig. 15.5, Fig 15.6a, Fig 15.6b © 2010, The Health and Social Care Information Centre.

Fig. 15.4 © Crown copyright.

About the authors

Editors

Paul Linsley (MMedSci(Hel), BMedSci(Nur), RGN, RMN, RNT, AdipAcutePsyh, DipMHS) began his nursing career as a general nurse working within acute medicine. Following conversion to mental health nursing he gained valuable experience in a variety of clinical settings. Paul is registered as a clinical specialist in acute psychiatry and is trained in cognitive behavioural therapy. As a senior lecturer at the University of Lincoln he teaches on a number of courses, single and joint honours undergraduate programmes, research masters programmes and pre and post registration nurse training programmes. He has written on and has an interest in acute mental health and health informatics.

Roslyn Kane (PhD, MSc, BSc, RGN, RNT, FHEA) is a Senior Lecturer at the University of Lincoln. After working for some years as a nurse in women's health, she worked for ten years in the Department of Public Health and Policy at the London School of Hygiene and Tropical Medicine where she did her PhD. She has worked on many research projects, mainly around sexual and reproductive health, teenage pregnancy and service evaluation.

Sara Owen (PhD, BA, BEd, RMN, SRN, RNT) is Professor of Nursing and Dean of the Faculty of Health, Life and Social Sciences at the University of Lincoln. She has research interests in women and mental health, workforce issues, and evaluation of education and training.

Contributors

Iain Armstrong is a consultant in alcohol policy and workforce development in the substance misuse field and from 2005–10 has been an advisor to the Alcohol Policy Team in the Department of Health in England where he leads on training for health professionals to support policy implementation. He is Chair of the DOH Alcohol Improvement Programme Workforce Development Group, a member of the Steering group for the Substance Misuse in the Undergraduate Medical Curriculum project (International Centre for Drugs Policy) and was the Department's lead editor on a number of policy documents including: 'Safe, Sensible, Social: The next steps in the National Alcohol Strategy' (2007), and 'Models of Care for Alcohol Misusers' (2006).

From 1995-2004, Iain was Head of Training and Consultancy for Alcohol Concern and from 1998–2006 was a member of the Management Committee for the development of the Drugs and Alcohol National Occupational Standards (DANOS).

Sonia Budgen (RGN, DipN, MSc) is a clinical domain and solution specialist at Computer Science Corporation and until very recently has been maintaining her clinical practice as a Triage Nurse in an out of hours setting. She has actively been involved in the RCN Information in Nursing Forum since 2004; ensuring nurses are informed about the importance of information technology through workshops at the annual congress, articles in the nursing press and representation at various events. She has 27 years of experience in the NHS in various roles—latterly in management and the implementation of clinical information systems. Her dissertation explored a best way to implement clinical information systems with nurses. Her move from the NHS was to influence the design and implementation of clinical information systems to ensure they are useable at the coal face.

Andrew Finney (BSc, Dip, RN, PGCHE) is a Lecturer in Nursing at Keele University School of Nursing and Midwifery. He is also undertaking research at the Arthritis Research UK Primary Care Centre. Andrew has published a number of papers in nursing specific journals and has recently published a chapter in the text book 'Study Skills for Nurses' 4th edition (2010). Andrew is a reviewer for the journal 'Nurse Education Today'.

Nigel Horner (BA, MSW, CQSW, PGCE) is Deputy Head of the School of Health and Social Care at the University of Lincoln. He is the author of What is Social Work (2009, 3rd edition), co-author (with Steve Krawczyk) of Social Work in Education and Children's Services (2006) and co-editor (with Adam Barnard and Jim Wild) of The Value Base of Social Work and Social Care: An Active Learning Handbook (2008). He is currently working on an EU / TEMPUS project to support social work education in Russia.

John Hurley (PhD, MSc, RGN, RMN) is a Senior Lecturer in Mental Health nursing at the University of Dundee. He teaches on a number of pre and post registration courses and is vastly experienced in community and crisis intervention work. In addition, Dr Hurley is a qualified counsellor and gestalt therapist. He maintains links with the mental health services within his home country of Australia, as well as advising and helping shape mental health services in Scotland.

Maria Joyce (MSc, BSc, RHV, RM, RGN, RNT, CPT, FHEA) is a Senior Lecturer in nursing at the University of Lincoln. With extensive experience as a health visitor working in both inner city and rural locations, she specializes in teaching public health. She is currently a doctoral student in the Centre for Education and Research undertaking qualitative research. She has a particular interest in narrative methods, particularly in women's experiences of educational leadership and is a member of a variety of narrative research groups. Her current role involves managing the extensive Learning Beyond Registration programme which provides continuing professional education for registered health professionals.

Jill Ladlow (RGN, RM, MSc, BSc (Hons), PGCE) is a Nurse Consultant for Sexual Health in the Northern Lincolnshire and Goole Hospitals NHS Foundation Trust, where she has worked since January 1984 in all areas of midwifery practice and now within the field of Sexual Health. Jill works closely with a dedicated sexual health team, to assist the implementation of the National Strategy for Sexual Health and HIV, working together with hospital services and primary care to meet sexual health needs of people. Raising awareness of 'Safer Sex' Messages and Sexual Health Promotion are important aspects of the role, reaching people of all ages and cultural groups. Jill is also family planning trained and a non-medical prescriber and developed guidelines, patient group directions and scope packages to facilitate nurse-led activity within the local Contraception, Advice and Sexual Health (CASH) Services.

Vicki Linsley (Dip Resp Dis Man RGN) is COPD Nurse Specialist at Grantham and District Hospital. She has experience of working in intensive care and acute medicine prior to her current role of COPD Nurse Specialist. This role for the last 5 years has involved COPD supported discharge, admission avoidance and involvement in pulmonary rehabilitation. She is currently undertaking a degree in long-term conditions with Nottingham University.

Ian Loveday (MSc, PGCert, Bsc (Hons), BA (Hons), RN) is an Emergency Care Practitioner for DHU working in out of hours primary care in Derbyshire. He has been published on issues relating to prescribing and emergency care. In the past he has worked in A&E and at Sheffield Hallam University as a senior lecturer in nursing. He still holds a position as an associate lecturer in nursing at Sheffield Hallam University and lectures on a range of subjects.

Sian Maslin-Prothero (RN, RM, DipN, CertEd, MSc, PhD) is Professor of Health and Ageing and former Dean of the Graduate School and Professor of Nursing at the Keele University, Staffordshire in the United Kingdom. She has worked in academia, education, clinical nursing and midwifery in a variety of settings in both the United Kingdom and Australia. Sian is Conjoint Professor at the University of Newcastle, New South Wales and Adjunct Professor at Edith Cowan University, Perth, Australia. She has a Masters of Science degree from the University of Bristol and a Doctor of Philosophy from the University of Nottingham. Her research interests include user and carer involvement in health and

About the authors

social care, and older people. She is widely published, with many of her books being translated into other languages, such as 'Bailliere's Study Skills for Nurses and Midwives' now in its 4th edition, and 'Blackwell's Dictionary of Nursing' with Dawn Freshwater. She is the Associate Editor for Nurse Education Today and a member of the editorial board for the European Journal of Cancer Care.

Abigail Masterson (MPA, MN, BSc, RN, PGCEA, FRSA) has been running her own consultancy company since 1998. She has carried out many policy orientated projects for professional organizations, regulatory bodies and Government departments. She has had a long interest in health policy and politics and has edited several books and written many articles in these areas.

Sheena MacRae (BSc, MA) is Programme Co-ordinator for Sexual Health in the Specialist Health Promotion Service of North East Lincolnshire Council. She works collaboratively with a range of practitioners around sexual health, promoting sex education for all, training for professionals, working in partnership to develop projects supporting positive sexual health, providing advice and guidance on policy and practice. Previously Sheena worked in the drugs field in peer-led harm reduction, community rehabilitation and as a Trainer and Project Consultant with HIT in Liverpool, a company specializing in public health inverventions and social marketing.

John McKinnon (MSc, PGDip, BA (Hons)) is a Senior Lecturer in Nursing at the University of Lincoln. He is currently a doctoral student with the University of London. He has been a registered nurse since 1979 qualifying and practicing across adult, mental health and public health branches of Nursing and Midwifery Council Register. Throughout the 1990's he pioneered a range of public health initiatives. He is a former non-medical prescribing lead and the editor of 'Towards Prescribing Practice'. His experience as a nurse specialist in child protection and child rights advocate has led him to write a number of papers on safeguarding children and he has published widely on intuitive knowledge and the ethics of the nurse patient relationship.

Damian Mitchell (RGN RMN, MHEA) is the National Improvement Lead for the Alcohol Improvement Programme, Department of Health. He has previously held the posts of Senior Consultant with the Care Services Improvement Partnership, National Lead, Health and Social Care in Criminal Justice Programme, Subject Lead for Mental Health, Justice and Offender Services within the School of Interprofessional Care, National Health Service University and Head of Healthcare Training for the Prison Service (England and Wales) and is a former Lecturer in Mental Health Nursing at the University of Nottingham. Damian has published numerous journal articles on Mental Health and is the co-editor of 'Mental Health Nursing: From Acute Concerns to the Capable Practitioner' (London: Sage Publications). He has a degree in Applied Social Science, a Post Graduate Certificate in Academic Practice (PGCAP) and a Masters degree in Applied Research and Quality Evaluation and is a member of the Higher Education Academy.

Alison Mostyn (BSc, PhD, PGCHE, FHEA) is a Lecturer in Comparative Cellular Physiology at the School of Veterinary Medicine and Science at the University of Nottingham. She is the author of many peer reviewed journal articles on adipose tissue physiology and the impact of size at birth upon future health. Alison has been the academic advisor for the Nottingham city based childhood obesity programme 'Go 4 It' since 2005.

Dilip Nathan (BMedSci (Hons), BMBS, MRCP, FRCPCH, MMedSci) is a consultant community paediatrician who helped establish a Nottingham City wide obesity intervention programme. He continues to conduct research within obesity involving both preschool and in older children. He is an NHS consultant at the Nottingham University Hospitals Trust, UK and in addition to clinical responsibilities as Team leader of the Nottingham City Central area, is also the Designated Paediatrician for Unexpected Death (Nottingham), undergraduate coordinator for Community Paediatrics at Nottingham University and has a part time appointment within a specific project for child obesity within the Collaboration for Leadership in Applied Research and Care (National Institute for Heath Research). He was formerly the Academic Convenor of the British Association of Community Child Health.

Tracy Pilcher (MSc, RGN, PGDip Autonomous Practice, DipHe Critical Care) is Deputy Chief Nurse at the United Lincolnshire Hospitals Trust. She is responsible for workforce development and education. Tracy has an extensive clinical background in critical care and is currently the Chair of the British Association of Critical Care Nurses. She has published predominantly in the field of critical care leadership and practice.

Dianne Ramm (MSc, RGN, Dip. DN) is a Senior Lecturer in Nursing at the University of Lincoln, leading on the development of clinical skills within the undergraduate nursing programme (Adult Branch). Dianne has a district nursing background and a specialist knowledge of continence care, and was formerly employed as Clinical Nurse Specialist/Countywide Professional Advisor for Continence for Lincolnshire Community Health Services. She is currently undertaking her Post Graduate Certificate of Education at the University of Lincoln.

Ruth Reilly (MMed. Sci. BA, RGN RHV FHEA) is a Senior Lecturer in Nursing at the University of Lincoln. Ruth has been a nurse, health visitor and practising educationalist in excess of thirty years. Previously she was part of the multi professional collaborating group of commissioners and service colleagues who developed the BSc (Hons) Public Health programme currently being delivered at the University. Her teaching and research interests are in health inequalities, clinical governance and mentorship in nursing practice.

Laura Serrant-Green (PhD, MA, BA, RGN, PGCE) is Professor of Community and Public Health Nursing at The University of Lincoln. She has extensive experience in public health research, teaching and policy development nationally and internationally. She is a visiting professor at the University of the West Indies (School of Advanced Nursing education) and was part of the Prime Minister's commission on the Future of Nursing and midwifery in England 2010.

Trevor Simpson (BSc, PGDE RN) is a Lecturer in Nursing at the University of Lincoln where he is a member of the programme team for the BSc (Hons) Nursing. He has extensive experience in critical care nursing and inter-professional learning and working in practice. He has a special interest in the use of alternative media to promote clinical skills learning for health and social care students. He is currently undertaking a Masters Programme in Clinical Research.

A. Niroshan Siriwardena (MBBS, MMedSci, PhD, FRCGP DCH, DRCOG) is a General Practitioner and Professor of Primary and Pre-hospital Care at the University of Lincoln. His interests centre on quality improvement in primary and pre-hospital care. He is editor of the international journal Quality in Primary Care and co-editor of "The Quality and Outcomes Framework: QOF—Transforming General Practice" (2010).

Grace Spencer (BSc (Hons), RN (adult), MPH, MRes) is a postgraduate researcher at the Thomas Coram Research Unit, Institute of Education. Her research interests include the investigation of young people's perspectives on health and health related risks. Her current research examines concepts of empowerment in relation to young people's health and health promotion and she has published in this field in a number of nursing and health related journals. As a qualified nurse and Lecturer in Public Health, she has worked on community health development projects in Australia, Tanzania, South Africa, Brazil, and the UK.

Rachael Spencer (MSc, BSc, RGN, RM, RHV, RNT) is an experienced nurse, midwife and health visitor, who is currently working as a Senior Lecturer in Nursing at the University of Lincoln. Rachael has an undergraduate degree in public health nursing, a Masters degree in health care education, and is currently writing up her doctoral thesis "An exploration of breastfeeding experiences". Rachael teaches research methods and methodology, public health, and ethical, legal and professional perspectives of health care across a range of undergraduate and postgraduate programmes.

List of abbreviations

AAF	Alcohol Attributable Fractions
ABV	Alcohol by Volume
ADHD	Attention Deficit Hyperactivity Disorder
AIDS	Acquired Immunodeficiency Syndrome
AL	Activities of Living
ALC	Alcohol Learning Centre
ANARP	Alcohol Needs Assessment Research Assessment Project
ANMC	Australian Nursing and Midwifery Council
APHA	American Public Health Association
ARC	Arthritis Research Campaign
ASH	Action for Smoking and Health
AUDIT	Alcohol Use Disorder Identification Test
BASHH	British Association for Sexual Health and HIV
BMI	Body Mass Index
BNF	British National Formulary
CAF	Common Assessment Framework
CAIPE	Centre for the Advancement of Inter-professional Education
CCF	Congestive Cardiac Failure
CDC	Centre for Disease Control
CDSS	Clinical Decision Support Software
CDX	Community Development Exchange
CEIMH	Centre of Excellence in Inter-Disciplinary Mental Health
CfH	Connecting for Health
CHAI	Commission for Health Care Audit and Inspection
CHD	Congenital Heart Disease
CIS	Clinical Information Systems
CMO	Chief Medical Officer
CNO	Chief Nursing Officer
COPD	Chronic Obstructive Pulmonary Disease
CPAG	Child Poverty Action Group
CPD	Chronic Pulmonary Disease
CSDH	Commission on Social Determinants of Health
CSP	Chatered Society of Physiotherapists
CT	Cystic Fibrosis
CTQ	Critical to Quality
CUILU	Combined Universities Inter-professional Learning Unit
DCSF	Department for Children, Schools and Families
DES	Directed Enhanced Services
DFFP	Diploma of the Faculty of Family Planning and Reproductive Health Care

DFLE	Disability-free Life Expectancy
DHSS	Department of Social Security
DHSSPS	Department of Health, Social Security and Public Safety (Northern Ireland)
DH	Department of Health
DWP	Department of Work and Pensions
EC	European Community
ECC	European Economic Community
ECDL	European Computer Driving Licence
EPA	Environmental Protection Agency
EPS	Electronic Prescription Service
EU	European Union
EWTD	European Work Time Directive
FAS	Foetal Alcohol Syndrome
FFFP	Fellow of the Faculty of Family Planning and Reproductive Health Care
FFPRHC	Faculty of Family Planning and Reproductive Health Care
FHEA	Fellow of Higher Education Academy
FPA	Family Planning Association
FVC	Forced Vital Capacity
GCS	Glasgow Coma Scale
GHS	General Household Survey
GMC	General Medical Council
GMS	General Medial Service
GP	General Practitoner
GROS	General Register Office for Scotland
GSF	Gold Standards Framework
GUM	Genito-Urinary Medicine
HDA	Health Development Agency
HES	Hospital Episodes Statistics
HFA-DB	European Health for All Database
HIV	Human Immunodeficiency Virus
HLE	Healthy Life Expectancy
UNHA	Health of the Nation
HNA	Health Needs Assessment
HPA	Health Protection Agency
HPC	Health Professional Council
HPV	Human Papilloma Virus
HRP	United Nations system for research in human reproduction
HRSA	Health Resources and Services Administration
HSC	Health Select Committee
HSE	Health Survey England
IBA	Identification and Brief Advice
ICN	International Council of Nurses
ICT	Information and Communications Technology
ID	Indices of Deprivation
IDUs	Intravenous drug users
IG	Information Governance

List of abbreviations

INR	International Normalized Ratio
IPP	Inter-professional practice
ISC	Intermittent Self-catheterization
IUD	Intrauterine (contraceptive) device
IUS	Intrauterine (contraceptive) system
LARC	Long-acting reversible contraceptive
LE	Life Expectancy
LHO	London Health Observatory
LHP	Local Health Profiles
LOC	Level of Consciousness
LS	Longitudinal Study
LSP	Local Service Provider
LTC	Long-term Conditions
LTCA	Long-term Conditions Alliance
LTCANI	Long-term Conditions Alliance Northern Ireland
LTCAS	Long-term Conditions Alliance Scotland
LTCC	Long-term Conditions Collaborative
LVP	Liverpool Care Pathway
MDoH	Minnesota Department of Health
MDT	Multidisciplinary Team
MedFASH	Medical Foundation for AIDS and Sexual Health
MFFP	Member of the Faculty of Family Planning and Reproductive Health Care
MMR	Mumps, Measles and Rubella
MoCAM	Models of Care for Alcohol Misusers
MRSA	Methicillin Resistant Staphylococcus Aureus
MSM	Men who have sex with men
MUST	Malnutrition Universal Screening Tool
NAAFA	National Association to Advance Fat Acceptance
NCMP	National Child Measurement Programme
NCSP	National Chlamydia Screening Programme
NGO	Non-Governmental Organisation
NHS	National Health Service
NHS CRS	NHS Care Record Service
NICE	National Institute for Health and Clinical Excellence
NIMHE	National Institute for Mental Health in England
NISRA	Northern Ireland Statistics and Research Agency
NMC	Nursing and Midwifery Council
NPC	National Prescribing Centre
NPfIT	National Programme for Information Technology
NRT	Nicotine Replacement Therapy
NSAID	Non-steriodal Anti-inflammatory Drugs
NSF	National Service Frameworks
ONS	Office for National Statistics
OPSI	Office of Public Sector Information
OT	Occupational Therapist

OTC	Over the Counter
PABCAR	Public Health Decision-making model
PACS	Picture Archiving and Communications Systems
PCT	Primary Care Trust
PDA	Personal Digital Assistant
PDSA	Plan, do, study, act
PE	Physical Education
PEC	Professional Executive Committee
PEG	Pecutaneous Endoscopic Gastrostomy
PGDs	Patient Group Directions
PHO	Public Health Observatories
PID	Pelvic Inflammatory Disease
PPI	Proton Pump Inhibitor
PSA	Public Service Agreement
PSHE	Personal, Social and Health Education
QNI	Queen's Nursing Institute
QOF	Quality and Outcomes Framework
RBAC	Role Based Access
RCGP	Royal College of General Practitioners
RCN	Royal College of Nursing
RCOG	Royal College of Obstetricians and Gynaecologists
SALSUS	Schools Adolescent Lifestyle and Substance Use Survey
SBI	Screening and Brief Intervention
ScotPHO	Scottish Public Health Observatory
SE	Scottish Executive
SEAL	Social and Emotional Aspects of Learning
SEU	Social Exclusion Unit
SIPS	Screening and Intervention Trailblazers Research Programme for Sensible Drinking
STIs	Sexually Transmitted Infections
TCS	Transforming Community Cervices
TUILIP	Trent University's Inter-professional Learning in Practice
UAI	Unprotected Anal Intercourse
UK	United Kingdom
UKCC	United Kingdom Central Council
UKCRC	United Kingdom Clinical Research Collaboration
UNDP	United Nations Development Programme
UNFPA	United Nations Population Fund
UPSI	Unprotected Sexual Intercourse
USA	United States of America
WHO	World Health Organization
WMRO	West Midlands Regional Observatory

How to use this book

Nursing for Public Health explores what public health means for the nursing profession and outlines the skills required by nurses to promote good health. This brief tour shows you how to get the most out of this textbook package.

Case Study 4.1: The Hardy family

David and Rose Hardy are in their seventies and live in a council owned bungalow on the Travis estate. David has smoked since his teens and now has **Congestive Cardiac Failure**. He seldom leaves the bungalow as he finds physical effort such as walking makes him very breathless and

Case studies link public health theory, policies and models to nursing practice and everyday nursing care through patient scenarios and nursing projects.

Activity box

Look up the term **Caldicott Guardian**. Find out why this is important to the health care organizations. Are you able to identify the Caldicott Guardian for your organization?

All clinical staffs are bound by the Caldicott Principles which are:

Activity boxes ask you to think about ideas particular to each chapter and to develop appropriate nursing skills.

Discussion points

Many recent studies highlight the above as indicators of likely health inequality.

1. Studies have shown that many economically poorer people have to decide whether they can afford to collect a prescription or to take time off work when ill, as they will lose money. Statutory sick pay will usually not fully compensate

Discussion points explore key issues for nursing by providing critical analysis and guidance for practice.

Nursing Practice box

How to measure BMI

First measure height using a stadiometer; feet should be flat on the base and heels hard against the back of the stadiometer, the person being measured should be looking straight ahead while height is assessed. Secondly,

Nursing Practice boxes highlight specific skills, tools or knowledge for practice; for example how to recognise signs of mental health issues or how to measure BMI.

Learning recaps are provided by quick chapter summaries, helpful for consolidating what you've learned and handy for revision.

Summary

This chapter has explored definitions of obesity and examined the epidemiological evidence on the prevalence of obesity in the UK and how to measure obesity in adults and children. It has examined some of the causes of obesity and its impact, both at individual and societal level. Local and national strate-

Technical terms are highlighted in blue and bold and are explained in the glossary at the back of the book.

The first of these, **empowerment** describes a social action process through which individuals, organizations, or communities gain confidence and skills to improve their quality of life. **Community capacity** refers to characteristics of a community that allow it to identify social problems and address them (e.g., trusting relationships between neighbours, civic engagement). **Participation** in the organizing process helps community members to gain leadership and problem-solving skills.

Online Resource Centre

Nursing students need to put public health theory into practice on placement and stay up to date with this constantly evolving area of healthcare—this book has a dedicated website to help you get started! Just bookmark the address and go there when instructed to in the book:

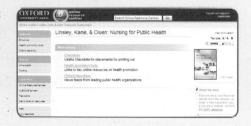

 www.oxfordtextbooks.co.uk/orc/linsley/

Students can:

- Stay up to date with developments in public health by signing up to our RSS feeds – frequently updated content from key healthcare organisations can be found on the website
- Download practical checklists and assessments for placement
- Look at interactive health promotion tools which have been recommended by the authors
- Get ahead with 'insider' sources of further information and guidelines.

For lecturers – you can use all of the above and download the figures for the book.

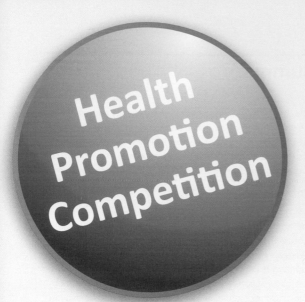

Health Promotion Competition

Oxford University Press and the authors of *Nursing for Public Health* have teamed up to offer an exciting competition for nursing students. We are looking for the **best health promotion poster presentation produced by student nurses**.

Posters should demonstrate understanding of **public health theory** and a critical analysis of a **health promotion intervention or educational material**. Students are invited to submit posters which have been specifically created for a module assignment.

At the end of the academic year, OUP and the authors of *Nursing for Public Health* will choose the entry considered the best.

The winning entrant will receive **£250 cash**, a **certificate** and have **their material published by Oxford University Press** on the online resource centre for the book.

For full details of the competition, including eligibility, closing dates, how to submit work, what the judges are looking for and terms and conditions please go to:

www.oxfordtextbooks.co.uk/orc/linsley/

Introduction

Paul Linsley, Roslyn Kane and Sara Owen

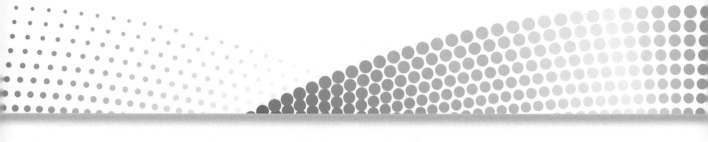

The opportunities afforded by public health to nursing and health care are substantial. Recent years have seen a shift in the delivery of health care and in the role of health care professionals. The new public health agenda emphasizes the role and practice of the nurse and challenges nurses and those they work with to engage in a number of new initiatives aimed at promoting health and well-being. Like all new opportunities within health, these will not be reached without examining and adapting the way in which nurses currently work, the nature of their education and how health care is delivered.

Two major factors can be identified as having influenced this change of focus. Firstly, the role of preventative health has gained increasing importance and, secondly, there has been a parallel shift in the locus of care with much more emphasis on caring for people in their own homes, rather than in the acute hospital setting. Combined, these forces have necessitated a change in the way nurses think and deliver care. Consequently a change in the content and nature of pre-registration nurse education programmes now equip students with a firm understanding of the fundamentals of public health.

One result of these influences has been the expansion of the nurses' role in the delivery of care. Whilst nurses have always cared for people who are ill, they are now increasingly involved with promoting the health and well-being for all, whether in a hospital or community setting. The idiom 'prevention is better than cure' is a central message in many public health interventions.

This book examines the policy context underpinning these changes and celebrates the many contributions that nurses can make to the health and well-being of the society in which they live and work. It recognizes the changing role of the nurse and acknowledges the new skills and understanding required to deliver care in contemporary society and within the context of the ongoing development of the profession.

A central tenet of the book is the increasing need for nurses to be aware of the importance of developing their skills to support their increasing contribution to public health and the reduction of health inequalities. Nurses also need to be aware of the complex socio-economic, cultural and environmental influences on health. A good education and a safe environment are important determinants of positive health status, alongside healthy behaviours such as a good diet and taking plenty of exercise. Our health is strongly linked to where we live, how we care for each other and our sense of community.

The concepts and ideas presented in this book provide a basis for appraisal of the contrasting perspectives of public health. It is hoped that this will encourage a greater level of awareness of, and sensitivity to, the nursing role and its part in delivering the public health agenda.

A plethora of approaches is necessary to meet the diverse health needs of the population and while this book is about the nursing profession, it also has wider relevance to the other professionals in the field of public health. However, it is not possible for one book to cover adequately all aspects of what is a wide area of interest and it is not our intention to attempt to cover all aspects of public health. Instead, the book concentrates on selected topics of particular relevance to nursing and which illustrate key points and matters of interest within the field.

How this book can help nurses to deliver the public health agenda

The book is divided into four discrete but interrelated sections. Part 1 examines the impact of the new public health agenda on the delivery of nursing care, necessitating a departure from the traditional model. Part 2 addresses the changing role of the nurse to accommodate this. Part 3 looks at key skills fundamental to public health practice. Lastly, Part 4 explores how nurses can begin to address key areas of health need by working with individuals and communities.

Chapter introductions provide a brief outline to the key themes of the chapter. The student is invited to test their knowledge and learning at various stages. This is done through a series of activities aimed at promoting critical thought and debate.

Questions and tasks are embedded within the text and encourage the student to complete an activity or to take pause and think about what they have learned. Review and discussion questions help the student to assess their understanding of the topic and aim to stimulate further investigation. At the same time they encourage students to integrate the material presented in the chapter with their own current understanding and experience of the world of nursing and public health.

Case studies are provided within chapters to provide insight into an element of practice or to demonstrate the specific skills needed in particular situations. Throughout readers are also encouraged to complement their reading by drawing upon their experiences in clinical practice.

Figures and tables illustrate key statistics, concepts and processes, visually reinforcing the students' learning whilst key terms are highlighted in the text when they first appear. These terms are also included in the Glossary at the end of the book.

The references and web links at the end of each chapter are to encourage the student to pursue further any issues of particular interest. Health care practice continually develops and new guidelines and evidence emerge on a steady basis. To help readers stay current with the latest developments in each subject area, and to support e-learning seen in all universities today, this book has a dedicated Online Resource Centre at http://www.oxfordtextbooks.co.uk/orc/linsley/

Part 1

What is the new public health agenda and why does it matter?

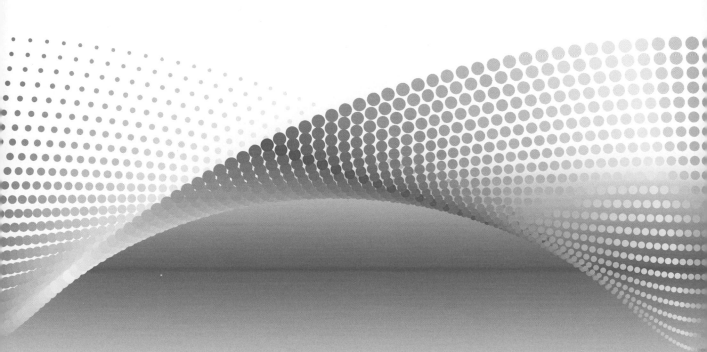

Part 1

Chapter 1

The context and direction of health care

Sara Owen and Ruth Reilly

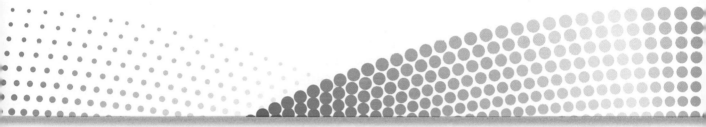

Introduction

'People in the twenty-first century expect services to be fast, high quality, responsive and fitted around their lives. All public services should put the person who uses them at their heart. This applies especially to health and social care because all care is personal'
DH, 2006a.

The statement above neatly encapsulates the vision for contemporary health care in the United Kingdom. It also highlights the changes that have taken place in the way services are delivered since the inception of the National Health Service (NHS). The purpose of this chapter is to provide the policy context to this change and to highlight how this in turn has impacted upon and influenced the changing role of the nurse. We have adopted a broad public health perspective throughout in order to demonstrate the increasingly important role and contribution of public health to the prevention of illness and the promotion of well-being. There is a large and growing body of literature on health policy, public health policy and its implications for the future roles of health and social care professionals. We have therefore selected and summarized the key policy documents to illustrate the important messages within them. This will provide a broad context for understanding the subsequent chapters in this book, where specific policy initiatives are presented with reference to particular debates and health issues.

The policy content

Background

The NHS was created in 1948 and in its earliest years, faced significant challenges providing basic care when people fell sick and tackling **communicable diseases**. Nowadays, diseases such as measles, polio and diphtheria, previously common and deadly to the post-war generation, are rare and preventable, thanks to vaccination, and treatable, thanks to advances in research and technology. The NHS in the twenty-first century faces a very different set of challenges and these include:

- rising public and patient expectations,
- demographic change,
- continuing development of an 'information' society,
- advances in treatment,
- changing patterns of disease,
- changing expectations of the health workplace.

Despite its many achievements, the NHS had not kept pace with the huge changes that had taken place in contemporary society since 1948. For example, particular areas of concern included patients experiencing long waiting times for consultation and treatment, and unacceptable variations in the standards of care provided across the country. This was compounded by historical and financial constraints, resulting in pressurized working conditions for staff with insufficient time and resources to provide the best possible service.

In 2000, the Government published *The NHS Plan* (DH, 2000); an ambitious ten-year programme of reform and investment. Its aim was to address the systematic weaknesses inherent in the NHS, to tackle the challenges which chronic under investment had created, and to provide a health service designed around the needs of the patient. The first years focused on building an infrastructure fit for the twenty-first century. For example, recruiting more doctors, nurses and **allied health professionals**, and radically reviewing pay and conditions. With more staff, the NHS could set about meeting one of the main concerns of patients and the public — improved access to health care with less time to wait. The second phase concerned updating and reviewing systems and processes in the NHS to make it more responsive to a modern consumer society both knowledgeable and opinionated about how health care should be provided (Maben and Griffiths, 2008).

The NHS is currently moving into the third phase of reform that will focus on improving the quality of care provided. That is, to progress from an NHS that has focused on increasing the quantity of care to one that focuses on improving the quality of care. The aim is to transform the NHS into a high quality, high performance system engaged in a continuous cycle of improvement, whose staff readily evaluate and raise their performance, so that the best care is available to all. The vision for this third phase of reform is set out in the NHS Next Stage Review publications; *High Quality Care for All* (Darzi, 2008a), *A High Quality Workforce* (Darzi, 2008b), and *Our Vision for Primary Care* (Darzi, 2008c). The vision is structured around four main themes:

- High quality care for patients and the public — an NHS that works in partnership to prevent ill health, providing care that is personal, effective and safe.
- Quality at the heart of everything we do — high quality care throughout the NHS.
- Freedom to focus on quality — putting frontline staff in control.
- High quality work in the NHS — supporting staff to deliver high quality care.

In summary, the NHS is slowly being transformed into a service that will meet the demands and expectations of patients in the twenty-first century. This has been achieved through significant investment, reform of the way the service is delivered, and an emphasis not only on the quantity and type of care delivered but on its quality. Perhaps one of the biggest shifts has been the increased emphasis on the

prevention of illness and the maintenance of good health rather than cure, and the move to provide more care in the community rather than in hospital-based facilities. The next section of this chapter explains the reasons for this shift and introduces the key policy documents that are driving the change.

Tackling inequalities in health

The Government in the United Kingdom has prioritized the need to tackle the causes and consequences of health inequalities as part of its commitment to deliver economic prosperity and social justice. Action to break the cycle of deprivation and its impact on avoidable ill health is at the heart of this endeavour. Preventing avoidable illness will also allow concentration of resources on other conditions. The Government's aim is to reduce health inequalities by tackling the wider social determinants of health such as poverty, poor educational outcomes, unemployment, poor housing, homelessness, and the problems of disadvantaged neighbourhoods.

The issue of health inequalities is covered in some detail in Chapter 14. In brief, to understand better the causes of health inequalities, and how to tackle them, the Government established the *Independent Inquiry into Inequalities in Health* (Acheson, 1998), chaired by Sir Donald Acheson. The inquiry came to a similar conclusion as the *Black Report* (DHSS, 1980), that there were health inequalities in the United Kingdom and that poverty was a significant determinant of health. Drawing on a wide range of evidence, the inquiry highlighted that although average mortality had fallen over the past fifty years, unacceptable inequalities in health persisted. For many measures of health, inequalities have either remained the same or have widened in recent decades. These inequalities affect the whole of society and they can be identified at all stages of the life course from pregnancy to old age. Drawing on a socio-economic explanation of health inequalities, the inquiry traced the roots of ill health to such social determinants as income, education and employment as well as to the material environment and lifestyle. The inquiry also identified a range of areas for future policy development including:

- poverty,
- income,
- tax and benefits,
- education,
- employment,
- housing and the environment,
- mobility,

- transport and pollution,
- nutrition.

Areas are also identified by the stages of the life course:

- mothers,
- children and families,
- young people,
- adults of working age,
- older people.

In order to tackle health inequalities, there needs to be a shared understanding of what is meant by 'inequity' and unfairness in health and health care. Some health inequalities are to be expected, for example, older people are more likely to become ill, and so can be expected to consume more health service resources. Others however cannot be accounted for by a difference in need. Inequalities exist throughout the health system from causes to outcomes and include:

- Health outcomes in disease or life expectancy,
- Access to services such as health care,
- Lifestyle factors which influence health, such as smoking or diet.

Within any level in the system, inequalities may also be found between many types of community or population group, but Government policy focuses on a few important dimensions including:

- Socio-economic status such as income, and area based measures of deprivation,
- Ethnicity,
- Gender,
- Age,
- Disability.

The Acheson inquiry largely influenced the Government's initial policies to address health inequalities including the Green Paper *Our Healthier Nation* (DH, 1998), the White Paper *Saving Lives* (DH, 1999), *Well being in Wales* (Welsh Assembly Government, 2002), *Improving Health in Scotland* (Scottish Executive, 2003), *A Healthier Future: a 20-year vision for health and well being in Northern Ireland 2005– 2025* (Department of Health, Social Services and Public Safety, 2004), *Delivering for Health* (Scottish Executive, 2005) and *Better Health, Better Care: Action Plan* (The Scottish Government, 2007). These and subsequent policies have sought to influence change through three key strategies, namely:

- Setting targets,
- Changing the locus of care,
- Influencing individual and public behaviour.

These three strategies will now be considered in turn.

Setting targets

As identified in the previous section, a programme of addressing inequalities in health was initiated in England by the **Acheson Report**, which triggered a series of key policy documents that have brought health inequalities forward as a cross-government priority. Government-wide targets known as PSA or Public Service Agreement targets set in 2001, aim for faster improvement in health outcomes in the fifth of areas with the worst health and deprivation indices (in life expectancy, death from heart disease and stroke, and cancers). These areas are known as 'Spearhead Authorities'.

The last Labour government's key targets for reducing health inequalities are summarized in Box 1.1. The main focus is on physical health and on geographical and socio-economic inequalities. Mental health is the focus of separate targets on suicide reduction and reducing ethnic disparities in mental health care.

Box 1.1 Public Service Agreement (PSA) targets to reduce health inequalities (DH, 2002)

The single overall target:

- Reduce health inequalities by 10% by 2010 as measured by infant mortality (from a 1997-99 baseline) and life expectancy at birth (from a 1995-97 baseline).

The single target is supported by the following two specific targets:

- Starting with children under one year, by 2010 to reduce, by at least 10%, the gap in mortality between 'routine and manual' groups and the population as a whole.
- Starting with Local Authorities, by 2010 to reduce by at least 10% the life expectancy gap between the fifth of areas with the worst health and deprivation indicators and the population as a whole.

Supporting targets:

- Substantially reduce mortality rates by 2010 from heart disease and stroke and related disease by at least 40% in people under 75 with a 40% reduction in the inequalities gap between the fifth of areas with the worse health and deprivation factors and the population as a whole.
- Substantially reduce mortality rates by 2010 from cancers by at least 20% in people under 75 with a reduction in the inequalities gap of at least 6% between the fifth of areas with the worse health and deprivation factors and the population as a whole.
- Reduce adult smoking rates to 21% or less by 2010, with a reduction in prevalence among routine and manual groups to 26% or less.

To support the challenge of meeting the above targets, *Tackling Health Inequalities: a Programme for Action* (DH, 2003) set out a comprehensive programme across a range of policies and services. The aim was to show what needed to be done to meet the 2010 national targets on life expectancy and infant mortality as well as the actions that needed to be set in motion to insure against a continuation of health inequalities into the future. Many of these actions rely on strong and effective partnership working with local authorities and other key partners. Specifically the document sets out the key NHS interventions that will help achieve these targets, achievement being underpinned by the availability of good quality primary care. These plans were further developed in *Choosing Health* (DH, 2004) and its subsequent delivery plan (DH, 2005).

It is recognized however that action on a range of fronts, within and outside the NHS, at national, regional and local level, is needed to tackle health inequalities and deliver on these targets. Local agencies will need first to understand their local health inequalities, which determinants and services are most influential locally in producing unequal outcomes, and the most appropriate interventions. This is a complex task that requires considerable resource and expertise. In order to assist with this there is a wealth of local and national resources to support local action to understand, prioritize and reduce health inequalities. For example, the **Association of Public Health Observatories** together with the Department of Health holds and produces a range of materials to support local action. This includes the **Health Inequalities Intervention Tool** that can help local authorities and Primary Care Trusts understand the causes of their local life expectancy gap and to predict the impact of a number of evidence based interventions designed to reduce the gap. These resources are easily accessible from any of the Public Health Observatories' websites.

Changing the locus of care

The last few years has seen an unprecedented shift away from hospital to community based and primary health care. This shift reflects a global drive towards primary health care as an approach to achieving health for all (World Health Report, 2008). In the United Kingdom, the **Wanless Report** (Wanless, 2004), in setting out a framework and guiding principles for developing health and social care, stated the need for:

- The transferring of some services and activity out of **secondary care** into **primary care** (where clinically safe and economic).
- Investment in **intermediate** and **community care** to reduce admission rates to hospital and facilitate early discharge.
- Development of **integrated care pathways** to ensure that there is effective planning of health care and that treatment is in the right place, at the right time, by the right person.

This was followed by the White Paper *Our Health, Our Care, Our Say: a New Direction for Community Services* (DH, 2006a), which set out a new and ambitious vision and direction for the future of community services. This vision is also reflected in Scottish, Welsh and Irish publications (Farrell, *et al.* 2008, Scottish Executive, 2005, Scottish Government, 2007, Welsh Assembly Government, 2005). Together they emphasize the need for a radical and sustained shift in the way in which services are delivered to ensure that they are more personalised and can fit into people's busy lives. In the consultation and debates that preceded its publication, people identified that they wanted: seamless health and social care to support them to stay healthy and to lead independent lives, more services provided locally, and services that are fair to all, with more help for people who need them most. Acute hospitals should be places where people go when it is really necessary, not as a matter of routine. Community services therefore need to take centre stage in the health and social care system of the future. The White Paper has four main goals:

- Better prevention services with earlier intervention,
- Giving people more choice and a louder voice,
- Focusing on tackling inequalities and improving access to community services,
- Providing more support for people with long-term needs.

In order to achieve the above, two key strategies were recommended:

- Shifting resources into the prevention of illness.
- Undertaking more care outside hospitals and in the home. This included joining up of services at a local level, encouraging innovation, and allowing different providers to compete for services. The emphasis was on having more services available to people in their local communities or in their own homes to avoid unnecessary trips to hospitals.

Two years later, the **NHS Next Stage Review** (Darzi, 2008c), noted that when people think of health and health care, it is still hospitals that spring to mind. However over 90% of all contact with the NHS now takes place outside hospital with primary care staff. This document sets out the vision for how services will continue to grow and develop over the next ten years, within the broad context and acknowledgement that the provision of health care is constantly evolving.

The review argues that primary and community care should increasingly play a vital role in helping people live healthy lives. For example, we can do far more to embed health promotion in the millions of daily contacts with family doctors, community nurses, pharmacists and other community-based staff. We can also do more to promote health at all stages of life and more systematically identify and support those individuals most at risk of ill health. To support this there should be increasing access to services that help people maintain and improve their health and well-being.

Whilst the demand for primary and community care services will grow over the next ten years, the nature of this demand will also change. For example;

- People increasingly expect public services to do more to treat them as whole individuals rather than isolated symptoms, listen to their needs, and tailor services to meet those needs.
- Continuing advances in technology and medical treatments will allow more and more people to receive care in community-based settings (rather than travelling to hospital) or in their own homes. For example, new technologies have allowed people to take physical measurements such as blood sugar and blood oxygen at home and allow those to be monitored remotely by a community matron who can then take swift action if there is cause for concern.
- An ageing society, with the number of people over 85 set to double by 2029, will lead to increasing demand for primary and community care.

The review also emphasizes that improving health and reducing inequalities will only be achieved by primary and community health services working with other organizations. Our health and lifestyle choices are influences by a wide range of factors rooted in local communities, including how we develop in school, the quality of social care when we need it, access to leisure facilities, and the quality of our environment including housing, transport, planning and amenities. Primary and community health services will need to work ever more closely with local authorities and develop innovative partnerships with third sector organizations to forge common goals for improving the health and well-being of local communities. Third sector organizations include voluntary and community groups, social enterprises, charities, cooperatives and mutuals.

Influencing individual and public behaviour

Since the 1980s, the growing field of population health has broadened the focus of public health from individual behaviours and risk factors to population-level issues such as inequality, poverty and education — as previously discussed. Modern public health is often concerned with addressing determinants of health across a population, rather than advocating for individual behaviour change. There is a recognition that our health is affected by many factors including where we live, genetics, our income, our educational status and our social relationships, these are commonly referred to as 'social determinants of health'. The statement below however clearly shows that the Government is taking a two-pronged approach to promoting health and reducing inequalities in the United Kingdom by emphasizing both individual and government responsibility. These will be considered in turn.

'We each have a responsibility for our own health and well being throughout our lives. At the same time, the government has a role in promoting healthier, longer lives lived to the full.

We will build on and strengthen the opportunities for improving the health of the population first set out in the document *Choosing Health*'
DH, 2006a.

Helping people look after their own health and well-being

The emphasis on individual responsibility for health and well being was highlighted in the document ***Saving Lives*** (DH, 1999), by asserting that people can make decisions about their and their families' health, which can make a difference. It suggested that people can improve their own health through physical activity, better diet and quitting smoking. In order to do this, people need to be properly informed about the risks to make decisions about their behaviour.

The White Paper ***Choosing Health*** (DH, 2004) builds on this theme of individual responsibility by setting out the key principles for supporting people to make healthier and more informed choices regarding their health. The principles of this new public health approach include informed choice and personalization. Informed choice is an acknowledgement that people want to make their own decisions about choices that impact on their health and to have credible and trustworthy information to help them to do so. Personalization is an approach that supports the notion that some people want support in making healthy choices, but particularly in deprived groups and communities, find current services do not meet their needs or are difficult to use. To be effective in tacking health inequalities, support has to be tailored to the reality of individual lives, with services and support personalized sensitively and provided flexibly and conveniently.

More recently, ***Our Health, Our Care, Our Say*** (DH, 2006a) argues that the best way of empowering people to take charge of their own health and well-being is to focus on the major risk factors that may affect their health. These include obesity, smoking, alcohol misuse, mental health problems and stress-related conditions, and sexually transmitted infections. One intervention that has been developed is the new NHS 'Life Check' service to help people, particularly at critical points in their lives, to assess their own risk of ill health . The tool is based on a range of risk factors, and on family history. The NHS 'Life Check' is a personalized service in two parts:

- an initial assessment for people to complete themselves,
- offers of specific advice and support on the action people can take to maintain and improve health.

It is also anticipated that the introduction of non-professional **health trainers** who come from within local communities to offer support to individuals with such complex conditions may succeed where traditional approaches have been less successful.

Finally, the important issue of access to services is addressed in the *NHS Next Stage Review: Our Vision for Primary and Community Care* (Darzi, 2008c). The report stresses the importance of people being able to easily access extra support for healthy living when they need it, whether it is to help give up smoking, control their use of alcohol, or improve diet or exercise. Pharmacies, community health clinics, third sector organizations and others are providing an increasing range of these services. The review explores how to make more services available on an 'open access' basis to ensure that the public can easily use them when required.

Government responsibility

Tackling Health Inequalities: a programme for Action (DH, 2003) set out a strategy for tackling health inequalities. This established the foundations required to achieve the challenging target for 2010 to reduce the gap in infant mortality across social groups, and to raise life expectancy in the most disadvantages areas faster than elsewhere.

For the 2010 target, a number of specific interventions were identified that were most likely to have an impact amongst disadvantaged groups. The key interventions for closing the life expectancy gap are:

* Reducing smoking in manual social groups.
* Preventing and managing other risks for coronary heart disease and cancer such as poor diet and obesity, physical inactivity, and hypertension through effective primary care and public interventions, especially targeting the over-50 year olds.
* Improving housing quality by tackling cold and dampness, and reducing accidents at home and on the road.

To close the gap in infant mortality, key short-term interventions include:

* Improving the quality and accessibility of antenatal care and early years support in disadvantaged areas.
* Reducing smoking and improving nutrition in pregnancy and early years.
* Reducing unwanted teenage pregnancy and supporting teenage parents.
* Improving housing conditions for children in disadvantaged areas.

Five discrete principles were suggested to guide how health inequalities are tackled in practice:

* Preventing health inequalities getting worse by reducing exposure to risks and addressing the underlying causes of ill health .
* Working through the mainstream by making services more responsive to the needs of disadvantaged populations.

* Targeting specific interventions through new ways of meeting need, particularly in areas resistant to change.
* Supporting action from the centre by clear policies effectively managed.
* Delivering at a local level and meeting national standards through diversity of provision.

Our Health, Our Care, Our Say (DH, 2006a) devotes a whole chapter to enabling health, independence and well being. It builds on and strengthens the opportunities for improving the health of the population set out in *Choosing Health* (DH, 2004) and argues that public bodies can and should do more to give everyone an equal chance to become and stay healthy. There is a specific focus on childhood, people of working age, older people, and disabled people and people with high support needs; each with aims and suggested actions. For example the aims for promoting health and well being in old age are:

* To promote higher levels of physical activity in the older population.
* To reduce barriers to increased levels of physical activity, mental well-being and social engagement among excluded groups of older people.
* To continue to increase uptake of evidence-based disease prevention programmes among older people.

In this section, we have explored a number of policy approaches to influencing the health and well-being of individuals and populations. The White Paper *Choosing Health* (DH, 2004) and *Saving Lives* (DH, 1999) however also want to see a new balance in which people, communities and the government work together in partnership to improve health. The government and individuals alone cannot make progress on healthier choices. Real progress depends on effective partnerships, which must engage with service users and their carers across health and social care communities, including local government, the NHS, business, advertisers, retailers, the voluntary sector, the media, faith organizations and many others. Government policy documents are necessary to provide strategic direction, inform service provision and promote partnerships; however, as we have seen, that alone is not enough to make national **health gain.** We all need to take our health and the health of our families seriously; and most people are prepared to engage constructively in this shared effort.

A summary of progress

The final status report, *Tackling Health Inequalities: 2007 Status Report on the Programme for Action* (DH, 2007a) was published in March 2008. This showed progress against the Government's Public Service Agreement (PSA) targets to reduce health inequalities, with almost all of the commitments wholly or substantially achieved. Overall since 1997, there have been significant absolute improvements in the health of disadvantaged groups and areas. The key progress in absolute health inequalities outcomes include:

- The 2004–2006 infant mortality rate for routine and manual groups is the same as the rate for the whole population in 1997–1999.
- Life expectancy for men in the target Spearhead group has increased by over two and a half years in the period since 1995–1997, and by over one and a half years in women.
- Heart disease and cancer mortality rates for those under 75 have fallen fastest in the Spearhead areas — by 32% for heart disease and 11% for cancer.

There is however an expected differential progress, as the causes of health inequalities vary from area to area. The report shows that, despite the absolute improvements, inequalities remain stubborn and persistent. This picture is also reflected in recent publications in Scotland, Ireland and Wales (Farrell *et al.*, 2008, Scottish Government, 2008, Welsh Assembly Government, 2005).

The nursing contribution to the new public health agenda

Nurses have an increasingly important role to play in the public health arena. In this section we will explore how and why public health and health promotion has become a central activity for all nurses, rather than the specific remit of those nurses who work primarily in community-based settings. We will also highlight and summarize the key documents that have attempted to identify the key elements of this public health role.

There has been for some time a formal policy commitment to enhancing the contribution of nurses to public health. Since the publication of the *Independent Inquiry into Inequalities in Health* (Acheson, 1998), the need for a radical approach to improving the health of the population has been recognized. In 1998 the European and Chief Nursing Officers made an official statement of intent to analyse and strengthen the work of nurses within the public health arena. This was reinforced in the June 2000 Munich Declaration, when Ministers of Health of the European region of the World Health Organization pledged to 'enhance the role of nurses and midwives in public health, health promotion and community development' (WHO, 2000). They believed that:

'nurses and midwives have key and increasingly important roles to play in society's efforts to tackle public health challenges of our time, as well as ensuring the provision of high quality, accessible, equitable, efficient and sensitive services, which ensure continuity of care and address people's rights and changing needs'
WHO, 2000.

More recently a report produced by the International Council of Nurses emphasizes the leading role nurses should play in the broad public health arena with particular reference to primary care (International Council of Nurses 2008). This report analyses the evolution of primary health care, articulates nursing roles, highlights many examples of nurses delivering primary health care, and provides a glimpse into the future.

The UK Government also recognized that the rapid change in the direction of health care, discussed in the earlier sections of this chapter, would not be possible without an accompanying shift in the focus of the workforce. *Choosing Health* made direct reference to the need to:

'develop training and support for all NHS staff to develop their understanding and skills in promoting health and to foster and expand a comprehensive range of community health improvement services'
DH, 2004:14.

More recently the *NHS Next Stage Review* (DH, 2008b and d) clearly states that nurses play a vital role in the NHS, as they will always be at the heart of shaping patient experience and delivering care. The review aspires to the quality of nursing care in the UK being recognized as excellent, to continue to attract highly motivated and talented individuals and to support nurses in leadership roles at all levels in the NHS. More specifically it emphasizes that health care services play a central role in helping people live healthy lives, and argues that health promotion should be embedded in the millions of daily contacts between clinical staff and patients. More needs to be done to promote health at all stages of life and more systematically identify and support those individuals most at risk of ill health. There should be increasing access to services that help people maintain their health and well-being. Primary and community clinicians can enhance their role in promoting equality of opportunity and equality of health outcomes. There will be expanded and new opportunities for nurses in promoting health and well-being and reducing health inequalities. In addition, nurses will play a key role in care planning for the 15 million people with long-term conditions, helping people take more control over their health and care.

Recent high profile documents about the future role of the nurse also reflect the changes in health care policy. The *Modernising Nursing Careers: Setting the Direction* (DH, 2006b) document reinforces many of the arguments set out in recent health policy. For example, the view that health care must respond to the global shift in the burden of disease that is seeing a rise in the numbers of people affected by one or more long-term condition. It also identifies that health inequalities persist despite all efforts to reduce the gap. As well as the disadvantaged, many of those whose physical health is poorest have long-term and enduring mental health problems or learning difficulties. The document also goes on to argue that we must respond to a very different world where health care is designed around patients, where long-term conditions with their propensity for responding to preventative measures have a higher profile, where health promotion and self-care are recognized as the bedrock of a healthier society and where services are offered nearer to home. The Modernizing Nursing Careers programme is working to equip nurses with the skills and capabilities for their roles by:

- Creating a more flexible and competent workforce,
- Updating career pathways and choices for nurses,
- Better preparing nurses to lead in a changed system,
- Updating the image of 'the nurse'.

It also highlights that support for careers in health promotion is needed to enable nurses to play a full role in health promotion and in maximising health potential for people, families and communities.

Other key documents include *The Future Nurse: the Future for Nurse Education* (RCN, 2007a), which clearly maps out the contribution of nurses to improving the health of the public and argues for the strengthening of nurses' position so that they can better influence the health of communities. This is echoed in the consultation document, *Towards a Framework for Post Registration Nursing Careers* (DH, 2007b). It suggests that all nurses should contribute in some way to public health via short opportunistic or planned health promotion or educational interventions. The future emphasis will be on intervening at a population level in working in partnership to address the determinants of health. Health needs assessments for populations, communities, groups, families and individuals will be a key component and will provide the basis for intervention to improve health, reduce health inequalities and support for vulnerable families and individuals.

Despite the many indicators for the future direction and focus of nursing identified above, some concerns still exist within the profession that nursing has lost its way and that there are still unacceptable variations in the quality of care. The National Nursing Research Unit at King's College London is currently leading work with the Department of Health, partners and employers to reaffirm the role of the nurse. Their report sets out a view of the modern nurse, rooted in the values of the nursing profession and the NHS (Maben and Griffiths, 2008). The recommendations set out to restore public confidence in the profession, define what patients and nurses want in terms of good quality care in all health care settings and identify a range of measures to secure a step change in the quality of care. In the past, the registered nurse's role within the team has often been as a practitioner, an expert in their clinical discipline. Yet frontline nurses have the talent to look beyond their individual clinical practice and act as partners

and leaders of care and service. This report defines registered nurses as:

- Skilled and respected **practitioners** providing effective high quality health care across a range of settings.
- Vital and valued **partners** in the delivery of health care — partners in the multidisciplinary team, coordinating different resources and skill sets to ensure high quality care, partners with patients and carers in delivering personalized care, and responsible members of the broader health care system taking personal responsibility for efficient and effective functioning.
- Confident and effective **leaders** and champions of care quality with a powerful voice at all levels of the health care system, from policymaking to the frontline.

The practitioner, partner, leader vision is rooted in the core values and ethos that underpin the profession but also recognizes the dynamic and changing nature of nursing and health care that will shape the future.

In this section we have discussed the expectation that nursing roles will need to change and continue to develop to reflect the public health agenda outlined in recent and current health policy. We have also highlighted that these expectations have raised some concerns among the profession about the collective will and ability to deliver this ambitious agenda. It is evident however, that further work needs to be done to clarify the role of nurses in public health and health promotion. The work streams arising from the *NHS Next Stage Review* (DH, 2008d), including the work from the National Nursing Research Unit at King's College London (Maben and Griffiths 2008), are currently working in partnership with professional bodies, employers and other stakeholders to define the unique role and contribution of each of the health care professions and how their roles are changing across the pathways of care.

In the meantime there is a useful document that has endeavoured to map out the key elements of the nursing role in public health. The *Nurses as Partners in Delivering Public Health* (RCN, 2007b) document states that the aims of delivering public health through nursing services are to:

- Increase life expectancy by influencing healthy behaviours.
- Reduce health inequalities, for example, by targeting vulnerable populations to improve health outcomes and access services.
- Improve population health, for example, reducing obesity, alcohol abuse, and unwanted poor sexual health outcomes including unwanted pregnancy and sexually transmitted infections.
- Increase the awareness of positive healthy behaviours in communities
- Promote and develop social capital.
- Engage with individuals, families and communities to influence the design and development of services.

This can be achieved through a range of interventions in a wide spectrum of services, see Box 1.2 for more detail.

Box 1.2 Public health nursing interventions (RCN, 2007)

- Identify individual and population health need, using assessment.
- Target their services at vulnerable individuals and communities.
- Contribute to and develop services that protect the public's health, for example, immunization, emergency planning and communicable disease prevention.
- Share health information to encourage individuals, families and communities to become more active in developing healthy lifestyles.
- Prevent ill health and promote health enhancing activities by working with families and individuals.
- Promote and develop action to tackle the underlying causes of ill health.
- Lead partnership working for health with other key organizations.
- Advocate for health gain in relation to all public activities, for example, housing, leisure, transport, shopping and the environment.
- Be catalysts for health, creating new resources and collaboration to sustain good health in local groups and communities, such as schools and prisons.
- Challenge vested interests that threaten public health.
- Access hard-to-reach groups, engaging them around their hopes and fears.

Summary

As a nation we are healthier that we have ever been. Nationally life expectancy has improved year-on-year over the past decade. However, the health of the most disadvantaged has not improved as quickly as that of the better off. Inequalities in health persist and, in some cases, have widened.

The recent document, **Health Inequalities: Progress and Next Steps** (DH, 2008e) outlines the approach to hitting the 2010 health inequalities Public Service Agreement Targets. It also assesses what interventions have and have not worked, and sets the direction of travel beyond 2010. As we have discussed in this chapter, the current strategy on health inequalities focuses on the wider social determinants of health, the lives people lead and what the NHS can do. The last Labour government plans to continue on this path, as set out in **Tackling Health Inequalities: a Programme for Action** (DH, 2003).

There will be strengthened support to meet the 2010 Public Service Agreement Targets, and more action on the factors that drive inequalities. Beyond 2010, the Government has new ambitions for reducing health inequalities along with the structures, systems and actions to sustain their long-term delivery.

To support these ambitions, the Government appointed Professor Sir Michael Marmot, Chair of the World Health Organization Commission for Social Determinants, to lead a Post 2010 Strategic Review of Health Inequalities. The aim of the Review was to devise an evidence-based strategy for reducing health inequalities from 2010 that included policies and interventions that address the social determinants of health inequalities.

The review entitled **Fair Society, Healthy Lives**, published in February 2010 (**The Marmot Review, 2010**), provides a thorough and comprehensive analysis of the state of health inequalities in England. It acknowledges the nature, sustainability and intensity of government policies over the years towards improving social justice and equity, and identifies key areas for future action across the social determinants of health. These include action on:

- the early years,
- education,
- skills and life chances,
- work,
- a healthy standard of living,
- sustainable communities,
- prevention.

The review's advice will contribute to the development of a cross government health inequalities strategy post-2010, to build on the current national PSA targets on health inequalities when they expire in 2011. Work has already begun on addressing the review's recommendations. What is certain is that nurses will be required to play a continuing and increasingly important and pivotal role in creating the opportunities for people to live positive healthy lives, prevent ill health, and by influencing public and health policy.

 Online Resource Centre

For more information on the context and direction of health care visit the Online Resource Centre —
http://www.oxfordtextbooks.co.uk/orc/linsley/

References

Acheson, D. (1998). *Independent Inquiry into Inequalities in Health Report*. London: The Stationery Office.
Darzi, A. (2008a). *High Quality Care for All: NHS Next Stage Review*. London: DH.

Darzi, A. (2008b). *A High Quality Workforce: NHS Next Stage Review*. London: DH.

Darzi, A. (2008c). *NHS Next Stage Review: Our Vision for Primary and Community Care*. London: DH.

Darzi, A. (2008). *NHS Next Stage Review: Our Vision for Primary and Community Care: What it means for nurses, midwives health visitors and AHPs*. London: DH.

Department of Health (1998). *Our Healthier Nation: a Contract for Health*. Cm3852, London: DH.

Department of Health (1999). *Saving Lives: Our Healthier Nation*. London: The Stationery Office.

Department of Health (2000). *The NHS Plan: a Plan for Investment, a Plan for Reform. Cm4818-I*. London: The Stationery Office.

Department of Health (2002). *Tackling Health Inequalities through Local Public Service Agreements*. London: DH.

Department of Health (2003). *Tacking Health Inequalities: a Programme for Action*. London: DH.

Department of Health (2004). *Choosing Health: Making Healthier Choices Easier*. London: DH.

Department of Health (2005). *Delivering Choosing Health: Making Healthier Choices Easier*. London: DH.

Department of Health (2006a). *Our Health, Our Care, Our Say: a New Direction for Community Services*. London: DH.

Department of Health (2006b). *Modernizing Nursing Careers: Setting the Direction*. London: DH.

Department of Health (2007a). *Tackling Health Inequalities: 2007 Status Report on the Programme for Action*. London: DH.

Department of Health (2007b). *Towards a Framework for Post Registration Nursing Careers: Consultation Document*. London: DH.

Department of Health (2008). *Health Inequalities: Progress and Next Steps*. London: DH.

Department of Health and Social Security (1980). *The Black Report*. London: DHSS.

Department of Health, Social Services and Public Safety (2004) *A Healthier Future: a twenty-year vision for health and well being in Northern Ireland 2005–2025*. Belfast: DHSSPS.

Farrell, C., McAvoy,H. & Wilde,J. (2008). *Tackling Health Inequalities. An All-Ireland Approach to Social Determinants*. Ireland: Institute of Public Health.

International Council of Nurses (2008). *Delivering Quality, Serving Communities: Nurses Leading Primary Health Care*. Geneva: International Council of Nurses.

Maben, J. & Griffiths, P. (2008). *Nurses in Society: Starting the Debate*. London: National Nursing Research Unit, Kings College.

Marmot Review (2010). *Fair Society, Healthy Lives: Post 2010 Strategic Review of Health Inequalities*. London: UCL Research Department of Epidemiology and Public Health.

Royal College of Nursing (2007a). *The Future Nurse: the Future for Nurse Education*. London: RCN. .

Royal College of Nursing (2007b). *Nurses as Partners in Delivering Public Health: a Paper to Support the Nursing Contribution to Public Health*. London: RCN.

Scottish Executive (2005). *Delivering for Health*. Edinburg: Scottish Executive.

Scottish Executive (2003). *Improving Health in Scotland: The Challenge*. Edinburh: Scottish Executive.

Scottish Government (2008). *Equally Well: Report of the Ministerial Task Force on Health Inequalities*. Edinburg: Scottish Government.

Scottish Government (2007). *Better Health, Better Care*. Edinburg: Scottish Government.

Wanless (2004). *Securing Good Health for the Whole Population (The Wanless Report)*. London: DH.

Welsh Assembly Government (2005). *Inequalities in Health: The Welsh Dimension 2002–2005*. Cardiff: Welsh Assembly Government.

Welsh Assembly Government (2002) *Well being in Wales*. Cardiff: Welsh Assembly Government.

World Health Report (2008). *Primary Health Care: Now More Than Ever*. Geneve: World Health Organization.

World Health Organization (2000). *Munich Declaration: Nurses and Midwives: a Force for Health 2000*. Geneva: World Health Organization.

Chapter 2

Influences on health and the causes of ill health across the lifespan

Laura Serrant-Green

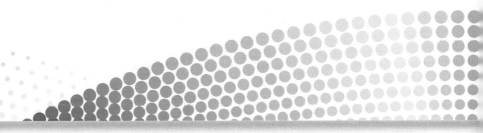

Introduction

In June 1946 at the International Health Conference, New York, as a preamble to the Constitution of the World Health Organization (WHO), health was identified as being:

'A state of complete physical, mental and social well being and not merely the absence of disease or infirmity'
WHO, 1948

This now famous declaration of what it means to be healthy was formally adopted at the conference in June 1946; signed on 22 July 1946 by the representatives of 61 States and came into force on 7 April 1948. This original and well quoted definition remains unchanged as the foundation to our understanding of health and being healthy.

The declaration was a catalyst for a shared understanding of the nature of health and what it means to be healthy. It has since formed the basis of many local, national and international strategies to improve the health and life chances of people who make up populations in society. However, in the time since the declaration it has become increasingly apparent that the health of indi-

viduals and communities in any given society is also dependent on a range of contextual factors, which directly or indirectly affect their chances of reaching optimum physical, mental (emotional) or social well-being. In addition it is acknowledged that 'one size does not fit all' and at different stages in the lives of individuals, the impact of these factors on health chances, the ability of the individual to influence their own health and the consequences for their communities vary greatly.

This chapter focuses on the factors influencing health and the causes of ill health across the lifespan. The impact of lifestyles, poverty, education, culture and the environment are explored. It considers health influences over the age range, including longevity and the impact this has for planning health and care services. The chapter will help you to understand how and why individuals at different stages of life will exhibit different health needs and may hold variable attitudes towards their personal health. It will analyse the widely held view that these needs and attitudes are not solely related to the physical process of moving through identified age ranges associated with a particular stage in life and related disease patterns, but also to social and environmental influences.

The chapter concludes by considering the implications for nursing practice and public health nursing in particular, through a brief introduction to the National Service Frameworks (NSF) for older people, and for children, young people and maternity services.

The variable nature of health and well-being

The twenty-first century has been preceded by decades in which the advances in science, care practice and medical knowledge have resulted in an increase in lifespan as well as a reduction in global ill health. Many of the diseases and illnesses which claimed the lives of people in the last century have been eradicated, while in many societies the number of children living healthy lives beyond childhood has increased immensely. There is a general optimism in relation to health in many countries and particularly in Western countries ill health is deemed to be an incidental or occasional aspect of people's lives rather than a determining factor. Health could be said to be 'booming' relative to times past.

Each year the WHO produces a report reflecting the state of health across the world in relation to a specific aspect of health. The report includes a detailed expert assessment of global health in richer and poorer nations, supported by the latest related statistical data. The report aims to provide the countries themselves, associated agencies and international organizations with the evidence they need to underpin health care policy decision making and service planning as well as providing an indirect general overview of the impact of implemented strategies to improve health. The report provides a good basis therefore for assessing the current health of populations on a global scale.

In addition to this individual countries also maintain their own internal regular monitoring of the health of their people by gathering health intelligence through their own national screening initiatives, public health monitoring and health profiles. For example in England, **The Health Profile of England** produced by the **Public Health Observatories** (PHO), provides a collated report of national and regional health data reflecting key health concerns and disease profiles across age, gender and economic status. These data provide a baseline against which data from Local Health Profiles (LHP) from one region can be easily compared with another. They also enable the reader to gain insight into how health varies across a region in relation to a specific health concern. Since 2008 the online report also contains updatable tables showing regional comparisons and national trends for those health concerns represented by indicators presented in **Local Health Profiles**. There is also a small section on the report providing some international comparisons of the same health indicators. This provides a useful snapshot of public health and well-being in England and a brief insight into international comparisons.

The availability of such a wide range of data sources means that health care practitioners and the general public have access to a wealth of reports and information as to the health of their specific local population and the wider national and international community. However, when we investigate the 'health boom' in greater depth through these reports the picture is neither as clear nor as optimistic as it first appears. Despite the overall increase in the availability of treatments and care for many illnesses that could potentially severely restrict health, research across societies reveals that health is unequally distributed within and between populations (Nazroo, 2001; Aspinall and Jacobson, 2004; WMRO, 2007). While there is some variation in the degree of disparity in different countries dependent on the nature of the health care conditions discussed, the important fact is that the greatest burden of ill health is borne by the marginalised groups in societies worldwide (Marmot, 2005; Futterman and Lemberg, 2007).

The **Office for National Statistics (ONS)** for example, regularly publishes reports and tables comparing life expectancy **(LE)**, healthy life expectancy **(HLE)** and disability-free life expectancy **(DFLE)** at birth and at age 65 for populations in the UK, Great Britain, England, Wales, Scotland and Northern Ireland. The 2008 quarterly health report found that for the three year period 2004–06, people born in Scotland could be expected to live approximately 2 years less than their peers when compared to the UK as a whole. In addition, their HLE at birth was also judged to be lower than that for the rest of the UK, significantly so for males. Moreover if the life expectancy of people post state retirement age (over 65) was compared with the rest of the UK, it was also lower in Scotland (by 1 year) for both males and females (ONS, 2008). The data therefore suggests that that the lower LE predicted in newborn babies in Scotland compared to the rest of the UK is not simply due to higher risk of death at younger ages, but also inequalities in older age. A fact which is quite startling if we consider that in comparison to many areas of the world, the UK is perceived to be a relatively affluent society where free and equitable health care is available to all.

This raises the question as to how and why health and indeed life chances vary. In a study funded by the Joseph Rowntree Foundation, Mitchell *et al.* (2000) found that an individual's risk of premature death was strongly related to their age, sex, social class and employment status. The researchers calculated the number of premature deaths, which could be expected in each parliamentary constituency in Britain based on these characteristics. Their calculations were based on national mortality statistics, census data and statistical models, using data from 1981–85 and 1991–95. The impact of any changes in the cultural, social or economic environment of the individuals on their life expectancy was then calculated to illustrate how external factors e.g. health and employment policies could have an affect on the life expectancy of the individual. For example, their studies demonstrated that for a middle-aged, long-term unemployed man, the effect of returning to work under conditions of full employment would be to lower his risk of premature mortality. They concluded that changes in economic circumstances alone could result in about 37% of 'avoidable' deaths in poorer areas being prevented (Mitchell *et al.,* 2000). The issue of health inequalities is discussed in more depth in Chapter 14.

Since the initial definition of health by WHO stated earlier, it has been recognized that health is determined by more than just the physical condition of a human being. Increasingly it is recognized that the cultural, social and environmental contexts in which health or ill health is experienced, has a major impact on health and life chances (Aspinall and Jacobson, 2004; Healthcare Commission, 2005). These contextual factors which influence health are often collectively known as the social determinants of health and refer to the social and economic conditions in which people live that impact (directly or indirectly) on their health. These are the confounding factors which affect health 'risks' in their broadest sense, that is the nature of the illness a person may be more likely to be exposed to, their ability or willingness to adhere to recommended treatments and their degree of **self agency** .

The social determinants of health are by nature not completely divorced from the individual's personal choices. As such, how or why they impact on health cannot simply be understood in isolation from the cultural, social and environmental contexts in which people live their lives and manage their health. There are many sociological and anthropological texts which critically explore the various aspects and uses of the terms culture, social contexts and environment in their purest sense and the aim here is not to repeat or review those debates in depth. However, they are recommended for detailed discussion of the use and meanings of these terms (Denzin, 1992; Bhopal, 1997; Polaschek, 1998). What follows here is a brief overview of the key issues as they relate to public health nursing.

The influence of culture on health

Culture may be understood as a shared system of meanings, values and beliefs learned through socialization (Haralambos and Holborn, 2008). In its simplest sense it may be viewed as the 'rules of behaviour and the expectations of us' that we learn in particular social situations or at different stages of our lives. For example, as we grow up in our families from babies to adults we learn the 'rules' of behaviour and what is expected of us from our parents. As nursing students you learn skills relating to practice as well as expectations of professional conduct laid out in the Code of Professional Conduct for Nurses and Midwives (Nursing and Midwifery Council, 2007).

Culture may be seen as universal in some sense in that it is an aspect of life for all people while at the same time it varies between individuals and groups and may be modified over time through legislative, political or social action. For example, in the last few years smoking in public has become less socially

acceptable in British culture as a result of increased knowledge about the dangers of passive smoking and the risks to individual health, resulting in legislation to ban it in public places. This is a far cry from the 1940s when open promotion of smoking in the film, sport and advertising media was acceptable. Thus what is accepted as a cultural norm today may not exist or be demonstrated in the same way in the future.

Cultural beliefs and cultural learning occur on both an individual and group level. Some values and beliefs that make up our culture may be personal to us as individuals while others reflect the expectations of a social group (for example, families, communities, religious affiliation).

Individual and group cultures are an essential part of a person's world view as they may impact on how we live our lives and indeed how we make sense of the world and our place in it (Haralambos and Holborn 2008). Our beliefs about health, what it is and how we maintain or measure our health are informed by our culture and the influence of the groups we belong to. It is the close relationship between culture, the individual and their community which explains why health is so frequently affected by it.

'Culture has a significant contribution to make to health, not least because in all its forms it helps to provide the social fabric of communities, making them 'communities' in the real sense and sustaining the individuals within them'
London Health Commission, 2002

The interdependent nature of the relationship between cultural beliefs and health means that the choices, opportunities and actions arising as a result are subject to variability between individuals and groups as well as over time. Therefore in practice while 'health' beliefs can be found to exist in all cultures, their meanings and importance to individuals and groups in differing societies are not universal. In addition, the increasing ethnic diversity and globalization which exists in the twenty-first century means our health beliefs and behaviours are also influenced by exposure to cultures which differ from our own. Thus health is experienced and influenced within the complex and varied relationships existing within and between groups from the same and differing cultures in all societies, which in turn modify health outputs.

Variations in culture between and within social groups may have an effect on:

- Understandings of health — how we understand 'health' and 'ill health' at different stages in the lifespan, what our expectations are in relation to our health.

- Health behaviour — how we act to promote or maintain our health (diet, exercise) and that of others in our care (children, patients, dependants, peers).

- Illness behaviour and expression — how we act at times of illness, whether and when we seek support to manage illness, how we expect others to behave when they are ill (seek medical help, self care, take time to recover).

The factors identified above may impact on the willingness and ability of an individual or group to access health care services and to accept the care available. This is often dependent on the degree of congruence between the culturally determined health beliefs of the individual in relation to these factors and the available health care service or recommended practice. For example the religious restrictions on blood transfusions for Jehovah's Witnesses may affect the willingness of a patient to consent to certain types of procedures or require the health care providers to consider alternative options when advising a patient.

The key issue when considering the impact of culture on health is to understand that complex and varied belief systems around specific aspects of health exist in and between cultural groups. These belief systems may be evidenced in patient or client health behaviours such as:

- Willingness to seek early advice or care for health concerns,
- Expressing or demonstrating doubts about the need for medical intervention or procedures for specific health concerns,
- Degree of compliance with medical advice or treatment.

It is important that nurses appreciate the role of culture as a contextualizing factor in a person's health and use this knowledge to inform assessment of their needs. This will form the basis of a process by which they can work to minimize cultural conflicts in advice given to patients and optimize the success of care provision.

The influence of poverty, education and social environment on health

The quote from the London Health Commission in the last section identifies the close association between culture and communities. Culture however is not the only thing which unites social communities and impacts on health. Communities in a physical sense are often viewed as comprising of neighbourhoods of people who often have similar facilities and amenities in their locality. In relation to public health, neighbourhood mapping collates information concerning the relative affluence of populations with and between geographical areas. Health maps of these localities have revealed health inequalities existing across and within communities; research has continued to identify the cause and effect of these inequalities in the population. The results of these ongoing investigations demonstrate that poverty, educational attainment and social environments are some of the key factors, which have the greatest impact on community health. Poverty, education and social environment are very closely related and impact directly and indirectly on each other in the life chances of the individuals who make up a community.

There has been much debate about the definition of poverty and how we determine when someone is in poverty. A useful definition of poverty which takes into account the impact on the daily lives of individuals and their communities was provided by Professor Peter Townsend who conducted a survey on poverty in the UK in 1979:

'Individuals, families and groups in the population can be said to be in poverty when they lack the resources to obtain the types of diet, participate in the activities, and have the living conditions and amenities which are customary, or are at least widely encouraged and approved, in the societies in which they belong.'
Townsend, 1980:31

Poverty is a central concern in public health. The effects of poverty on the health of individuals, families and communities are well documented and make sombre reading. Research has firmly established that families living on low incomes have a lower health status than those with higher incomes (Hirsch and Spencer, 2008). This is not restricted to one country but a worldwide phenomenon. People living in poverty have a reduced life expectancy and experience poorer health than the rest of the population in all societies worldwide (Isaacs and Schroeder, 2004; Schulz and House et al., 2008). In some senses poverty is an 'equal opportunity' risk factor for health, the pattern of worsening outcomes for those living in poverty is evidenced for the majority of health risk factors and diseases, remaining applicable across a range of racial and ethnic groups (Schulz et al., 2008).

One of the major ways in which poverty affects health is that it increases the exposure to living environments that increase the risk of ill health (such as poor housing, adequate sanitation or overcrowding) while at the same time reducing the ability of individuals to meet some of the economic challenges to maintain their own health. For example, limited budgets may mean buying inexpensive foods, which are more likely to be processed, fatty, and lacking important nutrients. The situation is compounded by the fact that they are also more likely to live in poor environmental situations with limited local health care resources, thus incurring additional 'costs' in accessing health care.

Poverty has also been found to impact on the mental and social aspects of health as well as the physical. The Child Poverty Action Group identifies that the impact of poverty goes beyond simply 'being on a low income and going without'. They stress the social and emotional 'costs' of living in poverty such as powerlessness, loss of respect, higher rates of poor educational attainment, loss of self-esteem and social isolation (Hirsch and Spencer, 2008).

Educational attainment is directly linked to employment prospects and the earning potential of an individual in British society. The majority of high earning jobs require more than a basic level of education and training. This has the obvious impact of reducing the chances of living in poverty and minimizing exposure to some of the health risks earlier. This summation is reinforced by research, which has directly compared the health outcomes for individuals by educational attainment. For example a study by Higgins *et al.*(2008) presents a range of international evidence, which indicates that lower educational attainment is related to reduced life expectancy, increased risk of premature death and increased likelihood of living with poorer health compared with those with higher levels of education. In particular, the findings report associations between educational level and death from lung cancer, stroke and cardiovascular disease as well as increased risk of diabetes, asthma, dementia and depression.

The link between poverty and low educational attainment has a negative impact on society as well as the individual. The overall affect is to reduce the pool of potential employees with the appropriate skills available to employers. This in turn has the effect of impeding economic growth in a country. This was well illustrated in a study on child poverty, which found that the cost to Britain of the failure to achieve a good level of general education by significant sections of the population was at least £25 billion a year (Hirsch, 2008).

The social environment comprises the groups and communities in which people live and social networks within them. The social networks in a community exist at an individual and group level and are important aspects of the ability to maintain health along with family structure, culture, access to facilities, economic status and the physical neighbourhood. The consequences of living in poverty or relative wealth and low educational achievement versus higher level qualifications combine with these other aspects of an individual's life to underpin the social environment in which they live. It is in this social context that health chances are determined, experienced and managed by an individual through their lifespan. Consequently it is important for nurses to remain aware that the affects of poverty, educational achievement and the social environment act as modifying factors influencing the health of individuals, families and communities.

The contexts of health — influences across lifespan

The lifespan provides a useful framework for exploring the challenges and opportunities influencing public health needs and the causes of ill health. From a life course perspective it is possible to reflect on the current and future key concerns over health of the public in a given society. As indicated in the previous discussions concerning culture and the social contexts of health, these influences are highly contextual and variable at an individual and group level. These are often linked to the incidence and prevalence rates of specific illnesses, diseases and health indicators in the population at different stages of

the lifespan. The major challenges to public health also vary across countries so it is important when considering these issues to ensure the context is clearly articulated. What follows next is a broad overview of health and ill health in Britain during the major developmental milestones: childhood and adolescence, adulthood and older age.

Health in childhood and adolescence

Childhood represents the stage in life when there is the greatest degree of physical, emotional and social growth and development. This is characterised by many developmental milestones through which the initially highly dependent newborn baby becomes a fully functioning physically independent human being. Childhood health in Britain covers the needs of children from pre-birth (antenatal period) to 18 years — the legal age of adulthood. The WHO and its partners, charge all societies to take seriously the importance of ensuring the healthy growth and development of their children in order to safeguard the future health and well-being of their population (WHO and UNICEF *et al.*, 2002).

According to the 2001 census, children make up on average 25% of the population in England (ONS, 2001). When compared to the health of children in developing countries, child health in the UK is relatively good with the infant mortality rate steadily falling since the inception of the NHS and increased availability of high quality maternity services and child health provision. However, there are some aspects of child health which continue to challenge health care providers and the public. Health data reported by the NHS indicates that:

- Almost 10% of children aged 15–16 years are diagnosed with a mental health disorder.

- There are an estimated 700,000 disabled children under 16 years in Great Britain

- A pre-school child will see a GP about six times a year.

DH, 2004

When considering the influences on health in childhood it is important from a public health perspective to acknowledge the degree to which child health is impacted on by the social contexts in which they live and in particular the health behaviours of their parents and others on whom they are dependent. Poor health choices made by expectant mothers (such as diet, smoking, alcohol intake) or inadequate attendance for antenatal care can affect the health of children even before they are born. Newborns and young children are particularly vulnerable to malnutrition and infectious diseases, many of which can be effectively prevented through use of immunization programmes or treated if appropriate medical advice is accessed in time. The decisions and willingness to make such positive health choices are closely aligned to the importance of education for health as discussed earlier. Research has shown that the educational level of the parent has a significant impact on their willingness to access preventative services and follow healthy living advice (Hirsch and Spencer, 2008).

One very important aspect of child health is the far reaching affects of poverty on children. This has been shown to result in not only the experience of poorer health during childhood but research shows that the effects are likely to last throughout their lives (WHO and UNICEF et al., 2002). The **End Child Poverty Campaign** (2008) millennium cohort study found that in households with annual incomes below about £10,000, three year old children were 2.5 times more likely to suffer from long-term chronic illnesses than children in households with incomes above £52,000. Further evidence of the impact of poverty on child health is found in the infant mortality rates. Not withstanding the falling mortality rates for children over the last decades, within group comparisons in the UK reveal that the risk of mortality is higher for children living in poorer households. These were reported to be 5.9 infant deaths per 1,000 live births, a rate which was 20% higher than the average 4.9 per 1,000 (DH, 2007).

This suggests that public health initiatives to improve the health outputs of children must be focussed on more than simply disease recognition and treatment. They must take into account the influences of the social and cultural environments which impact on their life chances.

Worldwide it is estimated that one in every five people are aged between 10–19 years — the period of transition from child to adult known as adolescence (WHO and UNICEF et al., 2002). Adolescence is identified as one of the most turbulent periods of human development characterised by a period of major physical and psychological change, at the same time as cultural shifts in expectations, social interactions and relationships (British Medical Association, 2003).

In British society, adolescence is seen as a generally healthy period of development, free from the helplessness of childhood or the pressures of adulthood. However, ill health and mortality are still evident in this stage of life. Many adolescents still die as a result of preventable or treatable conditions related to poor health choices or lack of awareness of health risks. The death rates in adolescence due to accidents, suicide or violence may reflect the pressures of trying to manage this challenging stage of development alongside the complexities of life in the twenty-first century (British Medical Association, 2003). The public health impact of other influences on adolescent health may not emerge or affect the individual until later in life. The long-term effects of untreated sexually transmitted infections on fertility or increased risk of premature death due to alcohol abuse stemming from binge drinking in adolescence are two such examples (Viner and Taylor, 2007). It is also important to note that in addition to increased mortality rates many of the life limiting consequences of long-term chronic illness in adult life result from poor self care in adolescence (Twisk et al.,2002).

Chronic illness and disability are equally part of the profile of adolescent health as for other stages in human development. This often brings with it additional dimensions in relation to family health needs as many such adolescents require direct family care beyond the normal developmental age. In relation to public health this means the burden of care for families is extended along with the economic costs of caring for a child with additional health needs. When this is viewed in the context of the impact of poor educational achievement and family poverty on life chances, it suggests that the health of adolescents living with disability or chronic illness and their families may be further compromised.

The health of adolescents in any society also has an effect on that of future populations as the prospective parents of the next generation. Research illustrates that babies born to adolescent parents have a higher risk of perinatal mortality and of suffering from low birth weight (WHO and UNICEF et al., 2002; Higgins et al., 2008). The high levels of teenage pregnancy in the UK adds a further dimension in that the effects on the next generation are likely to be seen before the parents reach adulthood themselves. The WHO for example identifies that preventing teen pregnancy and improving the nutritional status of girls before they enter pregnancy could reduce maternal and infant mortality, and contribute to breaking the cycle of inter-generational malnutrition (WHO and UNICEF et al., 2002). In addition, as with other children their future life chances are also likely to be determined by the social environment and any social or economic disadvantages of their parents. In the case of teen parents, the disadvantages are likely to be greater as their young age, coupled with their parental responsibilities precludes them from full time employment and may impede high educational achievement (Higgins et al., 2008).

The needs of children and adolescents can be seen to have important consequences for them at the most vulnerable phases in their development. The personal, social and economic case for optimizing the focus on health in childhood and adolescence is compelling. The consequences of ill health or increased risk in this age group could impact on the child, their family and the wider community. In supporting children and their families to live healthy lives, health care professionals can influence public health in both current and future populations.

Health in adulthood

Adulthood covers the greatest period of time in the lifespan. It is a time of social independence and optimal autonomy in British society. Many of the issues affecting public health reported and recorded through health data relate to adult populations. As previously discussed, through variations in culture, education, poverty and social environments a range of diverse factors impact on health in adulthood between and within social groups in every society.

Adulthood is also in some sense a 'determining' stage in relation to health of individuals and communities. The consequences of life experiences or health care decisions made during childhood and adolescence often fully emerge in adult life. Furthermore, the independent decisions and social context in which health is experienced in adulthood, has also been found to significantly affect life expectancy in older age as well as future quality of life (London Health Commission, 2002).

The key messages relating to factors impacting on health were discussed at the beginning of this chapter and all relate in some way to public health needs in adulthood. It is therefore vitally important that public health nurses are able to understanding the broad factors influencing health discussed earlier and can relate these to the health experiences of the adults in their care. Adults are frequently responsible for the health of others as well as their own. Good health in adulthood not only increases the individual's chance of a healthy, more productive life, but will also directly impact on the health and life chances of their children. The majority of public health work at this stage of human development relates to providing effective health education to help inform adults about the factors impacting on their health in order that they can make informed choices for themselves and their dependants.

Conversely public health in adults is also concerned with supporting and maintaining the health of those living with chronic illness or disability. This brings with it particular challenges as these members of the population may be unable to fulfil their social roles in society due to ill health. This can impact on emotional or mental health and may be associated with depression and further risk of social isolation (Morris, 2004). The challenge to public health here is to support adults living with chronic illness or disability to remain fully engaged with society by optimizing their self agency and independence. This may involve seeking ways to support their carers and families who bear the brunt of the economic and emotional costs of caring as well as providing for the physical health care needs of the individual.

Health in older age

The success of strategies to improve health and well-being through public health initiatives is reflected in the increase in life expectancy. The number of people in the population aged over 60 years is growing faster than any other age group in almost all countries worldwide (WHO, 2000). However, the increasing longevity of the population also brings with it challenges to ensure that the older population in society experience better quality of life and good health along with the increase in number of years of life.

Good health is an essential prerequisite for older people to remain independent in order that they can continue to care for themselves and play an active part in family and community life (Swedish National Institute of Public Health, 2007). It is therefore of particular importance in this age group that health care initiatives support them to maintain their capacity to engage in society by maximizing their physical functioning and social engagement. Research has shown that onset of non-communicable and chronic diseases, such as heart disease, stroke and cancer can be prevented or delayed in the older population through use of health promotion activities and disease prevention strategies (DH, 2001).

Ill health or reduced functioning is experienced by many people as a consequence of the aging process. Some of the health problems many older people face may be directly or indirectly linked to health choices made in earlier life. However, when physical health is impaired in older people, it is imperative that accessible, integrated and regular care is provided as the consequences for the older person extend beyond the physical into the social and emotional aspects of their health. The time taken to recover from bouts of illness is extended in older age and the risk of developing chronic health complications and being socially isolated as a result is increased (Cacioppo and Hawkley, 2003). The health of the older person therefore requires strategies which unite their health and social care needs in order to minimize the development of associated disabilities and negative effects on their quality of life.

In relation to public health the older population should not always be viewed as a drain on the resources of a society. Many aspects of the social functioning of a healthy community, which is central to public health, are sustained by the activities of older people. For example, in Britain, older people play a central and crucial role in sustaining the social environment of communities through volunteering, transmitting experience and knowledge and helping their families with caring responsibilities (Wheelock and Jones, 2002; Lie et al., 2009). In addition, since the change in equality laws regarding age of employment, many have continued to contribute to the economic health of society by increasing their participation in the paid labour force (Ball, 2009).

Implications for care practice — National Service Frameworks (NSFs)

The influences and causes of ill health in a population are often reflected in public health policies or health care strategies reflecting the greatest threats to life or maintaining good health at a particular stage of life. These policies and strategies are used to inform and guide best practice in relation to the health of the population. They link closely to the cultural and social functioning of a society and beliefs about the part played by health care providers in sustaining and supporting health. A driving factor in contemporary practice in public health is a belief that effectively applied skills and interventions at the individual level can collectively have a positive impact on population health.

One of the most recent strategic approaches over the last decade which focussed on the optimization of health care in the UK was the introduction of the **National Service Frameworks**. The National Service Frameworks came into being in the mid-2000s and were devised as a systematic approach for meeting the agenda of improving standards and quality across health care sectors throughout the country. NSFs recognized the cultural and social contexts of care provision for the population and the importance of taking this into account when devising health care plans to meet the needs of individuals, groups and communities. They were therefore implemented in partnership with social care and other organizations to enable the diverse factors impacting on health to be addressed.

The NSFs reflect the areas of greatest concern to the health of the public in the 21ˢᵗ century. There are specific frameworks relating to the key health challenges of particular illnesses such as cancer, heart disease and long-term conditions, as well specific stages in the lifespan e.g. older age, childhood. However, all the NSFs were devised to fulfil the same shared objectives. They:

- set national standards and define service models for a service or care group,
- put in place programmes to support implementation,
- establish performance measures against which progress within agreed timescales would be measured.

DH, 1998

The two NSFs which relate to lifespan are the National Service Framework for older people (DH, 2001) and the National Service Framework for children, young people and maternity services (DH, 2004). Full details of all the NSFs and their recommendations were published by the Department of Health. A brief summary of these two NSFs is given below.

The National Service Framework for older people

The national service framework for older people was launched in 2001 and presents eight standards, which form the focus for a ten year programme of action to meet the health needs of older people. The eight standards detailed in the document cover:

- rooting out age discrimination; person-centred care,
- intermediate care; general hospital care,

- stroke,
- falls,
- mental health in older people,
- the promotion of heath and active life in older age.

It provides directives for linking health and social care services to support independence in the elderly, emphasizing the move to promote good health and provision of specialised services for key conditions (DH, 2001). The standards also embody the fundamental principles of equality by championing care based on clinical need, not age. They take into account the issues relating to emotional and social health needs at this stage in the life course by requiring that care services treat older people as individuals, with equal emphasis being placed on promoting their quality of life, independence, dignity and autonomy in relation to making decisions about their own care.

The NSF for older people sets out specific goals for addressing some of the greatest challenges to health and longevity in older people. In addition it also addresses the needs for support and personalized care in community settings through prioritization of intermediate care facilities. Intermediate care has been shown to accelerate discharge from hospital for older people and increase their ability to manage at home or in supported community settings (Swedish National Institute of Public Health, 2007). Effective provision of care closer to home has the added benefit of helping the elderly to avoid personal health related crises and emergency hospital admissions by offering more timely and personalized care (Garasen *et al.,* 2007).

The National Service Framework for children, young people and maternity services

The National Service Framework for children, young people and maternity services launched in September 2004, sets out the quality of services that children, young people and their families have a right to expect and receive. Like the NSF for older people it presents a ten year programme of strategies for development and delivery of long-term and sustained improvement through high quality care.

The NSF for children, young people and maternity services takes into account the needs of children and their families at this very vulnerable stage in life. The recommendations and targets outlined in the NSF include provision for children and their families in partnership with the range of health and social care services that support them. The NSF for children, young people and maternity services recognizes the importance of the social environment and wider cultural influences in the antenatal and adolescent phases of development on health and life chances. It sets out to address these by ensuring that fair, high quality and integrated health and social care, is available for children and families from pregnancy through to adulthood.

This NSF is published in three parts and contains standards closely aligned to the 'Every Child Matters' agenda, a UK government initiative aimed at improving children's overall health and well-being as well as ability to make a positive contribution to society (Barker, 2009).

The framework was developed as a partnership between health and social care and other stakeholders in the health and well-being of children and families. The cultural shift in relation to this NSF is the importance placed on including children in the decision-making process relating to their care. This is especially important in the UK context where legal status of children has historically marginalised their involvement making choices about their care (DH, 2004; Barker, 2009).

Summary

In summary it can be seen that sustaining and improving the health of the population through the lifespan is about valuing diversity and difference within and between social groups. This requires public health practitioners to appreciate how health needs change over the lifespan and incorporate this knowledge into care planning, needs assessment and service delivery to maximize the health and life chances of an individual, group or community.

 Online Resource Centre

For more information on the influences on health and the causes of ill health across the lifespan visit the Online Resource Centre —
http://www.oxfordtextbooks.co.uk/orc/linsley/

References

Aspinall, P. & B. Jacobson (2004). *Ethnic disparities in health and healthcare: A focused review of the evidence and selected examples of good practice*. London: London Health Observatory.

Ball, C. (2009). 'Ageing and work'. *Quality in ageing and older adults* 10(2): 47–53.

Barker, R. (2009). *Making Sense of Every Child Matters — Multi - professional practice guidance* London: Policy Press.

Bhopal, R. (1997). 'Is research into ethnicity and health racist, unsound, or important science?' *British Medical Journal* 314: 1751

British Medical Association (2003). *Adolescent Health*. London: British Medical Association: 66.

Cacioppo, J. & L. C. Hawkley (2003). 'Social Isolation and Health, with an Emphasis on Underlying Mechanisms.' *Perspectives in Biology and Medicine* 46(3) Supplement:. S39–S52.

Denzin, N. K. (1992). *Sybolic interactionism and cultural studies*. Oxford: Blackwell.

Department of Health (1998). *A first class service: Quality in the new NHS*. London: DH.

Department of Health (2001). *The National Service Framework for older people*. London: DH.

Department of Health (2004). *National Service Framework (NSF) for Child Health and Maternity services*. London: DH.

Department of Health (2007). *National Service Framework (NSF) for Children, Young People and Maternity services. The Mental Health and Psychological Well Being of Children and Young People*: Standard 9. London: DH.

Futterman, L. G. & L. Lemberg (2007). 'Inequalities in the Healthcare System: A Problem, Worldwide'. *American Journal of Critical Care* 16: 617–620.

Garasen, H., R. Windspoll, *et al.* (2007). Intermediate care at a community hospital as an alternative to prolonged general hospital care for elderly patients: a randomised controlled trial.' *BMC Public Health* 7: 68.

Haralambos, M. & M. Holborn (2008). *Sociology, themes and persectives*. London:Collins Educational.

Healthcare Commission (2005). *Count me in: Results of a national census of inpatients in mental health hospitals and facilities in England and Wales*. London: Commission for Healthcare Audit and Inspection: 44.

Higgins, C., T. Lavin, *et al.*(2008). *Health Impacts of Education: a Review*, Institute of Public Health in Ireland.

Hirsch, D. (2008). *Estimating the Costs of Child Poverty*. London: Joseph Rowntree Foundation.

Hirsch, D. & N. Spencer (2008). *Unhealthy Lives: Intergenerational links between child poverty and poor health in the UK* London: End Child Poverty Campaign.

Isaacs, S. L. & S. A. Schroeder (2004). 'Class — The Ignored Determinant of the Nation's Health'. *New England Journal of Medicine* 351: 1137–1142.

Lie, M., S. Baines, *et al.*(2009). 'Citizenship, volunteering and active ageing' *Social Policy and Administration* 43(7): 702–718.

London Health Commission (2002). *Culture and health: Making the link 2002*. London: London Health Commission: 20.

Marmot, M. (2005). 'Social determinants of health inequalities'. *The Lancet*, 365(9464): 1099–1104.

Mitchell, R., D. Dorling, *et al.*(2000). *Reducing health inequalities in Britain*, London: Joseph Rowntree Foundation.

Morris, J. (2004). *People with physical impairments and mental health support needs: a critical review of the literature*. York: Joseph Rowntree Foundation. Nazroo, J. Y. (2001). *Ethnicity, class and health*. London: Policy Studies Institute.

Nursing and Midwifery Council (2007). *The Code: Standards of conduct, performance and ethics for nurses and midwives*. London: Nursing and Midwifery Council UK.

Office for National Statistics. (2001, 01/11/05). 'Census England and Wales 2001'. Retrieved 03/04/10, 2010.

Office for National Statistics (2008). *Health Statistics Quarterly*. Newport. 40 Winter 2008.

Polaschek, N. R. (1998). 'Cultural safety: A new concept in nursing people of different ethnicities'. *Journal of Advanced Nursing* 27(3): 452–457.

Schulz, A. J., House, J. S., Israel, B. A., Mentz, G., Dvonch, J. T., Miranda, P. Y., Kannan, S., & Koch, M. (2008). 'Relational pathways between socioeconomic position and cardiovascular risk in a multiethnic urban sample: complexities and their implications for improving health in economically disadvantaged populations'. *Journal of Epidemiology and Community Health* 62: 638–646.

Swedish National Institute of Public Health (2007). *Healthy ageing — A challenge for Europe*. Stockholm: Swedish National Institute of Public Health.

Townsend, P (1980) *Poverty in the United Kingdom: A Survey of Household Resources and Standards of Living*. London: Penguin Books.

Twisk, J., & H. Kemper, *et al.*(2002). 'The Relationship Between Physical Fitness and Physical Activity During Adolescence and Cardiovascular Disease Risk Factors at Adult Age. The Amsterdam Growth and Health Longitudinal Study'. *International Journal of Sports Medicine* 23(S1): 8–14.

Viner, R. M. & B. Taylor (2007). 'Adult outcomes of binge drinking in adolescence: findings from a UK national birth cohort study'. *Journal of Epidemiology and Community Health* 61: 902–907.

Wheelock, J. & K. Jones (2002). 'Grandparents are the Next Best Thing': Informal Childcare for Working Parents in Urban Britain'. *Journal of Social Policy*, 31(3): 441–464.

WMRO (2007). *State of the Region Report Update 2007*. West Midlands: West Midlands Regional Observatory.

World Health Organization (1948). *Preamble to the Constitution of the World Health Organization*. International Health Conference, New York: WHO.

World Health Organization (2000). *Social Development and Ageing: Crisis or Opportunity?* Geneva, WHO

World Health Organization & UNICEF, *et al.*(2002). *A healthy start in life: Report on the global consultation on child and adolescent dealth and development*, Geneva: WHO: 40.

Chapter 3
Health promotion theory

Paul Linsley

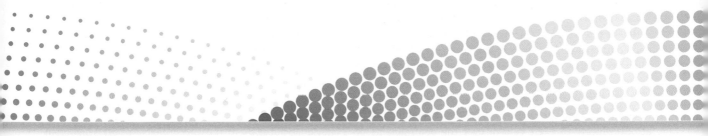

Introduction

This chapter introduces the reader to the field of health promotion and provides an overview of key health promotion definitions and concepts. It examines a range of models and theories of health promotion, which have helped shape health promotion practice. The chapter helps the reader to understand the complexities of delivering health promotion activities both at an individual and community level and looks at the role of the nurse in supporting this activity. This overview of approaches to working with individuals and communities to improve health demonstrates the breath of action and knowledge characteristic of current health promotion thinking. Taken together these approaches provide valuable guidance on how healthy public policy is developed to meet the changing demands of the general public and their perceptions of health.

Defining health promotion

Over the past three decades, the field of health promotion as emerged and provided a new way of thinking about the root causes of health and well-being. This thinking has sparked the development of new approaches to improving the health of individuals and communities. Before we can begin to look at health promotion however we need to be clear what we mean by the term health, the thing that we are trying to promote. Health has been described as:

'... a state of complete physical, mental and social well being, and not merely the absence of disease or infirmity, is a fundamental human right and that the attainment of the highest possible level of health is a most important worldwide social goal whose realization requires the action of many other social and economic sectors in addition to the health sector.'
WHO, 1978

Contained within this definition is the concept of positive health. This is used to describe not only physical fitness but the ability to meet mental stresses (see Chapter 17), solve life problems, and maintain emotional stability, as well as an individual's ability to improve his or her own well-being (Jadad and O'Grady, 2008). Achieving this requires the adoption of a social model of health recognizing a holistic and positive approach and highlighting socio-cultural, economic, political and key environmental determinants of health. Health promotion has been defined as:

'the process of enabling people to increase control over, and to improve, their health'
WHO, 1985: 5

Furthermore, in order to:

'reach a state of complete physical, mental and social well being an individual or group must be able to identify and to realize aspirations, to satisfy needs, and to change or cope with the environment. Health is, therefore, seen as a resource for everyday life, not the objective of living. Health is a positive concept emphasizing social and personal

resources, as well as physical capabilities. Therefore, health promotion is not just the responsibility of the health sector but goes beyond healthy lifestyles to well being'.
WHO, 1986a: 5

Goodstadt *et al.* (1987:61) extend this definition by describing health promotion as 'the maintenance and enhancement of existing levels of health through the implementation of effective polices, programmes and services. Whilst Tones, (1987:2) simply stated that health promotion is 'any planned measure which promotes health or prevents disease, disability and premature death'.

Health promotion is a process directed towards enabling people to take action. Thus, health promotion is not something that is done on or to people; it is done by, with and for people either as individuals or as groups. The purpose of this activity is to strengthen the skills and capabilities of individuals to take action and the capacity of groups or communities to act collectively to exert control over the determinants of health and achieve positive change (WHO, 1997a). It suggests that people and communities can bring about positive changes in their health and well-being: that improvement is achieved through personal endeavour and the support of others.

This provides an alternative to a traditional medical model of health care addressing the symptoms rather than the causes of ill health. It places medicine, and indeed health, in a wider social context. This context acknowledges, accepts and reveals the causes of ill health and health inequalities as not the sole responsibility of individuals or health care services but a range of public and private organizations including national and local government (Amos and Munro, 2002). It puts health on the agenda of policy makers in all sectors and at all levels, directing them to be aware of the health consequences of their decisions and to accept their responsibilities for health (Naidoo and Wills, 2000). This broadens the debate to include identification of problems and possible solutions for promoting health.

Health promotion distinguishes between those factors which are more within the control of individuals, such as individual health-related behaviors and the **use** of health services, and those factors which are outside the control of individuals, including social, economic and environmental, and the **provision** of health services (Tones and Green, 2004). Health promotion addresses both areas. It helps in providing individuals and groups with the knowledge, values and skills that encourage effective action for health (see Box 3.1). It also helps to generate political commitment for health supportive policies and practices, the provision of services and increased public interest, and demand for health.

Determinants of health

A number of prerequisites have been identified that are basic to good health within any society. These include peace,

---

Box 3.1 Health promotion programmes are aimed at:

- Whole populations,
- Communities,
- Individuals.

---

adequate economic resources (and their distribution) food and shelter, clean water, a stable ecosystem, sustainable resource use, and access to basic human rights (WHO, 2000). Recognition of these prerequisites highlights the inextricable links between social and economic conditions, structural changes, the physical environment, individual lifestyles and health. These links provide the key to a holistic understanding of health, and are meaningful to people's lives as they experience them. Such diversity reflects the fact that health promotion practice is not only concerned with the behaviour of individuals but also with the ways in which society is organized and the policies and organizational structures that underpin social organization (Tones and Green, 2004).

Determinants of health refer to the range of social, economic and environmental factors which determine the health status of individuals or populations (Nutbeam, 1998). These include:

- Income and social status,
- Social support networks,
- Education,
- Employment and working conditions,
- Physical environments,
- Social environments,
- Biology and genetic endowment,
- Healthy child development,
- Health services.

Nutbeam, 1998: 27

Health promotion practice is fundamentally concerned with addressing the determinants of health—including: the lifestyle factors related to the actions of individuals, such as health related behaviours (e.g., smoking, diet and physical activity); broader factors such as income, education, employment and working conditions, and social and physical environments. These factors, in combination, create the conditions determining health status at the individual and community level. Health promotion strategies can develop and change lifestyles, and the social, economic and environmental conditions which determine health.

Lifestyle is taken to mean 'a general way of living based on the interplay between living conditions in the wide sense and individual patterns of behaviour as determined by socio-cultural factors and personal characteristics' (Hood and

Leddy, 2003: 211). The range of behaviour patterns open may be limited by environmental factors and also by the degree of individual self reliance. The way an individual lives may produce behaviours that are beneficial or detrimental to health.

Often health promotion is seen as activities which focus on particular issues (see Box 3.2 for information on some of these issues). While this is one legitimate part of health promotion, it is much more than that. Health promotion also encompasses the principles that underlie a series of strategies that seek to foster conditions that allow individuals and populations to be healthy and to make healthy choices (Naidoo and Wills, 2004), for example, developing personal skills, strengthening community action, and creating supportive environments for health, backed by public health policy.

Box 3.2 Modern epidemics

The **World Health Report 2002** documented the public health impact of several major risk factors related to diet, nutrition, tobacco, alcohol, physical activity, hygiene, and unsafe sex. Failure to address these risks has led to cardiovascular and chronic respiratory diseases, diabetes, injuries and violence, several mental disorders and causes of substance dependence, HIV/AIDS and sexually transmitted diseases becoming major constraints to health development. Here is a list of health concerns currently occupying the British and other European and world governments:

- Obesity,
- Coronary heart disease,
- Diabetes mellitus,
- Long-term conditions,
- Disability,
- Suicide,
- Socially unacceptable behaviour.

All of these are amenable to health promotion interventions.

WHO, 2006

Good health is not equally shared however (Woodward and Kawachi, 2000) and health inequalities exist within and across communities and are influenced by social, cultural and economic factors (See Chapter 14). Health promotion aims at reducing differences in current health status and ensuring equal opportunities and resources to enable all people to achieve their fullest health potential (Lucas and Lloyd, 2005). Health promotion strategies and programmes should be adapted to the local needs and possibilities of individual countries and regions to take into account differing social, cultural and economic systems (WHO, 2006). This includes a secure foundation in a supportive environment, access to information, life skills and opportunities for making healthy choices.

Discussion point

- Does the government have the right to tell people how to manage their own health?
- Discuss the possible reasons for why some people might not be prepared or not be able to engage in initiatives and activities to improve their health.
- Do nurses have the right to judge people who have unhealthy lifestyles?
- Should nurses set an example to the public by adopting health lifestyles? For example, not smoking, taking plenty of exercise, and maintaining the correct weight.

The following extracts are from **The Wanless Report: Securing Good Health for the Whole Population (2004)** which sought to address the very questions posed in the discussion points box above:

7.3 Individuals are, and must remain, primarily responsible for decisions about their and their children's personal health and lifestyle. Individuals must be free to make their own choices about their own lifestyles.

7.4 If government or other bodies do intervene, it is essential that social welfare is improved and that personal freedoms are respected.

7.43 Individuals are primarily responsible for their own health and lifestyles. They are generally best able to make these decisions as they know more about their personal preferences and situation and generally are the best judge of their own health and happiness; and any intervention into an individual's lifestyle can raise legitimate questions of personal freedom.

7.29 Influencing and, over time, changing social attitudes to health and lifestyles is likely to be much more effective in the long run than a punitive approach that does not also aim for a change in attitude. Laws and regulations not accompanied by public support incur high enforcement costs, and could jeopardize the development of a consensus for future public health measures.

7.59 It is important that any government intervention is well managed, to protect against an inappropriate infringement of liberty or unintended consequences. To assist in the development of targeted interventions that increase both health and welfare, the following principles are suggested for adoption by government.

5 The right of the individual to choose their own lifestyle must be balanced against any adverse impacts those choices have on the quality of life of others.

8.7 Where regulation is enacted, it is important that it is both efficient and respects civil liberties.

8.13 In addition to public health campaigns, health professionals have a role in ensuring that citizens are more fully informed about ... alternative, less harmful, products and lifestyle choices they could make.

8.17 Taxes should therefore provide incentives for consumers either to lower consumption or to switch to less damaging products, thereby reducing demand for harmful goods to the socially optimal level. Furthermore, the suppliers of harmful products will have an incentive to produce less damaging goods, either through switching product mixes or investing in new technology.

Limits to government intervention:

8.42 Interventions to improve public health have the potential to reduce significantly personal freedoms. This is most clear when government acts explicitly to prevent or restrict individuals from behaving in certain ways, or from consuming particular goods.

8.43 In general, if the freedom to be curtailed or limited is a significant one and valued highly by the individual, the state would need strong reasons to impose its will over the individual on public health grounds. Usually, there should at least be a strong consensus, preferably public but certainly professional, that the public health measure is necessary to prevent harm to others. Government can of course legitimately intervene when one's freedom to act would infringe human rights for example, a person with a highly infectious disease may need to be quarantined without consent. In other cases, however, the mere fact of social or professional consensus may not provide sufficient justification for action.

8.44 Ideally, individual consent provides the strongest foundation for government action. However, in cases where it is only the individual's health that is at issue, the question of intervention without consent poses challenges. Nevertheless, there are examples where such measures have been enacted and have become accepted (for example, the restrictions on smoking see Chapter 13). First, individuals may already prefer not to be free to choose, and may accept restrictions. Second, they may come to accept the reasons behind the restrictions and no longer see them as an imposition. Nevertheless, it is important to recognize that measures should be justifiable in the public interest and to individuals as a reasonable restriction of their freedom.

The Ottawa Charter: The foundation for health promotion

The Ottawa Charter for Health Promotion was developed at the first International Conference on Health Promotion held in

Ottawa, Canada in 1986. This conference was primarily a response to growing expectations for a new public health movement around the world. Discussions focused on the needs in industrialized countries, but took into account similar concerns in all other regions. It built on the progress made through the **Declaration on Primary Health Care at Alma-Ata (1978)**, the World Health Organization's Targets for Health for All document published in 1985, and the World Health Assembly Report on intersectoral action for health (1986a). The Charter still represents consensus agreement on good health promotion practice and forms the basis of much health promotional work the world over. The action areas (discussed below) of the Ottawa Charter for Health Promotion (WHO1986b) are commonly used as a conceptual framework in health promotion programme development.

In tackling the determinants of health, health promotion will include combinations of the strategies first described in the Ottawa Charter (1986b), namely developing personal skills, strengthening community action, creating supportive environments for health, and reorientating health services towards health promotion, backed by healthy public policy.

Box 3.3 What makes good health promotion?

Build healthy public policy
Health promotion activities should encourage and support all agencies and workers to consider the impact of their decisions on health. Health promotion policy requires the identification of obstacles to the adoption of healthy public policies in non-health sectors, and ways of removing those obstacles. Joint action contributes to ensuring safer and healthier goods and services, healthier public services and cleaner, more enjoyable environments.

Create supportive environments
Health promotion activities recognize that health cannot be separated from other areas of life. They should aim to create ways of living, environmental conditions, working conditions and social structures which are safe, stimulating, enjoyable, satisfying and conducive to good health.

Strengthen community action
Health promotion activities should be developed in collaboration with the community to identify priorities for action and to develop strategies that will work. This involves supporting, encouraging, informing and skilling the community to take control of issues of importance to them and to define the way in which those issues are addressed.

Develop personal skills

Health promotion activities aim to support the personal and social development of individuals in their private and work lives so that they have the skills and information to make choices which will promote their health. This includes activities which will increase their capacity to undertake or facilitate actions in other areas. This enablement has to be facilitated in school, home, work and community settings. Action is required through educational, professional, commercial and voluntary bodies, and within the institutions themselves.

Reorient health services

Health promotion activities support the health system and all stakeholders in the system to move beyond clinical and curative services to services which aim at increasing and improving the health of the community. Health services also need to embrace an expanded mandate that is sensitive and respects cultural needs.

The Jakarta declaration on health promotion into the twenty-first century: building on the success of the Ottawa Charter

Participants, at the 4th International Conference on Health Promotion held in Jakarta in July 1997, confirmed the Ottawa Charter approaches and action areas:

'Research and case studies from around the world provide convincing evidence that health promotion works. Health promotion strategies can develop and change lifestyles, and the social, economic and environmental conditions which determine health. Health promotion is a practical approach to achieving greater equity in health'.
WHO, 1997b:3

To take health promotion into the twenty-first century and meet the new challenges, the conference participants prioritized five 'new forms of action' in addition to those cited in the Ottawa Charter which are as follows:

Promote social responsibility for health

The Jakarta declaration recommended the policies and practices should be pursued that:

- Avoid harming the health of other individuals,
- Protect the environment and ensure sustainable use of resources,
- Restrict production and trade in inherently harmful goods and substances.

Increase investments for health development

Investments for health should reflect the need to address health and social inequities, focusing on groups such as women, children, older people, indigenous people, those in poverty and marginalized populations.

Consolidate and expand partnerships for health

Health promotion requires health and social development partnerships among the different sectors at all levels of governance and society. Existing partnerships need to be strengthened and the potential for new partnerships should be explored.

Increase community capacity and empower the individual

Key strategies at a community level are:

- Strengthening advocacy through community action, particularly through groups organized by women.
- Enabling communities and individuals to take control over their health and environment through education and empowerment.
- Building alliances for health and supportive environments to strengthen the cooperation between health and environmental campaigns and strategies.
- Mediating between conflicting interests in society to ensure equitable access to supportive environments for health.
- Improving the capacity of communities for health promotion, which requires practical education, leadership training, and access to resources.
- Empowering individuals, which demands more consistent, reliable access to the decision-making process and the skills and knowledge essential to effect change.

Secure an infrastructure for health promotion

To secure an infrastructure for health promotion, new mechanisms for funding it locally, nationally and globally must be found. Incentives should be developed to influence the actions of governments, non-governmental organizations, educational institutions and the private sector to make sure that resource mobilization for health promotion is maximized.

'Settings for health' represent the organizational base of the infrastructure required for health promotion. New health challenges mean that new and diverse networks need to be created to achieve inter-sectoral collaboration. Such networks should provide mutual assistance within and among countries

29

and facilitate exchange of information on which strategies have proved effective and in which settings.

Training in and practice of local leadership skills should be encouraged in order to support health promotion activities. Documentation of experiences in health promotion through research and project reporting should be enhanced to improve planning, implementation and evaluation. All countries should develop the appropriate political, legal, educational, social and economic environments required to support health promotion. This requires countries and individual governments to work together in collaboration to meet the world wide health agenda.

The role of the nurse in health promotion

Whilst the health promotion function of nurses working in primary health care settings enjoys a longer tradition (Wass, 2000), it is only latterly that this has been applied to nurses working in hospital. Health promotion is an important part of the role of the nurse and one they are required to undertake as part of professional activity (NMC, 2008). Nurses are expected to participate in health promotion interventions by:

- Recognizing the role of the nurse in the promotion of health and self-care.
- Providing health promotion interventions.
- Being aware of the key health and social factors to be considered when carrying out an assessment of individual needs.
- Being aware of the contributions of other professionals to assessment and intervention.

Nurses, along with other professional and social groups and health personnel have a major responsibility to mediate between differing interests in society for the pursuit of health (Amos and Munro, 2002). The range of health promotion activities that nurses are currently involved in include:

- Supplying health education materials,
- Running public awareness and education programmes,
- Working with the mass media,
- Developing health promotions policies,
- Lobbying for healthy public policies,
- Coordinating/leading multi-agency work (healthy alliances),
- Community programme development within schools, workplaces etc.

Fundamental to the activities listed above is:

- The giving of information,
- Information gathering/consultation,
- Support,
- Advocacy for health,
- Initiation of services,
- Joint working.

Ewles and Simmett, 1999

Activity box

- What health promotion activities have you been involved in to date?
- You might like to reflect on these and their effectiveness.

Beliefs, attitudes and values

Psychological theories of health related behaviour have contributed a great deal to health promotion in the last two decades. The contribution of health psychology to health promotion is that it seeks to explain behaviour and offer ways of helping people to change their behaviour. Understanding the processes that take place in relation to health related behaviour is an important tool in planning health promotion activities (Tones and Green, 2004). There are a number of psychological theories that attempt to explain the different variables that exert influences on an individual's behaviour. Many of the above theories share similar components and terms:

- Beliefs — the information a person has about a particular object, it often links the object to some particular attribute. Information can influence beliefs which in turn can then influence behaviour.
- Values — Values are an integral part of every culture. They are acquired through socialization and are the emotionally charged beliefs about those things that a person regards as important. Values are often broad and influence the way we think about things in life, for example values relating to gender give rise to a number of attitudes to motherhood, employment for women etc.
- Attitudes — are more specific than values and describe relatively stable feelings towards particular issues or objects. The link between a person's attitudes and their behaviour is an unclear one. Sometimes changing attitudes may cause a behaviour change, and sometimes behaviour change may lead to attitude change (stop smoking for example).

McLeroy and colleagues (1988) identified five factors of influence for health-related behaviours and beliefs. These factors include:

(1) **Intrapersonal** or **individual** factors;

(2) **Interpersonal** factors;

(3) **Institutional** or **organizational** factors;

(4) **Community** factors; and

(5) **Public policy** factors. (See Table 3.1)

Table 3.1 Factors of influence

Concept	Definition
Intrapersonal factors	Individual characteristics that influence behavior, such as knowledge, attitudes, beliefs, and personality traits.
Interpersonal factors	Interpersonal processes and primary groups, including family, friends, and peers that provide social identity, support, and role definition.
Institutional factors	Rules, regulations, policies, and informal structures, which may constrain or promote recommended behaviors.
Community factors	Social networks and norms, or standards, which exist as formal or informal among individuals, groups, and organizations.
Public Policy factors	Local, state, and federal policies and laws that regulate or support healthy actions and practices for disease prevention, early detection, control, and management.

Health promotion theories and models

There are a number of significant **theories** and **models** that underpin the practice of health promotion. A theory is an integrated set of propositions that serves as an explanation for a phenomenon. The use of theory can help in the planning and delivery of health promotion programmes in several ways (Nutbeam and Harris, 2004). Theories and models:

• Help us understand better the nature of the problem being addressed.

• Describe and explain the needs and motivations of the target population.

• Explain or make propositions concerning how to change health status, health-related behaviours and their determinants.

• Inform the methods and measures used to monitor the problem and the programme.

A model is a subclass of a theory. It provides a plan for investigating and or addressing a phenomenon.

The main theories and models utilized are elaborated on below, but can be summarized as follows:

1. Those theories that attempt to explain health behaviour and health behaviour change by focusing on the individual. Examples include:
   • Health Belief Model,
   • Theory of Reasoned Action,
   • Stages of change Model,
   • Social Learning Theory.

2. Theories that explain change in communities and community action for health. Examples include:
   • Community mobilization.
      – social planning,
      – social action,
      – community development,
   • Diffusion of innovation

3. Models that explain changes in organizations and the creative of health supportive organizational practices. Examples include:
   • Theory of organizational change.

Health Belief Model

This model was originally designed to explain health behaviour by better understanding beliefs about health and Becker (1974), Kirscht, *et al.* (1970) and Rosenstock (1974) are proponents of this model. It is still one of the most widely recognized and used models in health behaviour applications. The rationale is that even though an individual recognizes the consequences of certain health behaviours his/her decisions to take action will be based on the following factors. The Health Belief Model addresses the individual's perceptions of the threat posed by a health problem (susceptibility, severity), the benefits of avoiding the threat, and factors influencing the decision to act (barriers, cues to action, and self-efficacy).

Susceptibility

The individuals belief about whether they are likely to contract the illness.

Severity

The degree to which an individual perceives the consequences of having the illness to be severe.

Together the two elements of susceptibility and severity comprise what is known as the perceived threat of illness, sometimes known as **vulnerability**.

The next two factors are concerned with the pros and cons of taking some action to combat the illness. What is to be gained? What do I have to pay?

Benefits

The degree of physical, psychological or financial benefit associated with any form of action *(benefits need to be achievable and assessable)*.

Barriers

Any decision to act will have a number of consequences. There may be a degree of physical, psychological or financial distress associated with any form of action.

The next two factors may stimulate action.

Cues to action

Cues are stimuli which can trigger appropriate health behaviour. They can either be internal (perception of bodily symptoms or states) or external (stimuli from the environment e.g. health professionals, media campaigns etc.).

Diverse factors

Includes things like environment, cultural, class and personality factors that may influence health behaviour.

Motivation

How predisposed a person is to engage in the health related behaviour, or how driven they are not to carry it out, for example the role that addiction plays in affecting behaviour change.

In order for a behavioural change to take place, an individual must:

• Have an incentive to change,
• Feel threatened by their current behaviour,
• Feel that change is beneficial in some way and have few adverse consequences,
• Feel competent to carry out the change.

The health belief model has been found most useful with preventative health behaviours such as screening and immunization. It has been less useful in guiding interventions to address more long-term, complex and socially determined behaviours such as alcohol and tobacco use (Glanz, Rimer, and Lewis, 2002). It has proved most useful as a planning tool for health education programmes intended to promote greater compliance with preventative health behaviours and health care recommendations (Nutbeam and Harris, 2004).

The theory of reasoned action and the theory of planned behaviour

Theory of Reasoned Action and the associated The Theory of Planned Behaviour (Fishbein and Ajzen, 1975; Ajzen and Fishbein, 1980; Ajzen and Madden, 1986) explore the relationship between behavior and beliefs, attitudes, and intentions. Both theories assume **behavioural intention** is the most important determinant of behavior. According to these models, behavioral intention is influenced by a person's **attitude** toward performing a behaviour, and by beliefs about whether individuals who are important to the person approve or disapprove of the behaviour **(subjective norm)**. The Theory of Planned Behaviour differs from the Theory of Reasoned Action in that it includes one additional construct, **perceived behavioural control**; this construct has to do with people's beliefs that they can control a particular behaviour. Azjen and Madden (1986) added this construct to account for situations in which people's behaviour, or behavioural intention, is influenced by factors beyond their control. He argued that people might try harder to perform a behaviour if they feel they have a high degree of control over it.

Stages of change model or transtheoretical model

The Stages of Change or Transtheoretical Model (Prochaska and DiClemente, 1983) was initially published in 1979 by Prochaska. In the 1980's Prochaska and DiClemente worked further on this model in outlining the stages of an individual's readiness to change, or attempt to change, toward healthy behaviours (Prochaska and Di Clemente, 1986). The Stages of Change Model evolved from research in smoking cessation and also the treatment of drug and alcohol addiction. More recently it has been applied to other health behaviours, such as dietary changes. Behaviour change is viewed as a process, not an event, with individuals at various levels of motivation or 'readiness' to change. Since people are at different points in this process, planned interventions should match their stage.

There are six stages that have been identified in the model:

1. **Pre-contemplation—(Not thinking about changing behaviour)** the person is unaware of the problem or has not thought seriously about change.

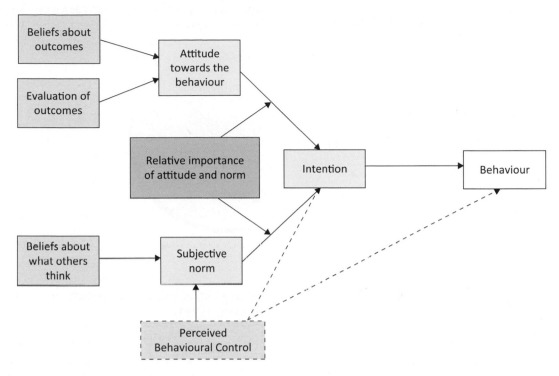

Fig. 3.1 Ajzen's theory of planned behaviour. Reproduced with permission from Ajzen, I. (1985).

2. **Contemplation—(Can stay at this stage for quite a while)**: the person is seriously thinking about a change (in the near future).

3. **Preparing to change**—the person is planning to take action and is making final adjustments before changing behaviour.

4. **Making the change**—the person implements some specific action plan to overtly modify behaviour and surroundings.

5. **Maintenance**—the person continues with desirable actions (repeating the periodic recommended steps while struggling to prevent lapses and relapse.

6. **Termination**—the person has no temptation and the ability to resist relapse.

Prochasaka *et al.* (1992) argue that whilst few people go through each stage in an orderly way, they will go through each stage, which is helpful as it enables us to understand that relapse is a part of the process and not necessarily a 'failure' on behalf of the person or health promoter. In fact individuals can go both backwards and forwards through a series of cycles of change — like a revolving door. For example, many people who give up smoking may actually stop and then relapse a number of times before they achieve the change permanently.

The prerequisites of change

It appears that there are certain minimum conditions required for change to take place:

1. The change must be self-initiated.

2. The behaviour must become salient (**must recognize that behaviour is harmful**).

3. The salience of the behaviour must appear over a period of time.

4. The behaviour is not part of the individual's coping strategy.

5. The individual's life should not be problematic or uncertain,

6. Social support is available.

The Stages of Change Model has become an important reference point in health interventions on a range of issues including smoking cessation, substance misuse, and weight control. Apart from the obvious advantage in health promotion of focusing on the change process, the model is important in emphasizing the range of needs for intervention in any given population, the changing needs of different populations and the need for sequencing of interventions to match different stages of change. It illustrates the importance of tailoring programmes to the real needs and circumstances of

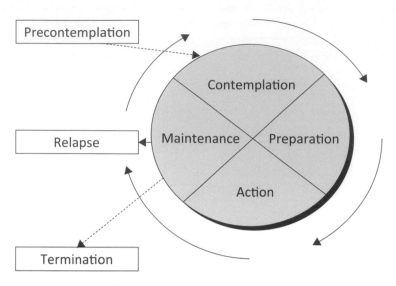

Fig. 3.2 Prochaska and Di Climente's Stages of Change Model. Reproduced with permission from Prochaska, J. O. and Di Climente, C. C. (1983).

individuals rather than assuming an intervention will be equally applicable to all. Above all, it recognizes that people are not always best placed to make changes and that the individual has the right to fail.

Social learning theory or social cognitive theory

Social learning theory (Rotter, 1954; Bandura, 1977), later renamed social cognitive theory, proposes that behaviour change is affected by environmental influences, personal factors, and attributes of the behaviour itself. Understanding of this interaction can offer important insight into how behaviour can be modified through health promotion interventions.

Of importance to this process is the belief in ones ability to successfully perform a behaviour. A person must believe in his or her capability to perform the behaviour (i.e., the person must possess self-efficacy) and must perceive an incentive to do so (i.e., the person's positive expectations from performing the behaviour must outweigh the negative expectations).

Additionally, a person must value the outcomes or consequences that he or she believes will occur as a result of performing a specific behaviour or action. Outcomes may be classified as having immediate benefits (e.g., feeling energized following physical activity) or long-term benefits

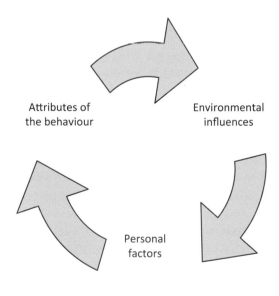

Fig. 3.3 Bandura's Model of Social Learning Theory. Reproduced with permission from Bandura A. (1977).

(e.g., experiencing improvements in cardiovascular health as a result of physical activity). Self-efficacy, that is individual's ability to carry out the desired change, is believed to be the single most important characteristic that determines a person's behaviour change. Self-efficacy can be increased in several ways, among them by providing clear instructions, providing the opportunity for skill development or training, and modelling the desired behaviour. To be effective, models must evoke trust, admiration, and respect from the observer; models must not, however, appear to represent a level of behaviour that the observer is unable to visualize attaining.

Taken as a whole, social cognitive theory provides a comprehensive theoretical basis for health promotion programmes. It recognizes the fundamental importance of individual beliefs, values and self confidence in determining health behaviour. It also explicitly identifies the importance of social norms and cues, and the environmental influences on health behaviour, and the continuous interaction between these variables.

The use of social psychology in health promotion has its critics. The main criticism is that behaviour is not the main determinant of health and that focusing on individual behaviour and attitudes minimizes the structural inequalities that limit people's potential for health. Nevertheless, attitude and behaviour change remain a significant aspect of many health promotion strategies, and many argue that as health promotion is a multi-dimensional concept there is room for attitude and individual behaviour change. The danger is that other structural elements that relate to health and the strategies to address them are not carried out in conjunction with attitude and behaviour change, particularly if we accept that external social factors play a crucial part in attitudes and behaviour anyway. Whilst they may not completely predict individual behaviour they can be helpful in planning programmes of health education by enabling health promoters to understand those factors which influence decisions.

Community organization and other participatory models

Having looked at the individual level models of change the chapter will now look at the community level of change models. Initiatives serving communities and populations, not just individuals, are at the heart of public health approaches to preventing and controlling disease. Community-level models explore how social systems function and change and how to mobilize community members and organizations. They offer strategies that work in a variety of settings, such as health care institutions, schools, worksites, community groups, and government agencies. Embodying an ecological perspective, community-level models address individual, group, institutional, and community issues.

Communities are often understood in geographical terms, but they can be defined by other criteria too. For instance,

there are communities of shared interests (e.g., neighbourhood watch; accident prevention; Slimmer's World) or collective identity (e.g., minority or ethnic groups, such as the African-Caribbean Community). When planning community-level interventions, it is critical to learn about the community's unique characteristics. This is particularly true when addressing health issues in ethnically or culturally diverse communities.

Community organizing is not a single mode of practice; it can involve different approaches to effecting change. Rothman and Tropman (1987) Tropman et al. (1995) produced the best known classification of these change models, describing community organizing according to three general types: locality development, social planning, and social action. These models sometimes overlap and can be combined.

- **Locality development**—(or community development) is process oriented. With the aim of developing group identity and cohesion, it focuses on building consensus and capacity.
- **Social planning**—is task oriented. It stresses problem solving and usually relies heavily on expert practitioners.
- **Social action**—is both process and task oriented. Its goals are to increase the community's capacity to solve problems and to achieve concrete changes that redress social injustices.

In a social action approach to community organizing, **self-interest** is seen as the motivation for action: community members become involved when they see that it will benefit them to take action, and targeted institutions are willing to make changes when they believe it is in their self-interest to do so. Community organizing seeks to expand participants' sense of self-interest to an ever wider sphere, from the individual or family level to their block, neighbourhood, city, region, and so on. Participants grow through this process, learning to take an active role in shaping the future of their communities.

Community organizing is a process through which community groups are helped to identify common problems, mobilize resources, and develop and implement strategies to reach collective goals. Comprehensive health promotion programmes often use advocacy techniques to help support individual behaviour change with organizational and regulatory change.

Even though community organization does not use a single unified model, there are several key concepts that are central to its practice to bring about change on the community level. The first of these, **empowerment** describes a social action process through which individuals, organizations, or communities gain confidence and skills to improve their quality of life. **Community capacity** refers to characteristics of a community that allow it to identify social problems and address them (e.g., trusting relationships between neighbours, civic engagement). **Participation** in the organizing process helps community members to gain leadership and problem-solving skills. **Relevance** involves activating participants to address issues that are important to them. **Issue selection** entails pulling apart a web of interrelated problems into distinct, immediate, solvable pieces. **Critical consciousness** emphasizes helping community members to identify the root causes of social problems.

In recent years, innovative tools and methods for evaluation and measurement have been developed to capture the successes of community-level health promotion efforts. Tobacco control/smoking prevention is one area where programs have been extensively evaluated. Local tobacco control initiatives typically pursue four concurrent goals:

(1) Raising the priority of smoking as a health concern,

(2) Helping community members to change smoking behavior,

(3) Strengthening legal and economic deterrents to smoking, and

(4) Reinforcing social norms that discourage smoking.

This multi-level approach has been proven very effective (see Chapter 13).

Diffusion of Innovations Theory

Diffusion of Innovations Theory (Rogers and Shoemaker, 1971) provides an explanation for how new ideas, products and social practices diffuse or spread within a society or from one society to another. Diffusion of Innovations Theory addresses how ideas, products, and social practices that are perceived as 'new' spread throughout a society or from one society to another. According to the late E.M. Rogers (1995), diffusion of innovations is 'the process by which an **innovation** is communicated through certain **channels** over **time** among the members of a **social system**.' Diffusion Theory has been used to study the adoption of a wide range of health behaviors and programs, including condom use, smoking cessation, and use of new tests and technologies by health practitioners.

Rogers described the process of adoption as a classic 'bell curve', with five categories of adopters:

1. *Innovators* (active information seekers of new ideas),

2. *Early adopters* (very interested in the innovation but not the first to sign up),

3. *Early majority adopters* (need external motivation to get involved),

4. *Late majority adopters* (are skeptics and will not adopt an innovation until most people in the social system have done so),

5. *Laggards* (last to become involved by a mentoring programme or through constant exposure and have limited communication networks).

When an innovation is introduced, the majority of people will either be early majority adopters or late majority adopters; fewer will be early adopters or laggards; and very few will be innovators (the first people to use the innovation). By identifying the characteristics of people in each adopter category, practitioners can more effectively plan and implement strategies that are customized to their needs.

Another aspect of time considers the **rate of adoption**, which is the speed in which an innovation is adopted by members of a social system. At the individual level, adopting a health behaviour innovation usually involves lifestyle change. At the organizational level, it may entail starting programs, changing regulations, or altering personnel roles. At a community level, diffusion can include using the media, advancing policies, or starting initiatives.

According to Rogers, a number of factors determine how quickly, and to what extent, an innovation will be adopted and diffused. Specifically:

- The relative advantage of an innovation shows its superiority over whatever it replaces.

- **Compatibility**—is an appropriate fit with the intended audience.

- **Complexity**—has to do with how easy it is to implement the innovation.

- **Trialability**—pertains to whether it can be tried on an experimental basis.

- **Observability**—reflects whether the innovation will produce tangible results.

By considering the benefits of an innovation, practitioners can position it effectively, thereby maximizing its appeal.

Organizational Change Theories

Among the many theories of organizational behaviour, two have shown special promise in the area of public health: Stage Theory and Organizational Development. Stage Theory of Organizational Change (Lewin, 1951; Zaltman, Duncan and Holbek, 1973; Beyer and Trice, 1978) helps to explain how organizations plan and implement new goals, programs, technologies and ideas. Organizations are believed to pass through a series of 'stages' with each stage requiring a unique set of strategies if the innovation is to progress. A strategy that may be effective at one stage may be wrongly applied at the next. An innovation's current stage of development must be correctly assessed and the proper strategies selected in order to be successful in the application of Stage Theory.

Stage Theory can be said to consist of four stages:

1. **Awareness**—problems are recognized and analyzed, and solutions are suggested and evaluated.

2. **Adoption**—policies are formulated, and resources for beginning change(s) are allocated.

3. **Implementation**—the innovation is implemented, reactions take place, and changes in roles occur.

4. **Institutionalization**—the policy or programme becomes an integral part of the organization, and new goals and values are a part of its structure.

These stages are 'in sequence'. However, movement can be forward, backward, or abandoned at any point in the process. There are some criticisms of Stage Theory. First, the stages need to be better defined. Second, the stage model is not yet complete since beyond institutionalization there should be renewal, when a well established program evolves to meet changing demands. Lastly, the factors known to contribute to the programme's development at each stage need to be expanded.

Organizational Development Theory

Human relations and the quality of life at work are often the targets of Organizational Development Theory (Lewin, 1951; Porras and Robertson, 1992). It has been divided into two main sections:

1. Change Process Theories,

2. Implementation Theories.

Change Process Theories deal with the underlying dynamics of change, whilst Implementation Theories are used to make sure the change is successful. Again, four stages can be identified for producing change in the organization:

1. **Diagnosis**—a specially trained person, usually an outside consultant, helps the organization identify its most striking problems which interfere with its functions.

2. **Action Planning**—strategies are developed for addressing these diagnosed problems.

3. **Intervention**—the consultant usually does not offer specific solutions but will aid in problem solving among the organization's members in group interactions.

4. **Evaluation**—the effort of the planned changes is assessed, and these changes in the organization are allowed to settle.

Generally speaking, Stage Theory and Organizational Development Theories have the greatest potential for creating positive health changes in organizations when used together. One example would be using consultation (Organizational Development) as the intervention in both the adoption and institutional stages (Stage Theory) in an organizational change.

Summary

Health promotion is complex and works on a number of levels and this is reflected in the health promotion theories and models discussed. Health promotion is directed toward action on the determinants or causes of health (e.g., food security, parenting skills, self-care skills, social support) and combines diverse, but complementary, methods or approaches including communication, education, legislation, fiscal measures, organizational change, community development and spontaneous local activities against health hazards. Nurses, as well as all health professionals and those working within the health and social arena, have an important role in nurturing, enabling and practicing health promotion.

 Online Resource Centre

For more information on health promotion theory visit the Online Resource Centre —
http://www.oxfordtextbooks.co.uk/orc/linsley/

References

Ajzen I. & Fishbein, M. (1980). *Understanding Attitudes and Predicting Social Behaviour*. Englewood Cliffs, NJ: Prentice-Hall.

Ajzen I. & Madden T. J. (1986). Prediction of goal directed behaviour: Attitudes, intention, and perceived behavioural control. *Journal of Experimental Social Psychology*, 22: 453–474.

Amos L. M. & Munro J. (2002). *Promoting Health: Politics and Practice*. London: Sage Publications.

Bandura A. (1977). *Social Learning Theory*. New York: General Learning Press.

Becker M. H. (1974). (ed.). The Health Belief Model and Personal Health Behavior. *Health Education Monographs* 2: 324–473.

Beyer J. & Trice H. (1978). *Implementing Change: Alcoholism Policies in Work Organizations*. New York: Free Press.

Ewles L. & Simnett I. (1999). *Promoting Health: A Practical Guide*, (4th ed.). Edinburg: Bailliere Tindall.

Fishbein M. Ajzen I. (1975). *Belief, Attitude, Intention, and Behaviour: An Introduction to Theory and Research*. Reading, MA: Addison-Wesley.

Glanz K., Rimer B. K. & Lewis F. M. (2002). *Health Behaviour and Health Education. Theory, Research and Practice*. San Francisco: Wiley & Sons.

Goodstadt M. S., Simpson R. I. & Loranger P. L. (1987). Health promotion: a conceptual integration. *American Journal of Health Promotion*. 1: 58–63.

Jadad A. R. & O'Grady L. (2008). How should health be defined? *BMJ*, 337: 2900.

Hood L. J. & Leddy S. K. (2006). *Conceptual Bases of Professional Nursing* (6th ed.) London: Lippincott, Williams and Wilkins.

Kirscht J. P., Haefner D. P., Kegeles S. S. & Rosenstock I. M. (1966). A National Study of Health Beliefs. *Journal of Health and Human Behaviour*, 7: 248–254.

Lewin K. (1951). *Field Theory in Social Science*. In D. Cartwright (ed.). New York: Harper.

Lucas, K. & Lloyd, B. (2005). *Health promotion: Evidence and Experience*. London: Sage Publications.

McLeroy K. R., Bibeau D., Steckler A., & Glanz K. (1988). An ecological perspective on health promotion programs. *Health Education Quarterly*. 15: 351–377.

Naidoo N. & Wills J. (2004). *Health Promotion: Foundations for Practice* (2nd ed.). London: Bailliere Tindall.

Nursing and Midwifery Council (2008). *The Code—standards of conduct, performance and ethics for nurses and midwives*. London: NMC.

Nutbeam D. (1998). Evaluating health promotion—progress, problems and solutions. *Health Promotion International*, 13: 27–43.

Nutbeam D. & Harris E. (2004). (2nd ed.). *Theory in a Nutshell. A practical guide to health promotion theories*. London: McGraw-Hill.

Porras J. & Robertson P. (1992). Organizational development: theory, practice, and research. In M. Dunnette, L. Hough (eds.) *Handbook of Industrial and Organizational Psychology* (2nd ed.) Palo Alto, CA: Consulting Psychologists Press, 3: 719–822.

Prochaska J. O. & Di Clemente C. C. (1983). Stages and processes of self-change of smoking: toward an integrate model of change. *Journal of Consulting and Clinical Psychology*, 51: 390–395.

Prochaska J. O. & Di Clemente C. C. (1986). Towards a comprehensive model of change. In: W.R. Miller & N. Heather (eds.), *Treating addictive behaviours: Processes of change*. New York: Plenum Press.

Prochaska J. O. & Di Clemente C. C. (1992). Stages of Change and the modification of problem behaviours. In M. Hersen, R. M. Eisler & P. M. Miller (eds), *Progress in behaviour modification*. Sycamore: Sycamore Press.

Rogers E. M. & Shoemaker F. F. (1971). *Communication of Innovations: A Cross-Cultural Approach* (2nd ed.). New York: The Free Press.

Rogers E. M. (1995). *Diffusion of Innovations.* (4th ed.). New York: Free Press.

Rosenstock I. (1974). Historical Origins of the Health Belief Model. *Health Education Monographs* 2: 4.

Rothman J. & Tropman J. E. (1987). Models of community organization and macro practice. In J. L. Erlich, F. Cox, J. Rothman, & J. E. Tropman (eds) *Strategies of Community Organization* (4th ed.). Itasca, IL: Peacock.

Rothman J. (1996). The interweaving of community intervention approaches. *Journal of Community Practice*, 4: 69–100.

Rotter J. B. (1954). *Social learning and clinical psychology.* New York: Prentice-Hall.

Tones B. K. (1987). Promoting health: the contribution of education. In *Education for Health in Europe: A Report on a WHO Consultation*. Edinburgh: Scottish Health Education Group.

Tones K. & Green J. (2004). *Health Promotion: Planning and Strategies*. London: Sage Publications.

Tropman J., Erlich J. & Rothman J. (1995). *Tactics and techniques of community intervention*. Itasca, IL: Peacock Publishers.

Wanless D. (2004). *Securing Good Health for the Whole Population*. London: Her Majesty's Stationery Office.

Wass A. (2000). *Promoting health: the primary health care approach* (2nd ed) Sydney: Harcourt Saunders.

Woodward A. & Kawachi I. (2000). Why reduce health inequalities? J Epidemiol Community Health, 54: 923–929.

World Health Organization (1978). *Primary Health Care: Report of the International Conference on Primary Health Care. Alma-Ata USSR. 6–12 September, 1978.* Geneva: WHO.

World Health Organization (1985). *Targets for Health for All: targets in support of the European strategy for Health for All.* Copenhagen: World Health Organization Regional Office for Europe. .

World Health Organization (1986a). *Intersectoral Action for Health — The Role of Intersectoral Cooperation in National Strategies for Health for All, background document for technical discussions*, Geneva: 39th World Health Assembly.

World Health Organization (1986b). *Ottawa Charter for Health Promotion*. WHO/HPR/HEP/95.1. Geneva: WHO.

World Health Organization (1997a). *Intersectoral Action for Health: A Cornerstone for Health for All in the 21st Century*. WHO/PPE/PAC/97.6. Geneva: WHO.

World Health Organization (1997b). *The Jakarta Declaration on Leading Health Promotion into the 21st Century*. HPR/HEP/4ICHP/BR/97.4. Geneva: WHO.

World Health Organization (2000). *Report of the Fifth Global Conference on Health Promotion*. Geneva: WHO

World Health Organization (2002). *Reducing Risks, Promoting Healthy Life*. Geneva: WHO.

World Health Organization (2006). *Working Together: The World Health Report 2006*. Geneva: WHO.

Zaltman G., Duncan R. & Holbek J. (1973). *Innovations and organizations*. New York: Wiley.

Part 2

Delivering public health: The role of nurses in the delivery of the new public health agenda

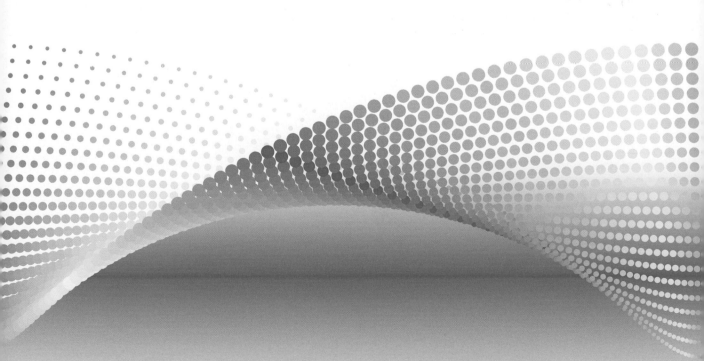

Chapter 4

The changing role of the nurse

Rachael Spencer

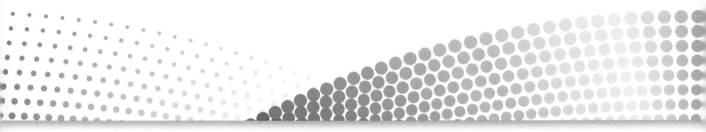

Introduction

Nursing practice in the UK has changed dramatically over the last 20 years, and this pace of change shows no sign of slowing down. Nurses in acute settings **manage an increasingly complex range of health care interventions that incorporate advances in technology and disease management, while nurses in** primary care settings **manage an increasing burden of** chronic diseases **and facilitate** patient self-management **of their health. The focus of health care has moved from hospital to community settings and has a far greater emphasis on health promotion for maintaining good health and well-being than has been seen previously.**

As outlined in Chapter 1, there has for some time been a formal commitment to increasing the contribution nurses make to public health but it is only now that it is starting to gain momentum. Since the publication of the Acheson report into health inequalities in 1988, the need for a radical approach to improving the health of the population has been recognized. In 1998 an official statement of intent to examine the role of nurses within the public health arena was published by the European and UK Chief Nursing Officers. This was later further enforced in the Munich Declaration (WHO, 2000), when ministers pledged to 'enhance the roles of nurses and midwives in public health, health promotion and community development'.

It was recognized however, that this would not be possible without an accompanying shift in the focus of the workforce. **Choosing Health** made direct reference to the need to 'develop training and support for all NHS staff to develop their understanding and skills in promoting health and to

foster and expand a comprehensive range of community health improvement services' (DH, 2004). This focus on prevention was further reiterated in a number of key policy documents including, **The Future Nurse: the RCN vision** (2004), **The Future Nurse: the future for nurse education** (2007a), and **Modernizing Nursing Careers: setting the direction** (2006).

This chapter will examine how the **new public health agenda** impacts on all nursing services, both those in hospitals and those in the community, and what it means for the nursing role. Key policy recommendations introduced in Chapter 1 and influences on the context of care and changing roles of nurses will be examined. The challenges facing nursing as a profession in the light of emerging responsibilities and opportunities will also be explored.

A case study ('the Hardy family') has been integrated throughout the chapter to illustrate key points raised in the text, in particular the role of the nurse in contemporaneous health care. The story of this family outlines their medical and social circumstances and is used also to illustrate the public health aspects of the role of the nurse.

Activity box

- What is nursing and what do nurses do?
- List ten activities that nurses undertake.
- Can you identify in your list whether those activities are undertaken by nurses working in an acute (hospital) setting, in a community setting, or both?

Discussion points

You could probably have listed hundreds of activities that nurses do, from bandaging someone's foot, to giving advice to a soon-to-be mother. Some of the things that you would have listed would be clinical skills, others would have related to managing care, whilst others still would have related to working as part of a health care team. Nurses work not only with sick people, whether those people are in hospital or in their own homes, but also with well people, to prevent them becoming ill.

But is nursing the same profession it was when it first emerged? What does the word 'nurse' mean to people? What image does the word 'nurse' conjure up to members of the general public, or even to nurses themselves?

Activity box

For one week, note how and in what context nursing or a nurse is mentioned in the media — for example in newspapers, on the television, magazine articles etc.

There are many common perceptions about the image of nurses. Nurses are often thought of as 'angels', 'doctor's hand-maidens', or even as 'battleaxes' or 'sex kittens'. This has largely resulted from the portrayal of nursing in the popular media. Are these accurate representations of the modern nursing role in the twenty-first century? The image of nursing has changed dramatically throughout the past fifty years or so from the media portrayal of the archetypal formidable matron played by the actress Hattie Jacques in **'Carry on Nurse'**, (1959) one of the now classic 'Carry On' comedy series of films from the UK. Whilst contemporary media examples of nurses portrayed on popular television programmes such as **'Casualty'** from the UK or **'ER'** from the USA differ, the common image is of nursing as being incredibly hard work, physically and emotionally, and often undertaken by virtuous altruistic women. Nelson and Gordon (2006) argue that presenting this image of nursing trivializes the education and experience required to practise complex skills.

A brief history of the nursing profession

Florence Nightingale 1820–1910

No outline of the nursing profession can be complete without consideration of the contribution of Florence Nightingale. Before the nineteenth century, there was no formal education or training for nurses, it was poorly paid and not considered a respectable occupation. As Florence Nightingale was to put it, nursing was left to those

'who were too old, too weak, too drunken, too dirty, too stupid or too bad to do anything else'.

In 1860, Florence Nightingale set up the first training school for nurses at St. Thomas' Hospital, London. Nightingale reformed conditions in hospitals throughout Britain, published two books, and raised the profile of nursing as a profession. She proposed five core concepts for nursing education and practice:

1. A theoretical basis for nursing practice.
2. Formal education for nurses.
3. A systematic approach to the assessment of patients.
4. An individual approach to the provision of care based on individual patient need.
5. Maintenance of patient confidentiality.

District nursing

Nightingale joined forces with a wealthy philanthropist, William Rathbone, to set up the first home nursing service in 1861. Recognizing that extra training for this role would be required (as these nurses would be in a position of great authority in comparison with their counterparts), a separate training scheme was established. The scheme was a success and Queen Victoria gave a significant proportion of the Women's Jubilee fund to extend the district nurses scheme. The district nurse became the Queen's Jubilee Nurse and later Queen's nurses.

Health visiting

A health visiting service was established in East London, in 1907 as a result of concerns over the high infant mortality rate, blamed at that time on a lack of maternal knowledge. Training courses were established to teach women about sanitation in homes, the management of the health of adults, women, infants and children. The child death rate halved in Ilford, London, during 1910–1912 following the appointment of the first health visitor in the area.

How much of this improvement in child mortality rates was attributable to the introduction of such interventions or the general improvements in living standards around this time is debatable. The historical analyses of Thomas McKeown attributed the modern rise in the world population from the 1700s to the present to broad economic and social changes rather than to targeted public health or medical interventions. His work generated considerable controversy in the 1970s and 1980s, and it continues to stimulate support, criticism, and commentary to the present day, in spite of his conclusions having been largely discredited by subsequent research, most notably in the work of Simon Szreter (1988; 2002). The ongoing resonance of his work is due primarily to the importance of the question that underlay it: are public health ends better served by targeted interventions or by broad based efforts to redistribute the social, political, and economic resources that determine the health of populations?

Regulating the profession

Over the next 40 years, training became longer, entry requirements more strict, including height and weight standards. By the end of nineteenth century there was a move for a nationally recognized certificate for all nurses led by Ethel Bedford Fenwick. As part of the campaign she lobbied parliament to introduce a law to control nursing and limit it to 'registered' nurses only. Previous to this, anyone could call themselves a nurse and care for the sick. Not everyone agreed with her views. Nightingale thought the profession was too young to be standardized and was suspicious of the 'stiff' examinations, rigid controls and high registration fee that was proposed by Bedford Fenwick. Bedford Fenwick was also involved in the suffragette movement, which alienated some of the support she had when the two campaigns became mixed.

In 1902, because of the concern about the deaths of women in childbirth, it was decided that midwives should be registered with a central board. Although the arguments for registration were different, the supporters of nurse registration saw this as an opportunity to persuade the government to set up a committee to investigate the registration of nurses. The committee agreed in principle but recommended two registers, one for those who had completed training and one for the less highly trained. In 1902, the Midwives Registration Act established the state regulation of midwives. Nurses Registration Acts were passed for England/Wales, Scotland and Ireland in 1919. These acts established the General Nursing Council for England and Wales.

What is a nurse in the twenty-first century?

Nursing as a profession has undergone many changes and evolved over time, not least since the inception of the National Health Service in 1948. In the United Kingdom, a nurse is expected to be a **'knowledgeable doer'**, to carry out practice that is underpinned by research, to be ethically responsible and accountable, and to be able to give individualized holistic care through caring and therapeutic interventions (UKCC, 1999). The mandate for qualified nurses is broadly similar throughout the world, as is their government through their

relevant professional body (for example in Australia Nursing and Midwifery is governed by the Australian Nursing and Midwifery Council [ANMC]). There are a number of key concepts and influences on the role of the nurse currently, particularly the new public health agenda — these will be discussed briefly below.

Key concepts and influences on the role of the nurse

Changing public expectations

Patients are no longer content to remain passive recipients of medical and nursing care. Long gone are the days when the hospital consultant stood at the end of the hospital bed and gave his orders to the nurse, who dutifully carried them out on the patient. Theoretical justification for service user representation is primarily in response to the need for health services to be accountable to users as taxpayers, voters and consumers. The NHS has sought to demonstrate 'user involvement' and patient centred care. Recent legislation, particularly Section 11 of the **Health and Social Care Act 2001** (Department of Health, 2001), mandates more direct forms of user involvement. This requires all NHS organizations to engage with users in service planning and evaluation, and facilitate participation in individual treatment decision-making.

Darzi Review

One of Gordon Brown's first actions when he took over as Prime Minister in June 2007 was to appoint a leading oncology (cancer) doctor, Lord Darzi, to undertake a review of the NHS. As discussed in Chapter 1, in October 2007, the interim report was published, and five areas for improvement were identified:

- A fair NHS in terms of access, outcomes and treatments.
- A personalized NHS, tailoring care to patient needs and preferences.
- An effective NHS, utilizing the latest techniques and technologies.
- A safe NHS, improving infection control.
- A locally accountable NHS.

Lord Darzi has emphasized the shift from acute hospital-based health care to primary (community) care, particularly for chronic conditions, proposing more primary care resources such as new health centres. However, the review has been criticized by nursing leaders such as Rosemary Cook CBE, Director of the Queen's Nursing Institute, for focusing on GPs and missing the potential of community-based nurses.

Case Study 4.1: The Hardy family

David and Rose Hardy are in their seventies and live in a council owned bungalow on the Travis estate. David has smoked since his teens and now has **Congestive Cardiac Failure**. He seldom leaves the bungalow as he finds physical effort such as walking makes him very breathless and light-headed. Rose is in good physical health, but sometimes feels hemmed in with her responsibilities for her husband and her grandchildren. Their eldest daughter is married and lives over 200 miles away with her husband and their three children. Their youngest daughter, Melanie is 33 and a single mother. She lives in a council-owned flat, also on the Travis estate. She has three children — Robbie, Dean and Amy. Robbie is 16 and has asthma. Dean is four and Amy 2 years old. Melanie left school pregnant at 16, with no educational qualifications. She now works every morning in the local supermarket whilst her mother (Rose) looks after Amy and Dean is at nursery. Robbie is in his final year at the local comprehensive school and is hoping to get an apprenticeship when he finishes his schooling.

David Hardy

David has been feeling progressively more short of breath, light-headed, dizzy and has difficulty sleeping as this seems to make his shortness of breath worse. For some years, David has been under the care of the cardiologist at a hospital which is twenty miles away for his home, and at his recent review appointment he was introduced to Nancy, a heart failure specialist nurse. Rose phones the heart failure nurse and they are offered a home visit the following day. Nancy evaluates David's medication and reviews the purpose, dosage and side effects of each drug. She spends time with him evaluating his dietary and exercise compliance, reiterating and discussing the importance of David weighing himself every day and its significance to treatment management. She spends some time discussing the importance of trying to stop smoking, and the benefits that this would have for David. Nancy encourages David to consider some of the smoking cessation support available, from nicotine replacement therapy to intensive support such as NHS Stop Smoking Services. Nancy arranges to visit him and Rose at home in a few weeks to discuss this again and ascertain his progress.

Box 4.1 Congestive Cardiac Failure

Congestive Cardiac Failure (heart failure) (CCF) accounts for approximately 5% of all medical admissions to hospital (DH, 2000). Its prevalence is expected to continue to rise due to decreased mortality from cardiovascular disease and a growing elderly population.

CCF can result from coronary heart disease, a culmination of long-standing hypertension, from advanced cardiomyopathy or valvular dysfunction (Connolly, 2000). Due to functional abnormalities the heart remodels itself by changing shape. In left ventricular systolic dysfunction, the myocardium of the left ventricle becomes thin and enlarged, whereas in left ventricular diastolic dysfunction the myocardium of the left ventricle becomes thick and noncompliant. Both types of left sided heart failure lead to symptoms of dyspnoea and fatigue. Other signs and symptoms include peripheral swelling, difficulty sleeping in a supine position, coughing, and the inability to perform normal activities of daily living and a sudden weight gain due to fluid retention. Light-headedness, dizziness and palpitations are also common and can indicate cardiac cachexia (Connolly, 2000).

Specialist nurse intervention

Patients with heart failure are heavy users of the health care system and therefore require close clinical management and encouragement to manage and identify their symptoms. The aim of the heart failure specialist nurse is to improve patient outcomes and decrease hospital admissions and therefore cost.

Patient attends the heart failure clinic, seen by a cardiologist who obtains a full history and performs a medical evaluation. The heart failure specialist nurse also sees them and the basics of heart failure reiterated. She also evaluates the patients' medication and reviews the purpose, dosage and side effects of each drug. The nurse spends time with the patient evaluating their dietary and exercise compliance, reiterating and discussing their daily weight monitoring and its significance to their treatment management. Risk factor management must also be maintained; that is, abstinence from smoking, maintaining a normal weight, healthy eating and healthy emotional coping strategies.

Home visits are offered as many of the symptoms of CCF can occur at rest, and therefore patents may find it difficult to function independently outside their homes, making clinic journeys difficult.

Summary

Congestive Heart Failure is a major public health problem. Hospital admissions are often unplanned readmissions, and have a high mortality rate. A coordinated disease management approach may be implemented that includes early assessment in the hospital, comprehensive education, and behaviour modification in order to improve disease management and improve patients' quality of life. Nurses are the integral providers involved in educating, monitoring and supporting patients and their families during the disease process.

Demographic changes

The people nurses care for are changing. People are prone to different illnesses at different times in their lifespan, and this has a direct impact on the provision of nursing care within these client groups. Certain groups have increased need for health care provision and services — infants aged less than one year, pregnant women, and the elderly. The demography of the western world is changing - there is a declining birth rate and a predicted rise in the numbers of elderly people. **Life expectancy** at birth has increased dramatically, with men in the United Kingdom now having a life expectancy of 77.5 years and women 81.7 years (ONS, 2009a).

The main causes of mortality in younger people are quite different from those in the middle-aged and elderly. Violent deaths, accidents and injury (external and self-inflicted) are major causes of death in younger people (Thomas *et al.*, 2007). Circulatory diseases, cancers and respiratory diseases are the most common causes of death in the older age groups (ONS, 2009b).

There are also important variations in mental illness between different age groups. In general, the elderly have higher levels of mental illness. Depression is common in the elderly, affecting 10–15% of the over 65s (Evans *et al.*, 1999). The UK has one of the highest rates of self harm in Europe and suicide is the most common cause of death for men aged under 35 (Department of Health, 2005a).

Studies of self-reported illness confirm the chronic nature of disease in older age groups. Although total life expectancy has increased, the prevalence of chronic illness and disability in old age remains at a high level, so that those additional years are often extra years with a disability, not of healthy life.

Health inequalities and long-term conditions

Box 4.2 Long-term conditions

The World Health Organization (WHO) defines long-term conditions (also called chronic diseases) as health problems that require ongoing management over a period of years. This includes a wide range of health conditions including non-communicable diseases (such as cancer and cardiovascular disease), communicable diseases (such as HIV/AIDS), certain mental disorders (for example schizophrenia, depression), and ongoing impairments in structure (for example blindness, joint disorders). According to the Department of Health, there are seventeen and a half million people in the country living with a long-term condition (DH, 2005b). Management of people with long-term conditions has recently become a focus of government; several policy documents have been published which set out current thinking for management of long-term conditions. The National Service Framework (NSF) for Long

Term Conditions was published by the Department of Health in March 2005 (DH, 2005c). The Public Health White Paper **Choosing Health: Making Health Choices Easier** (DH, 2004) discusses the introduction of community matrons to work with those with long-term conditions, providing personalized care and health advice for those with more complex problems. It is hoped that this could reduce the need for admission to hospital.

Social circumstances across the entire lifespan influence people's health and well-being. The characteristics of the areas in which people live, as well as their individual characteristics, influence their health (Dahlgren and Whitehead, 1991).

The mortality rate of men of working age is almost three times higher for those in routine occupations (such as bus drivers, road sweepers, labourers) as for those men working as large employers, higher managers (by National Statistics — Socio Economic Classification) (ONS, 2007). These growing differences are apparent for any of the major causes of death, including coronary heart disease, stroke, lung cancer and suicides among men (ONS, 2007), and lung cancer and ischaemic heart disease among women (ONS, 2009a).

Stillbirths, infant mortality and deaths of children are all more likely in social classes IV and V (Confidential Enquiry into Maternal and Child Health, 2006). A child born into a family where the father is an unskilled worker has twice the risk of being stillborn or of dying in infancy compared with one born into a professional family.

Although death rates have fallen and life expectancy increased, there is little evidence that the population is experiencing less morbidity or disability than 10–20 years ago. Rates of self-reported limiting longstanding illness in men and women vary considerably with class. The lowest rate of limiting longstanding illness was reported in the 2001 Census among those working in higher managerial and professional occupations (7 per cent), which was half that of those working in routine occupations (15 per cent). People who had never worked or were long-term unemployed had the highest rate of limiting longstanding illness (37 per cent) of any socio-economic group (ONS, 2001).

These issues are discussed in much more depth in Chapter 14 'Tackling health Inequalities'. However, there have been a number of policy and practice changes that have been introduced in an effort to address these inequalities in health care experience, many involving nurses developing a public health focus to their work, whether they are based in the acute (hospital) sector or in the community. There are many examples of community nurse initiatives in deprived inner city communities where nurses support people to access health care more effectively and contextualize health messages to reflect the local culture, thereby making it easier for people to participate in health enhancing activities. A recent initiative launched in

Hull is a structured twelve week weight management programme aimed primarily at overweight and obese men aged 40–65, backed by Hull City Football Club, and delivered by the Football Association qualified professional trainers at three sports clubs in Hull (NHS Hull, 2009).

Case Study 4.2: Rose Hardy

Rose Hardy has started to experience fresh rectal bleeding and is very anxious. As the main carer for David, she is especially worried about the possible consequences if this is something serious. She consults her family doctor (General Practitioner) who refers her to an **advanced nurse practitioner** for a flexible sigmoidoscopy. In the Outpatient Department two weeks later, she sees the advanced nurse practitioner who takes a comprehensive medical history, conducts a full physical examination, and performs a **flexible sigmoidoscopy**. On examination, some haemorrhoids are seen, but no other abnormalities. The advanced nurse practitioner takes time to sit with Rose and discuss her worries. She prescribes some haemorrhoidal cream and tells Rose how to use the cream when she has the symptoms. She also talks with Rose about diet and how high fibre foods such as wholemeal bread, drinking more fluids during the daytime, and increasing her intake of fresh fruit and vegetables will also help. In addition, Rose is given all this information in leaflets to take home and contact details for continued support should she feel this is necessary.

Body of knowledge — evidence-based practice, research, practice improvement

There is growing emphasis on evidence-based practice, research and practice improvement as contributing to the body of knowledge that defines nursing as a profession. However, there has been considerable discussion about the lack of research utilization in clinical practice, with nurses portrayed as intrinsically resistant to change (Willmot, 1998). Writers identity workplace culture, relationships between staff members, organizational structures and the perceived 'truth value' of the evidence as influencing nurses' willingness to change their clinical practice, and they emphasize the need for multiple strategies to achieve change (Rycroft-Malone *et al.*, 2004, Copnell and Bruni, 2006). Nurses are therefore urged to use research and best evidence findings to underpin safe and effective nursing practice. The move to an all-graduate nursing profession, the growing proliferation of nursing research facilitator posts across the United Kingdom, and the introduction of clinical academic career pathways can be seen as an attempt to develop a culture of research awareness amongst nurses, provide support and guidance in the development of research skills and the application of research in clinical practice.

Nursing career pathways

The Department of Health's **Modernising Nursing Careers** (DH, 2006a) recommended the development of new career paths for nurses in the UK. The following consultation, **Towards a Framework for Post Registration Nursing Careers**, (DH, 2007) proposed that nurses should 'major' in one pathway and 'minor' in the others. These five pathways are:

1. Children, family and public health.
2. First contact, access and urgent care.
3. Supporting long-term care.
4. Acute and critical care.
5. Mental health and psychosocial care.

All nurses would be expected to provide holistic care and possess skills in key areas such as health promotion, end-of-life care, prevention of long-term conditions and safeguarding vulnerable groups, but would also be able to move between pathways throughout their career. These five pathways reflect the current context and influences on health care and the future direction of nursing practice. What is apparent though is that the **new public health agenda** is key to the role of all nurses, whichever their chosen pathway, rather than solely the specific responsibility of those designated as public health nurses.

Case Study 4.3: Robbie Hardy

Robbie is doing work experience with an electrician in the nearby town of Dunston. Whilst on site one day, he falls off a stepladder and receives a cut to his forehead from a protruding nail in some plasterwork. He attends the local Minor Injuries Unit and is assessed by the nurse practitioner who cleans and sutures the wound and then administers a tetanus vaccine as Robbie is unsure of his immunization status. Within an hour he is back on site, but is tasked with making the teas and coffees for the rest of the day.

Challenges to health care delivery

Over recent decades we have seen an unprecedented rise in the number of techniques and technological advances in health care. However, the complexity of treatments, disease management of long-term conditions and the associated rise in health care costs have all impacted on the role and function of the nurse. These issues are discussed further below.

Disease management — long-term conditions

Over seventeen million people in the United Kingdom have a long-term health condition (previously referred to as chronic illness (DH, 2005b)). Examples include chronic obstructive pulmonary disease, diabetes and arthritis. Long-term conditions are discussed more fully in Chapter 19. It is estimated that up to 5% of these individuals account for 42% of annual hospital bed use (DH, 2005b). There is evidence that nurses who specialize in specific conditions can improve the health and quality of life of people with long-term conditions. For example, research has shown that when people with long-term conditions are followed up after discharge from hospital (by home visits, telephone support and nurse-led clinics), those patients have improved functional status or prevented deterioration and fewer hospital readmissions (Matheson and Porter, 2006). The Community Matron role has been recently introduced and the role is at varying stages of development in the different countries across the UK. In general they focus on the management of the care of people with long-term conditions, but as yet there is a lack of research evidence evaluating the effectiveness of specialist nurse-led services to these patients (Hutt *et al.*, 2004; McHugh *et al.*, 2009).

Workforce issues — recruitment and retention, role of unqualified workforce

Nationwide, the NHS employs about 400,000 qualified nurses and midwives, approximately one-third of the NHS workforce. There is growing concern about the numbers of nurses leaving the profession before retirement, and the percentages of those nearing retirement age. In addition, there are recruitment issues, particularly in high technology specialisms and in London and the South East. A number of initiatives have been established, including flexible working hours, family friendly policies such as on-site nurseries with subsidized places, zero tolerance policies for harassment and bullying, and greater emphasis on career development and further training.

There has been a raft of recent policy initiatives that are concerned with changing traditional working practices and professional boundaries. In England there are also initiatives to develop new health care worker roles, such as assistant health care practitioners. In general practice, nurses often manage their own clinics, and some nurses throughout the acute and primary care sector are now responsible for making diagnoses and (with further education and training) prescribing treatment. Over recent years many tasks and roles previously associated with and undertaken by doctors are becoming part of the role and function of the nurse. Likewise unqualified nurses (health care assistants, nursing auxiliaries) have taken on more roles previously undertaken by qualified nurses. In part this is due to the reduction of junior doctors' working hours, the result of a European Union Working Time Directive, and the Wanless Report (2002) recommended that there should be a full exploitation of the potential for a transfer of work from doctors to nurse practitioners in an attempt to ease the burden on medical staff.

Entrepreneurship

There are many opportunities for nurses to use their experience and skills outside of the National Health Service, setting up their own businesses to provide niche innovative healthcare services within primary care. The International Council for Nurses (ICN, 2004:4) defines a nurse entrepreneur as:

'a proprietor of a business that offers nursing services of a direct care, educational, research, administration or consultative nature. The self-employed nurse is directly accountable to the client, to whom or on behalf of whom, nursing services are provided.'

Although not a new concept to nursing (Mary Seacole, a contemporary of Nightingale, could be considered a nurse entrepreneur), entrepreneurship has seen a growth of interest in the last ten years. The current climate of patient choice, an increased range of providers and commissioning has provided opportunities for nurses to work as independent practitioners providing services to meet health care needs not provided for within the NHS. Examples of nurse entrepreneurs include a contraception and sex education resources company set up by an experienced nurse, or a nurse-led clinic established to help children with sleep problems, which is marketed back to the NHS so that parents living in deprived inner city estates can access the service free of charge.

Emphasis on public health

There is a current emphasis in health care policy and practice on public health and the role of the nurse in the prevention of illness. It has been influenced by key government documents such as the **Choosing Health: making healthy choices easier** (DH, 2004) the influential Wanless reports (2002 and 2004) and also reflects the direction of the government's public health agenda, addressing new initiatives such as those set out in the **Our Health, our care, our say: a new direction for community services** white paper (DH, 2006b). Traditionally, public health nursing was confined to the role of Specialist Community Public Health nurses (such as health visitors or school nurses) but the current drive is for all nurses, regardless of where they practise, with which client group or specialism, to have public health as a core component of their role. Recently the RCN publication **Nurses as partners in delivering public health** (May 2007) outlined the future responsibilities of nurses in delivering public health interventions. The five pathways outlined in the Department of Health's **Modernising nursing careers** (DH, 2006a) consultation each encompass aspects of public health. Nursing competencies can be mapped to the public health career framework, which is a competency based framework. Public health skills such as health profiling, building healthy alliances and policy development can now be seen as an integral compenent of **every** nurse's role, and current examples of this are explored in more detail in Chapter 14 of this textbook.

Case Study 4.4: Melanie Hardy

Melanie attends the health visitor's clinic one afternoon with Dean. She is concerned that Dean is constantly scratching his head and she thinks he might have got eczema on his scalp. Using a detection comb, the health visitor can see some living lice on the comb. She prescribes some head lice (insecticide) shampoo for Dean and talks to Melanie about head lice. The health visitor recommends to Melanie that every member of the family is checked, and treated if necessary. She also talks to Melanie about regularly checking for head lice and 'wet combing' with conditioner. The health visitor talks to Melanie about informing the nursery where Dean has been attending so that the other children can be checked too.

Policy drivers

A number of policies have been delivered over the past decade, emphasizing improved access and choice for patients, user / carer involvement, increased public expectations of improved public health, cost efficiency and measuring effectiveness, reducing variations in performance, improving productivity, incentive schemes and payment by results, practice based commissioning from an increased range of providers, revision of regulation of the health care professions in an effort to focus on quality and safety, and partnership working to coordinate effort between NHS and Social Services.

The principal emphasis of many of these policies has been the development of primary care in the drive to modernize the National Health Service. Public health policies vary between different parts of the United Kingdom due to political devolution which has led to variations in service developments (Hunter 2007). However, there is consensus that there is an expectation of a larger amount and greater variety of health care interventions being delivered in primary care and community settings that will require new roles and new ways of working by nurses in these settings. **'Liberating the Talents: helping PCTs and nurses to deliver the NHS Plan'** (DH, 2002) highlighted the need for a more flexible generalist nursing workforce in primary care and greater integration of hospital and primary care. There are numerous opportunities for nurses arising from both the new General Medical Service (GMS) and new Personal Medical Service (PMS) Contracts which emphasize the development of services to meet the needs of a specific population rather than focusing on the number of patients registered at a GP surgery. In 2006, a review of community nursing in Scotland was set up and a new model of community nursing is currently being tested in four

sites (Kennedy *et al.*, 2009). The Community Nursing Strategy in Wales (Welsh Assembly Government, 2009) proposes to introduce locality based nursing teams in an effort to meet the needs of patients, from ill health prevention to the management of complex needs. There are also new approaches to care and roles for nurses that are emerging as a result, for example in long-term conditions management, Sure Start, walk-in Centres and NHS Direct in England, well-being centres and NHS Direct Wales in Wales, and NHS 24 in Scotland.

Our Health...and patient-led NHS

The **Our Health, our care, our say: a new direction for community services** white paper (Department of Health, 2006b) set out a vision to provide people with good quality NHS and social care services in the communities where they live. The white paper emphasized patient choice and control over how and where their health and social care services would be provided, again reinforcing the government's commitment to a patient-led National Health Service.

Challenges for nurses

Responding appropriately — what are our core values?

Nursing is carried out in increasingly varied and complex environments. This includes an increasing need for flexibility and for multi-professional/multi-disciplinary working across traditional professional boundaries and the development of new roles.

Activity box

Make a list of the various health care professionals that work within the National Health Service.

Discussion points

You may have listed nurses, doctors, physiotherapists, occupational therapists, social workers, pharmacists, radiographers, and midwives. Did you list support staff such as medical secretaries, porters, estates officers, van drivers and receptionists? In taking care of patients, the nurse collaborates with other members of the health care team. The team is as big or small as the requirements and needs of the patient dictate.

What are the distinct qualities that nurses can bring to patient / client care?

The Future Nurse: the RCN Vision (RCN, 2004) outlined how nurses needed to adapt and rise to challenges while preserving their integrity and core values in an effort to meet public and patient need.

'The primary purpose of nursing is to provide holistic health and healthcare for patients, families, carers and communities. Registered nurses are responsible for maintaining all aspects of the health environment so that it is conducive to improving health, facilitating recovery from illness or rehabilitation, and where appropriate, achieving a dignified death'
RCN, 2004: 4

The vision reiterated that holistic patient-centred care must remain the core purpose of nursing, where patients are active participants in decisions about their care. It is clear that nursing care needs to be designed around the patient and the local community rather than being restricted by traditional boundaries and professional demarcations, and that the future qualified nurse will need to work at an advanced level to lead and coordinate such models of care. Nursing is an increasingly complex profession, requiring highly educated staff with a strong academic background (Hart, 2004). Whilst there is consensus in the literature about the need for an all-graduate nursing profession (Robinson *et al.*, 2003), findings from a recent study highlight the dichotomy expressed by some qualified nurses of wanting to advance in career terms in order to attain status rewards, financial rewards, increased responsibility and increased autonomy, but in the knowledge that this may possibly mean sacrificing patient contact (Spencer, 2006).

> **Box 4.3** What does the future hold for the direction of nursing?
>
> In February 2010 the Government launched Front Line Care: the future of nursing and midwifery in England — a Report of the Prime Minister's Commission on the Future of Nursing and Midwifery in England 2010.
>
> The Commission analysed nursing and midwifery today in the context of:
>
> - Socioeconomic, health and demographic trends.
> - The education, continuing professional development and supervision needed to meet future needs.
> - Management and workplace cultures.
>
> The report makes a number of recommendations which can be accessed using the following link http://cnm.independent.gov.uk/the-report/. This includes a video and a downloadable PowerPoint presentation. Take time out to study the report and its recommendations.

Summary

The chapter has examined how the **new public health agenda** impacts on all nursing services, whether acute or community, and what it means for the nursing role. Key recommendations from the Wanless reports (2002; 2004) and recent RCN documents on the changing roles of nurses have been examined. The emergence of new responsibilities and opportunities has also been explored. Although nursing as a vocation has been evident for many centuries, Florence Nightingale has largely been credited with developing education and training for nurses that evolved into a highly valued profession worthy of professional recognition through registration. Nightingale proposed five core concepts for nursing that included individualized patient care and a sound theoretical basis upon which to base that care. These core concepts would seem as relevant to nursing today as they were in Nightingale's era.

There have been a number of policy and practice changes that have been introduced in an effort to address inequalities in health care experience, and the growing elderly population, many involving nurses developing a public health focus to their work, whether they are based in the acute (hospital) sector or in the community. An ageing population with multiple long-term conditions leads to an increased demand for essential nursing care.

This is an exciting time for the nursing profession, with numerous opportunities to develop new ways of working, to develop nurse-led services and transform the public health agenda. Current workforce redesign has resulted in a proliferation of new advanced roles in nursing that include community matrons, consultant nurses and advanced nurse practitioners. Nurses are being given opportunities to work across traditional boundaries to improve patient care. Research is being undertaken to evaluate the impact of these new roles on efficiency and effectiveness, particularly in terms of comparing the impact of nurses with medical colleagues on aspects of care such as reducing unscheduled hospital admissions (Gardner and Gardner, 2005). Although the components of the nursing role have changed dramatically over time, there are some constants: to provide skilled care, particularly for the frail and the vulnerable in society, and it is these ideals that attract people into the profession — the desire to make a difference in people's lives and to contribute to society in meaningful ways.

 # Online Resource Centre

For more information on the changing role of the nurse visit the Online Resource Centre —
http://www.oxfordtextbooks.co.uk/orc/linsley/

References

Australian Nursing and Midwifery Council (ANMC) (2005). *National Competency Standards for the Registered Nurse*. Dickson: ANMC.

Barnet, M. (2003). 'A nurse-led community scheme for managing patients with COPD'. *Professional Nurse* 19: 93–96.

Confidential Enquiry into Maternal and Child Health, (2006) *Perinatal mortality Surveillance, 2004: England, Wales and Northern Ireland*. London: CEMCH.

Connolly, K. (2000). 'New Directions in Heart Failure Management' *The Nurse Practitioner* 25(7): 23–41.

Copnell, B. & Bruni, N. (2006). 'Breaking the silence: nurses' understandings of change in clinical practice.' *Journal of Advanced Nursing* 55 (3): 301–309.

Dahlgren, G. & Whitehead, M. (1991). *Policies and Strategies to Promote Social Equity in Health*. Stockholm: Institute for Future Studies.

Department of Health (2001). *Health and Social Care Act: Patient and Public Involvement*. London: The Stationery Office.

Department of Health (2002). *Liberating the Talents: helping PCTs and nurses to deliver the NHS Plan*. London: The Stationery Office.

Department of Health (2004). *Choosing Health: making healthy choices easier*. London: The Stationery Office.

Department of Health (2005a). *NHS Workforce Survey*. London: DH.

Department of Health (2005b). *National Service Framework (NSF) for Mental Health — Five Years On*. London: The Stationery Office.

Department of Health (2005c). *Supporting People with Long-term Conditions: An NHS and Social Care Model to Support Local Innovation and Integration*. London: The Stationery Office.

Department of Health (2005d). *National Service Framework (NSF) for Long Term Conditions*. London: The Stationery Office.

Department of Health 2006a). *Modernising nursing careers— setting the direction*. London: The Stationery Office.

Department of Health 2006b). *Our Health, our care, our say: a new direction for community services*. London: The Stationery Office.

Department of Health (2007). *Towards a Framework for Post Registration Nursing Careers*. London: The Stationery Office.

Department of Health (2007). *Our NHS. Our Future: NHS next stage review—interim report*. London: The Stationery Office.

Evans, O., Singleton, N., Meltzer, H., Stewart, R. & Prince, M. (2003). *The Mental Health of Older People*. London: Her Majesty's Stationery Office.

Gardner, A. & Gardner, G. (2005). 'A trial of nurse practitioners scope of practice.' *Journal of Advanced Nursing, 49, 135–145*.

Hart, C. (2004). *Nurses and Politics: The Impact of Power and Practice*. Basingstoke: Palgrave.

Hunter, D. (2007). 'Public health: Historical context and current agenda'. In: Scriven, A. & Garmen, S. (eds.) *Public Health: Social Context and Action*. Berkshire: Open University Press, 8–19.

Hutt, R., Rosen, R. & McCauley, J. (2004). *Case-managing long-term conditions*. London: King's Fund.

International Council of Nurses (2004). *Guidelines on the nurse entre / intrapreneur providing nursing service*. Geneva: ICN.

Kennedy, C., Elliott, L., Rush, R., Hogg, R., Cameron, S., Currie, M., Hall, S., Miller, M., Plunkett, C. & Lauder, W. (2009). *Review of community nursing: Baseline Study Research Findings 79/2009*. Edinburgh: Scottish Government.

Maben, J., Latter, S. & Macleod Clark, J. (2007). 'The sustainability of ideals, values and the nursing mandate: evidence from a longitudinal qualitative study.' *Nursing Inquiry*, 14: 99–113.

Matheson, F. & Porter, B. (2006). 'The evolution of a relapse clinic for multiple sclerosis: challenges and recommendations'. *British Journal of Neuroscience Nursing,* 2 (4): 180–186..

McHugh, G.A., Horne, M., Chalmers, K.I. & Luker, K.A. (2009). 'Specialist community nurses: a critical analysis of their role in the management of long-term conditions.' *International Journal of Environmental Research and Public Health*, 6 (10):2550–2567.

Nelson, S. & Gordon, S. (2006). 'Conclusion: Nurses Wanted: Sentimental Men and Women Need Not Apply'. In: S. Nelson, & S. Gordon (eds.) *The Complexities of Care: Nursing Reconsidered (The culture and politics of health care work)*. Ithaca, New York: Cornell University Press, 185–190.

NHS Hull (2009). *Final Call To The City's Heaviest Footballers*. Press Release. *http://www.hullpct.nhs.uk/templates/page. aspx?id=5588 Accessed 30 November 2009*.

Office for National Statistics (1998). *Living in Britain: results from the general household survey 1996*. London: The Stationery Office.

Office for National Statistics (2009a). *Health Statistics Quarterly 44 Winter 2009*. London: The Stationery Office.

Office for National Statistics (2009b). *Health Statistics Quarterly 43 Autumn 2009*. London: The Stationery Office.

Office for National Statistics (2007). *Health Statistics Quarterly 36 Winter 2007*. London: The Stationery Office.

Robinson, S., Murrells, T., Hickey, G., Clinton, M. & Tingle, A. (2003). *A Tale of Two Courses: Comparing the Careers and Competencies of Nurses Prepared via Three-year Degree and Three-year Diploma Courses*. King's College, London: Nursing Research Unit.

Royal College of Nursing (2004). *The Future Nurse: the RCN Vision*. London: RCN.

Royal College of Nursing (2005). *Maxi nurses: nurses working in advanced and extended roles promoting and developing patient-centred health*. London: RCN.

Royal College of Nursing (2007a). *The Future Nurse: the future for nurse education. A discussion paper*. London: RCN.

Royal College of Nursing (2007b). *Nurses as partners in delivering public health*. London: RCN.

Rycroft-Malone, J., Harvey, G., Seers, K., Kitson, A., McCormack, B. & Titchen, A. (2004). 'An exploration of the factors that influence the implementation of evidence into practice'. *Journal of Clinical Nursing* 13: 913–924.

Spencer, R.L. (2006). 'Nurses', midwives' and health visitors' perceptions of the impact of higher education on professional practice.' *Nurse Education Today*, 26: 45–53.

Szreter S. (1988). The Importance of Social Intervention in Britain's Mortality Decline c. 1850–1914: A Reinterpretation of the Role of Public Health. *Social History of Medicine* 1: 1–38.

Szreter S. (2002) Rethinking McKeown: The Relationship Between Public Health and Social Change. *American Journal of Public Health* 92(5): 722–725.

Thomas, J., Kavanagh, J., Tucker, H., Burchett, H., Tripney, J. & Oakley, A. (2007). *Accidental injury, risk-taking behaviour and the social circumstances in which young people live: a systematic review*. London: EPPI-Centre, Social Science Research Unit, Institute of Education, University of London.

United Kingdom Central Council for Nursing and Midwifery (1999). *Fitness for Practice, the UKCC Commissioning for Nursing and Midwifery Education.* London: UKCC.

Wanless, D. (2002). *Securing Our Future Health: Taking a Long Term View.* London: HM Treasury Public Enquiry Unit.

Wanless, D. (2004). *Securing Good Health for the Whole Population. Final Report.* London: The Stationery Office.

Welsh Assembly Government (2009). *A Community Nursing Strategy For Wales. Consultation Document.* Cardiff: Welsh Assembly Government.

World Health Organization (2000). *Munich Declaration. Nurses and Midwives: a force for health.* Copenhagen: WHO.

Willmot, M. (1998). 'The new ward manager: an evaluation of the changing role of the charge nurse.' *Journal of Advanced Nursing,* 28 (2): 419–427.

Chapter 5

Inter-professional practice and education in health and social care

Nigel Horner and Trevor Simpson

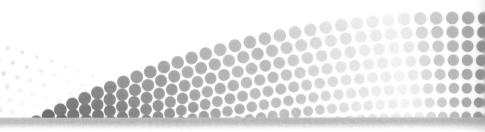

Introduction

The modern landscape within which nursing is undertaken has two interrelated defining features: firstly, the importance of putting the patient at the centre of all aspects of practice, and secondly, working in partnership with a whole range of human service organizations to provide a coherent, seamless service to the patient/service user (Secretary of State for Health, 2000). In this chapter we will examine the imperative for nurses to understand their roles and responsibilities in relation to both other health professionals and other professional or disciplinary groups, and we will consider how this understanding may be developed in both pre-registration training and in post-registration practice settings.

Almost without exception, politicians, professional lead bodies, academics and practitioners are in agreement that human services professionals from various disciplines need to be able to work effectively together. Why? Because the goal for all health professions should be to provide a seamless service for the patient or service user, to share standardized information to prevent patients and users of services having to endlessly repeat their symptoms and circumstances.

'People do not care about organizational boundaries when seeking support and help, and expect services to reflect this'
DH, 2006a

There is also a need to facilitate the through-care of patients and service users, to combine our efforts to best protect vulnerable children, young people and adults, and to make services optimally effective and (crucially) cost efficient.

'The creation of an organization defined by its client group rather than professional functions offers an important opportunity to involve children and young people in decision-making'
(DH, 2003: 78).

Nobody would argue against such a set of coherent and desirable outcomes — in fact, they have provided the cornerstone of health and social care policy for decades, and yet, one has to ask:

- If everyone has been in agreement about these goals for such a long time, then why does this revered Holy Grail of joined-up working remain so elusive in many practice situations?

- Why it is that the experiences of patients and users of care services are often so negative as they become caught up in the apparent failure of practitioners to keep the patient at the centre of their practice?
- Why is it that organizational ineptitude can appear to so often fail to protect children and vulnerable adults, sometimes with disastrous consequences?

As a response to these questions, it is our contention that such deficiencies are not the result of deliberate, conscious attempts to offer a poor service, nor do they necessarily stem from parochial, protectionist attitudes on the part of practitioners (although such unhelpful sentiments do indeed exist in some quarters). It is more likely that such difficulties arise from the inherent contradictions that are associated with modern practice. Nurses and other professionals are encouraged to establish and maintain a professional identity — with all that such an objective entails — whilst working within an environment of accelerating change in the structures of service delivery. A well documented response to precipitous change is retrenchment, and herein lays the contradiction of modernization processes.

Traditional service delivery settings, such as general hospitals, sanatoriums, infirmaries, the erstwhile psychiatric hospitals (asylums) and hospitals for people with learning disabilities were all institutions characterized by and structured around and by professional boundaries and role demarcation. Yet the focus of this book is public health, reflecting the modernizing health agenda, working in partnership with patients and service users, with their families and carers, in their own homes, within their localities, neighbourhoods and communities. In such a environment, traditional role demarcation becomes an impediment to delivering the goals desired by patients and service users, and will not facilitate the attainment political objectives such as those set out in the Department of Health paper, **NHS 2010–2015 : from good to great — preventative, people-centred, productive** (DH, 2009).

So, how might these tensions and contradictions be resolved? A useful start to our journey would be to explore definitions of *inter-professional working* and then to consider how education and infrastructure could enable a seamless service to be potentially realized for the benefit of patients. Most of the postmodern work in relation to this enviable question has been carried out in the theatre of higher education. CAIPE (2007) offer us the most commonly cited definition of what we seek when they describe *inter-professional education* as:

'Occasions when two or more professions learn with, from and about each other to improve collaboration and the quality of care'.

This mantra has been explicitly or implicitly at the centre of contemporary policy developments in health and social care teams for some time: the premise that could be drawn is that if two or more professions learn with, from and about each other then the next logical step would be for such learning to transpose into more effective inter-professional working. Within the health care landscape, 1999 saw the birth of several large multifaceted higher education based initiatives such as the **New Generation Project**, an innovative model aimed at developing common learning in higher education undergraduate programmes (O'Hallaran *et al.*, 2006). This work has been followed by several smaller scale projects such as the **Trent Universities Inter-Professional Learning in Practice** (TUILIP) project, which has a focus towards enabling learning for pre- and post registration learning and collaboration in the practice setting (Armitage *et al.*, 2009).

In this chapter we will examine the history of inter-professional working and remind ourselves of the policy imperatives to *work together*. We will examine definitions of inter-professional learning and working, and introduce the research evidence concerning the effective implementation of joined-up services. Finally, we will focus on the specific role of the nurse in the modernized and integrated health and social care landscape.

From fragmentation to integration

In terms of the history of human services and welfare provision, *inter-professional practice* is a relatively new concept but one that is fundamental and critical to the advancement of innovative policy within the varied and diverse milieu of contemporary practice for health and social care professionals. That said, the theoretical principle of working together for better health care provision has been a policy objective for several decades. The original movement concerning inter-professional working was almost entirely related to the practicalities of how to get a doctor, nurse and other health related professionals to work more closely towards patient care. In other words, the focus was on *intra-professional* cooperation within the health sphere. Keunssberg (1967), as part of a conference report for the Royal Colleges for General Practice, Midwifery and Nursing, cited the need for formal consideration of the working relationships between doctors, nurses and health visitors when they provide care for the family.

By the early 1990s, the attention of policy broadened to include the relationship *between* health professionals and the social care sector as the locus for change moved from within the institutional setting of the hospital to that of the wider community. The reforms of the National Health Service, as spearheaded by the introduction of the **NHS and Community Care Act 1990** (DH, 1989), heralded the convening of joint meetings between community nursing and social care teams to discuss the implementation of recommendations from the new Act. A core theme of the Act was to improve the joint planning of community based services, in part to reverse the undesirable yet emerging trend of older people requiring institutional care. A strategic approach to achieving such joint planning was through multi-disciplinary community services.

Over the past decade, the most significant New Labour policy agenda influencing the promotion of inter-professional learning has been the Government's explicitly stated **NHS Modernization Agenda** (DH, 1997). The policy drivers for this change were designed to streamline and modernize buildings and services, and to cut costs whilst transferring a significant investment to instigate new services, both in primary and secondary care. This new modernizing agenda resulted in financial encouragement by government for higher education institutions to incorporate inter-professional learning and working into the academic curricula for all health and social care professionals in training. This has been achieved in many universities successfully and the agenda now is to promote this new model of learning into the practice arena so that the qualified professional of tomorrow has been educated using the principles for inter-professional working.

Whilst these policy drivers have been emerging, the enquiries into the tragic and preventable deaths of children in England such as **Victoria Climbie** (DfES, 2003) and, most recently, **Baby Peter** (Ofsted, 2008) have stiffened the resolve of the Government to make the reforms work. Victoria Climbie was a vulnerable young girl who was subjected to physical and psychological abuse at the hands of her aunt. There were several missed opportunities for her life to have been potentially saved by intervention of health and social care professionals, but alas Victoria died. Baby Peter was a very similar case which occurred in the same London borough. Again, there were clearly identified opportunities for health and social care professionals to have recognized the signs of abuse, but they failed to prevent his death. Maria Colwell was a young girl who died in 1973 under very similar circumstances to the two cases above. Nearly thirty years after the death of Maria Colwell, the Climbie case in 2000 served to demonstrate the persistent failure of agencies to share information, to establish clarity of mutual responsibility and to thereby work towards the collective good. As the Laming Report succinctly concluded:

'.......effective support for children and families cannot be achieved by a single agency'
cited in Brammer, 2007: 202

Furthermore, the ensuing **Every Child Matters 2004** policy and the **Children Act 2004** resulted in the Common Assessment Framework (CAF) and integrated children's services. In spite of these developments, the **Baby Peter** case revealed further persistent failings in the capacity of agencies — community health professionals, paediatricians, police officers and social workers — to effectively share information as part of a comprehensive, coherent and robust safeguarding plan. The consequences of a further blow to public confidence in the child protection system in England may mean another

restructuring of professional roles and responsibilities. The **Social Work Taskforce Report**, published in December 2009, will herald a more robust inspection of social work qualifying and post-qualifying programmes, and a current review of nursing training in the United Kingdom may produce similar results.

In relation to all dimensions and arenas of working in nursing and allied sectors, it has long been recognized that change needs to produce a new generation of practitioner — one that is flexible and adaptable enough to respond to innovations and new directions in health and social care whilst retaining a sense of vocational identity, purpose and indeed loyalty. As we shall see, this is laudable vision, but one that is hard to translate into practice reality.

A global perspective

The World Health Report (2006) galvanizes understanding and respect for the challenges that lay ahead. The focus of Chapter 7 of the report is on enabling countries across the world to work together with the vision of health care working *'within and across countries'* (WHO, 2006). The report outlines that world health care provision is in crisis, particularly in relation to any organization's most valued resource — the workforce. The report outlined that there is a significant shortage of 4.3 million doctors, midwives, nurses and support workers worldwide. This heralded the launch of an ambitious ten year plan to enable workforce planning and health care provision restructuring, with the ultimate goal to achieve more **joined up and collaborative working** (our emphasis) within and across continents. This requires careful consideration of the provision of training and resource allocation for the ultimate benefit of communities. It is clear that many countries do not have the political infrastructure to achieve this ambitious goal, but the emphasis of this strategy is for more advanced countries to support their global partners to achieve greater unity.

Inter-professional working and learning is a key factor in this strategy because the restructuring of health services will also require a restructuring in the culture and working relationships that exist within the health sector across the world. We know from the work acknowledged by Barr (2001) that the one key change element is the recognition that good relations are attributed to parity of status and indeed inter-professional learning and working aids the transition of cultures towards this ethos.

The World Health Organization stipulates that for improved resourcing for health care in disparate countries across continents there needs to be an infrastructure aligned to policy, leadership, finance, education and partnership. They argue that this would then enable a situational analysis to begin an implementation process of a health system with the characteristics of equity, effectiveness, efficiency and quality (WHO, 1996). However, our contention is that this cannot happen without a foundation of understanding within and between countries about the need for inter-professional learning and working agendas to be at the heart of health care planning and delivery.

The contemporary policy drivers for inter-professional education and practice

Over recent years, the following policy directives have heralded the way forward for inter-professional working in England:

- National Service Plans (such as for Older People, for People with Learning Disabilities, for People with Mental Health needs, for Children, Young People and their Families),
- Working Together to Safeguard Children,
- The Framework for Long-Term Conditions,
- The Integrated and Qualified Workforce structure,
- Integrated Qualifications Framework (IQF).

All such policy directives assume that by putting the patient (or service user) at the centre of practice, problems of confusion, of miscommunication, of duplication and of inefficiency can be resolved. But this is to only state half of the story. Indeed, the well-being of the patient is our collective starting point. But how we achieve that goal requires much more than a statement of intent. As in most things, the devil lies in the detail. So, how do diverse teams work together?

The language of working together

The way in which NHS staff work, and how they collaborate with each other in effective teams, is key to the delivery of patient services in the NHS
DH, 2005a

One of the many conundrums when debating inter-professional learning is to decide what the term should describe and which term is the most appropriate to use to describe it. For example for several decades the terms *multi-disciplinary, multi-professional, multi-agency, inter-disciplinary* and *inter-professional* have been used almost interchangeably, and have been generally associated with the principle of *working together*. Indeed, Whittington (2003:15) refers to this as the 'lexicon of partnership and collaboration'. It is clear, however, that inter-professionalism either needs to be organically generated or institutionally demanded. To take this further, we need to consider three interrelated concepts:

Cooperation

This term commonly indicates assistance, help, support, teamwork and mutual aid. In a cooperative working environment, it is assumed that rigid procedures and protocols are unnecessary and that the spirit of cooperation will work best in an unregulated, unfettered creative milieu. The danger with organic cooperation is that it can be as easily dismantled as it can be generated. The Butler-Sloss Inquiry into child sexual abuse (Borough of Cleveland, 1988) indicated that Social Services and the Paediatric Service were indeed working very closely, but to the exclusion of the police and other agencies. Indeed, the Inquiry blamed the crisis on a lack of proper understanding by agencies of each others' functions, on a lack of communication between agencies and on differences of opinion by middle managers which were not recognized by senior staff and which then significantly, and adversely, affected those on the ground.

Collaboration

This term is associated with the positive notion of *working together*, but as an historical term it also has negative connotations, associated with the notion of cooperation with the 'enemy' (as in 'wartime collaborators'). This is important to recognize, as in a time of professional uncertainty, to be seen to be too close to another professional group can be seen as a betrayal of one's collective identity.

Partnership

This term is associated with legal relationships, as in civil partnerships, with mutualism (as in company partners), with a joint venture or project. To Whittington (2003) partnership indicates the formality of 'working together' arrangements.

Whittington (2003: 16) offers the following distinction:

'Partnership is a state of relationships, at organizational, group, professional or inter-professional level, to be achieved, maintained and reviewed; and collaboration is an active process of partnership in action.'

The language of learning together

As stated above, the term **inter-professional learning** is usually defined as 'occasions when two or more professions learn with, from and about each other to facilitate collaboration and the quality of care' (CAIPE, 1997, cited in Barr, 2002:6), whereas **multi-professional education** refers to 'occasions when two or more professions learn side by side for whatever reason' (CAIPE, 1997, cited in Barr, 2002:6).

These definitions epitomize all the principles related to the inter-professional learning and working movement throughout the world of health care: the challenge is to find the best way to facilitate two or more professionals learning about each other in order to work more closely with each other. The optimal prize is to achieve a higher quality of care delivery for the patient using the expertise and professional knowledge of each discrete professional group to maximize the benefit of care for patients and social groups.

The changing vocational landscape

As populations change, then so do the health and social care needs of shifting populations. Whilst the seventeenth century onwards was characterized by what Foucault (2001) defined as the 'great confinement', opportunities arose for nurses and doctors to acquire a professional colonization and monopoly of 'keeping and minding' functions (Scull, 2007) in relation to those defined as having mental health problems, as being people with learning disabilities, as children and adults with a whole range of physical disabilities and sensory impairments, or as older people. As society developed a range of medically run institutions for every kind of excluded difference, then so everyone needed to be nursed, treated or cured.

The health and social care epoch of progressive decarceration over the past forty years has witnessed the gradual but not insignificant erosion of the medical hegemony, and its replacement with an emerging and fledgling environment of negotiated complexity. This can be most clearly seen in the case of services for people with learning disabilities, who had indeed become the exclusive province of the medical profession, and their nursing associates, within the locale of grand, separated, total institutions. By the 1980s, nearly all such institutions had been closed under the aegis of the policy of **Care in the Community**, with the consequence of a lack of certainty as to the new role of nursing within learning disability services. As with other service scenarios, these developments have merited a radical reappraisal of the meaning of 'nursing' in

various ways, and requires 'health care' to be explored in relation to 'social care', and 'nursing' to be developed as a progressive community activity as distinct from an institutional function.

This development can be presented in three stages. Table 5.1 illustrates a contemporary contradiction.

The twenty-first century nurse is offered the chance to break through the medical ceiling and to acquire status through such activities as prescribing medicines at the same time as when the patient or health service user is being empowered to determine the service they wish to receive. In other words, the modern, specialized practitioner has to share their newly acquired status with the empowered patient in the pursuit of individualized care regimes in the name of 'personalization'. In this sense, the traditional authority of the institutionalized medical operative becomes replaced by the professionalized qualification — sanctioned authority of the professional in a negotiated milieu with the empowered, commissioning patient.

Case study 5.1: Jane

Jane is a 53 year old woman with a moderate learning disability. As a child she attended a special school and then was admitted to a hospital for people with a mental handicap (learning disability). At the age of 38, Jane moved back to live with her father and mother, and she attended a social education centre, as run by the former Social Services (now Adult and Community Services). Jane is currently undertaking a community-based education and training programme. Her home arrangements are proving to be progressively unsatisfactory, as Jane found her it very hard to adjust to her father's death and her mother has become progressively frailer. An assessment is being undertaken to consider current and future arrangements for Jane.

Question:
Who needs to be involved in this assessment process?

Table 5.1 The three stages of the development of nursing identity

Traditional nursing	Modern nursing	Post modern ursing
Hierarchical structure based upon a military model	Realignment of hierarchical structure	Democratic structure based upon civilian model
Institutional / hospital base	Shift towards community base	Community base
Tertiary care	Secondary care	Primary, secondary, tertiary care
Routinized, inherited and unquestioned knowledge	Research informed practice	Fluid, contested evidence-based practice wisdom
Doctor-led service	Nursing-led service	Patient / user led service

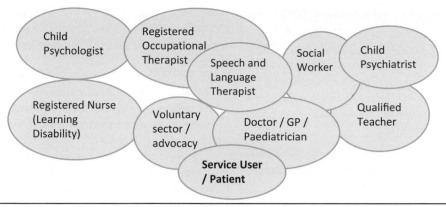

Fig. 5.1 The range of professionals involved in services for families with a child with a learning disability.

Discussion point

Clearly, the assessment process begins with Jane and her ideas about her current situation and what alternatives might be considered. The views of her mother and any other family or kinship member must also be encouraged and valued. Jane has a GP, a dentist, she works with social care staff in her community programme and she has some health difficulties that are being addressed by a learning disability nurse. Whilst enabling people to live as independently as possible, learning disability nurses are involved in promoting the health of their clients. As such, a key role is to engage in a variety of assessments regarding health needs such as epilepsy, screening and health education. Each of these professionals need to understand their role and that of others in order to provide the most effective service to Jane, her mother and other relevant parties (see Fig. 5.1 to see the range of professionals involved in learning disability services).

'We want to break down the professional boundaries that inhibit joint working,
(DfES, 2004: 12)

Professional identity in a modernized service

So, how can the new, modernized, flexible professional worker retain a sense of role identity, purpose, pride and distinctiveness whilst engaged in collaborative, fluid, postmodern, patient or service user-led negotiated programmes of activity, based upon the concept of personalization? Within any

inter-agency, multi-professional environment, the nursing profession needs to work on developing a coherent:

• Professional and role identity,

• Vision and leadership,

• Engagement and influence,

• Image and profile.

It is our contention that **learning together** encourages **working together**, and indeed recent empirical literature has suggested that shared learning is indeed beneficial and that it encourages collaborative working by promoting understanding across disciplines and professions (Barr, 2000; Morrison and Jenkins, 2007; Coleman *et al.*, 2008; Meads *et al.*, 2009).

Research studies by Miers *et al.*, (2008) conducted with adult nurses, physiotherapists, midwives and social workers attests to the desirability of such learning, even though the positive benefits may not be immediately apparent to the participants. Table 5.2 summarizes the opportunities as well as the challenges that inter-professional education presents.

Table 5.2 Inter-professional education (IPE): Opportunities v challenges

Opportunities	Challenges And Impediments
Acquiring shared visions, Talking the same language, Understanding each others' roles and responsibilities, Promoting flexibility and fluidity of response.	Segregated regulatory requirements, Professional idiosyncrasies, The specific nature of the qualifying Course content, Silo mentalities and professional jealousies.

Inter-professional practice (IPP)

We have considered how inter-professional education may enhance the potential of the practitioner to engage in mutually beneficial, collaborative practice, but training and education is only the starting point. The key issue is to consider and identify the key preconditions for the next step — integrated working. As Barr (2002: 7) notes:

'Team working, integration and workforce flexibility could only be achieved if there was widespread recognition and respect for the specialist base of each profession'.

So, what are the drivers and preconditions for effective partnerships and collaborative working?

To answer the question, we need to reflect upon how students will see the drive towards inter-professional education itself. Finch (2000) recognizes that inter-professional education could have different meanings for students: Indeed, is the object for students:

1. To know about the roles of other professions?
2. To be able to work with those others?
3. To be able to substitute for others? or
4. To find flexible career pathways?

Clearly, if students suspect the motivation as being Point 3 above, then they will see the training as either an opportunistic chance (to take work from others) or as a threat (to be encroached upon and even eclipsed by others). For students and practitioners to buy into a shared vision of integrated, collaborative working, they need to understand, accept and endorse the following preconditions for working together.

Preconditions for working together

- Clear roles and responsibilities,
- Reasons for intervention,
- Training about collaborative working and partnerships,
- Common goals and objectives,
- Consent, mandate and willingness to engage,
- Timescales and timely action,
- Sharing of information on a 'need to know' basis,
- Commitment to shared practice.

As Charles Handy notes, where no one has to lose there is more likely to be trust, collaboration, and mutual help (Handy, 1998).

Figure 5.2 sets out the four possible outcomes for the inter-relationship between inter-professional learning and inter-professional practice. Clearly, the goal for all is Type B, where shared learning leads to integrated practice. We will now look at a practice example of such a process.

Case Study 5.2: Inter-professional education and practice in action

The context

This case study relates to an orthopaedic ward in a medium sized provincial hospital that serves up to twenty-five patients, male and female, with an average age of 60 years.

The ward team comprises of physiotherapists, nurses, occupational therapists, social workers, doctors and a pharmacist. The ward is also populated with student nurses, physiotherapists and occupational therapists that access the ward as part of an experiential learning placement from various universities within the region.

The project

The ward has been selected to take part in a pilot project designed to promote inter-professional learning in practice and this consisted of a dedicated 'inter-professional learning in practice' facilitator joining the professional teams on the ward for a period of six months.

The inter-professional learning in practice facilitator is given the remit to design and implement new ways of learning and working in practice for all staff and students with the focus being on improving patient care.

In the early stages of the pilot project the facilitator found it very difficult to integrate into the team and although individual members of the team were attempting to be inclusive many did not see the relevance of the project and were reticent to accept the new outsider. In the initial stages the facilitator needed to be gain the trust and respect of the established team by working with them and proving their worth to the team and becoming valued by them.

This demonstrates an immediate barrier to making change in relation to inter-professional relationships and working, which is experienced by most newcomers to any group.

Once the team had verified the identity and validity of the facilitator they allowed them into the team ethic and this is when a drive towards inter-professional learning could begin. One of the first things the facilitator did was to survey the learning environment that existed for the students to enable an appreciation by all staff and students of the learning processes that existed and opportunities that could be utilized or adapted for the benefit of all.

The first signs of adopted change started to happen after approximately six weeks of the project commencing, however this perceived unused time served to create a solid foundation upon which to build a feeling of confidence and confidence is a major factor in this sustainable change.

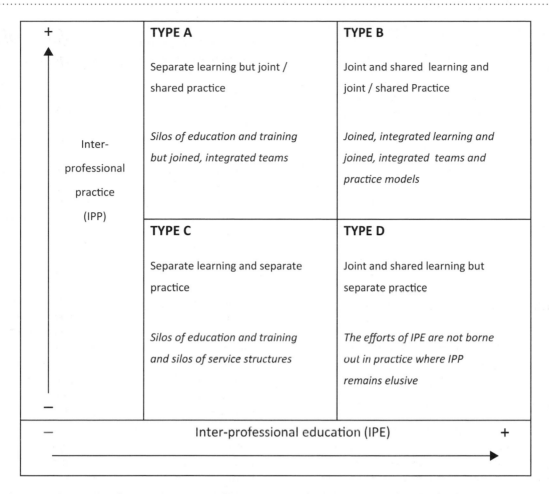

Fig. 5.2 Interrelationship between inter-professional education and inter-professional practice.

Tools for promoting inter-professional practice

Example 1

Using a simple action learning methodology, the facilitator created a tool named '*Word of the Week*'. A sheet of paper was mounted onto a board in the main corridor of the ward. Once a week a word would be placed onto the board by a member of the multidisciplinary team, which was accompanied by a question related to the word. This would remain for a week and the answer then posted by the originator. The process could then be repeated using a different word and a different question for the following week.

The staff and students embraced this idea fully and became confident in its simplicity and as it was a passive non-threatening tool most of the team were happy to become engaged in the learning because it was fun. The unexpected outcome was that members of the public became engaged too because they had read the question and then asked the members of staff for the answer which demonstrated a new dimension of engagement between staff, students, patients and members of the public accessing the ward.

Example 2

Students were set a project to complete during their placement and this was simply called '*Students Working Together*'. During this new approach students from the various professional groups attached to the ward were asked to complete a project in collaboration with each other.

For example a group of first year physiotherapists and nurses were set the task of creating a new patient information leaflet for a patient group that was relevant to the orthopaedic ward. The students chose the surgical operation 'total hip replacement' and they formed a working group to take the project forward. One of the major factors was for the facilitator to demonstrate how the mini project could help them satisfy the evidence requirements for one or more of their placement outcomes and once this was recognized by the students they embraced the idea fully. This again demonstrates the complicated intricacies of the change process and how individuals can be motivated.

The working group for the project designed a strategy for gathering information and opinion from the wider professional teams that contributed to total hip replacement.

The students approached individuals from the nursing, physiotherapy, occupational therapy, doctors, radiography, pain team, pharmacist, and the discharge liaison service. This immediately gave the students a broader perspective and understanding of the thought processes and priorities of each group with respect to caring for patients undergoing a total hip replacement.

In addition the students were encouraged by their mentors to approach patients who were experiencing the process related to total hip replacement to ask their opinion of the current provision of information, ease of understanding, did it meet their needs and what changes would they recommend.

Finally the students wrote up their findings and created a draft patient information leaflet that they presented to the group of mentors and patients.

These two examples were successful because of their ability to enable all students and staff to engage in the process and tailor their learning to the source available. The mentor team embraced the tools because they were simple and reusable that could be tailored to the learning needs of individual or groups of students.

Inter-professional learning in practice relies upon the desire or motivation for change and a use of media friendly sources that enables everyone to tailor their engagement to their needs with the significant addition of students and staff achieving this collaboratively and not in isolation.

As Goodman and Clemow note (2008: 118) 'inter-professional rivalry, tribalism and stereotyping exist and detract from effective care' and the above case study examples illustrate the ways in which such rivalries and tribalisms can be challenged and addressed.

Exercises:
- Could these techniques be used in other clinical areas within health and social care?
- Consider other examples that could be used to promote inter-professional learning in clinical settings within health and social care?

Discussion points

The examples portrayed in Case Study 5.2 could be adapted and developed to be used in almost any clinical area within health and social care. This is due to the relevance the exercises has to any clinician in most environments. Word of the week, for example could be adapted to be used online or in any clinical setting and students working together is in many situations a formalized exposure of what is happening anyway. The main significance of these two examples is that they are not profession specific or learner specific and therefore the main element for success is for mentors and supervisors to recognize the value of the examples and employ them in practice.

There are so many possible modes and practicum related to inter-professional learning in practice that the list is potentially endless. Several important elements to consider when designing such a tool is to avoid the tool being aimed at one professional group, ensure it enables group working across student professional groups, make it relevant to practice and the student must be able to instantly see its value in their learning.

In all inter-professional learning activities for students in practice the ultimate goal must be for the student to conceptualize their learning for the benefit of the care they will deliver in the future as health care professionals. We have made it clear earlier in the chapter that the emphasis should not be on simply blurring boundaries of care for professional groups and their patients, but rather for there to emerge a collaborative culture which is based upon mutual consent and respect for all professions. The key ingredient to achieve this is to devise a framework that enables an understanding of the skills required by an individual to achieve true understanding of inter-professional working and learning.

The work by Gordon and Walsh (2005) provides such a framework that has both theoretical underpinnings and a pragmatic use, and which evolved from mapping the practice skill and competency requirements of seven health and social pre-registration programme benchmark statements. These were provided by the Quality Assurance Agency, the Nursing and Midwifery Council, the General Medical Council and the Department of Health's Knowledge and Skills Framework. The framework was then utilized by the Combined Universities Inter-professional Learning Unit (CUILU) to enable a better understanding of the skills and attributes required by most health and social care students in the practice setting (CUILU, 2004).

The benefits of being able to measure at a practical level the ability of students to operate as knowledgeable inter-professional practitioners are significant, as in many cases these skills are transferrable into the specialist discipline within which the student is learning. It is established that there is a common ground of learning in the practice placement setting, which should drive the students to want to learn about each other and with each other.

Is the goal really about collaboration, integration or assimilation?

Nurses are not going to become social workers, physicians are not going to become teachers, but in the less clear arenas of modernized workforce innovation, the boundaries between doctors and nurses are blurring, the demarcation lines between the psychiatrist, the mental health nurse, the social workers, the graduate mental health worker and the social care support worker are up for grabs and contested. So, is integration of skills, knowledge and role within the wider health care team desirable? Table 5.3 lists the advantages and disadvantages of integration in the promotion of inter-professional working.

Table 5.3 The advantages and disadvantages of integration in the promotion of inter-professional working

Advantages	Disadvantages
Workforce fluidity, flexibility and economy, Facilitation of multi careers across skill mix teams, Capacity for rapid change, The service user gets the best service – from whoever is best able to deliver.	Fuzzy role definition and purpose, Potential for dangerous practice, Erosion of professional identity, self worth and pride, Loss of creative and critically dynamic tension between professions.

Summary

It is clearly the goal of the government to promote and develop a modernized, more flexible service, and a key plank of policy to achieve this objective resides in the arena of workforce reform:

'A better integrated workforce—designed around the needs of people who use services and supported by common education frameworks, information systems, career frameworks and rewards — can deliver more personalized care, more effectively'.
DH, 2006b: 185

Indeed, it has been suggested that in the future, skills to meet the needs of communities will be more important than titles, and thus professional groups may be required to relinquish the historic protectionism that has been a feature of the emergence of professional status.

In summary, it is instructive to reflect upon the **Ten Essential Shared Capabilities** as developed by NIMHE *et al.* (2004), for multi-professional mental health practitioners:

1. Working in partnership,
2. Respecting diversity,
3. Practising equality,
4. Challenging inequality,
5. Promoting recovery,
6. Identifying people's needs and strengths,
7. Providing service user centred care,
8. Making a difference,
9. Promoting safeties and positive risk taking,
10. Personal development and learning.

According to NIMHE (2004: 3) these capabilities provide the 'mental health specific context and achievements for education, training and continuing professional development at pre registration / qualification stage'. These capabilities are, significantly, not exclusive or specific to any professional group. If we start with the notion of what is required to be offered to service users, we are then left with the question of which professional groupings wish to claim competence to carry out such functions. It can be seen that inter-professional learning is seen as increasingly important across all health and social care qualifying and post qualifying programmes. As Whittington (2003) observes:

'Service users want social workers who can collaborate effectively with other professions and agencies; and strategies for service partnership and for the protection of children and vulnerable adults require it'

Almost without exception, politicians, professional lead bodies, academics and practitioners are in agreement that human services from various disciplines need to work effectively together. The agenda for more collaborative inter professional working and learning has received a raised profile in the last decade in the United Kingdom, with the release of policy such as **Every Child Matters** (2003), the **Victoria Climbie Inquiry** (2003), the **New NHS** (1997) and the OFSTED Report (2008) into the death of Baby Peter in the London Borough of Haringey.

A global perspective, centred on the **World Health Report (2006)** by the World Health Organization, suggests that human resource management in health care is in crisis. This was brought into sharp focus by the announcement that globally there is a shortfall of some 4.3 million health care workers. This report has sought to redefine how health care should be planned in a more collaborative way at a global level to encourage more advanced countries to enable their partners for the benefit of patient care.

The emergence of the need for a more public health focussed and practitioner-led services across the modernized world has required a change in the outlook, perspective and training of health care professionals. The need for a systemic transformation from an **illness** service to a **wellness** service has been a key focus for over a decade, both nationally and internationally. One important facet for this realization is the redefining of professional boundaries and skill sets and inter-professional learning and working agendas play a key role in this transformation.

The chapter has explored the language of working together that is often misunderstood and misinterpreted and so one facet of advancement could be to agree a common language for the phenomenon of inter-professional working and learning.

The chapter recognizes that in post modern times within health and social care, the learning and skills landscape is changing and is set to change again in years to come. Therefore the practitioner of today must be prepared in a way that enables an understanding of identity of themselves and of the other care professionals in a health and social care setting.

In conclusion, as graduates from professional qualifications — such as nursing, occupational therapy, social work and teaching — are increasingly entering professional worlds characterized by blurred boundaries, it is ever more essential that an understanding of the dynamics and complexities of inter-professional working becomes embedded in the pre-qualifying/pre-registration and post-qualifying/post-registration learning frameworks. We are all in this together.

 # Online Resource Centre

For more information on inter-professional practice and education in health and social care visit the Online Resource Centre — http://www.oxfordtextbooks.co.uk/orc/linsley/

Further reading

Journal of Interprofessional Care

The Journal of Interprofessional Care is a peer reviewed journal that is regarded as the authoritative scholarly publication in the field of inter-professional learning and working within a health and social care context.

Journal of Integrated Care

The Journal of Integrated Care facilitates the evidence-based integration of health, social care and other community services in order to benefit service users and patients, and transcend traditional service and professional boundaries.

www.integratedcarenetwork.gov.uk

The Department of Health Integrated Care Networks take the lead for the Putting People First team for integration and whole system reform, housing with care, assistive technology and partnership working.

www.caipe.org.uk

Founded in 1987, Centre for the Advancement of Inter-Professional Education is dedicated to the promotion and development of inter-professional education (IPE) with and through its individual and corporate members, in collaboration with like minded organizations in the UK and overseas.

References

Armitage, H., Pitt, R. & Jinks, A (2009). *Initial findings from the TUILIP (Trent Universities Inter-professional Learning in Practice) Project. Journal of Interprofessional Care* (23) 1: 101–103.

Barr, H. (2001). *Editorial: collaboration and conflict Journal of Interprofessional Care* 15 (1): 5–6.

Barr, H. (2002). *Inter-professional Education: Today, Yesterday and Tomorrow*. Occasional Paper No:1: March 2002. London: LTSN for Health Sciences and Practice, Kings College.

Barr, H. (2000). Working together to learn together: learning together to work together. *Journal of Interprofessional Care* 14 (2)Barr, H. (2005). *Inter-professional Education in the United Kingdom 1966 to 1997* Occasional Paper No: 7. London: The Higher Education Academy.

Barr, H. (2005). *The Theory-practice Relationship in Inter-professional I Education. Occasional* Paper. No: 9 London: The Higher Education Academy.

Barrett, G., Sellman, D. & Thomas, J. (eds) (2005). *Inter-professional Working in Health and Social Care.* London: Palgrave.

Brammer, A. (2007). Social Work Law. (2nd edn.) Harlow: Pearson Education.

Butler-Sloss, E. (1988). *The Cleveland Inquiry*. Middlesbrough: Cleveland County Council.

CAIPE (1997) *Inter-professional Education — A Definition*. London: CAIPE.

Coleman, M., Roberts, K., Wulff, D., Van Zyl, R. & Newton, K. (2008). Interprofessional ambulatory primary care practice-based educational program *Journal of Interprofessional Care* 22 (1): 69–84.

Combined Universities Inter-professional Learning Unit (2004). *Inter-professional Capability Framework* ONLINE: http://www.cuilu.group.shef.ac.uk/capability_framework.pdf (accessed 4/12/09).

Department for Education and Skills (2003). *The Victoria Climbie Inquiry: Report of an Inquiry by Lord Laming.* London: DfES.

Department for Education and Skills (2004). *Every Child Matters: Change for Children.* London: DfES.

Department of Health (1989). *The NHS and Community Care Act.* London. DH.

Department of Health (1997). *The New NHS: Modern, dependable.* London. DH.

Department of Health (1999). *Making a Difference.* London: DH.

Department of Health (2005a). *Independence, Well Being and Choice.* London: DH.

Department of Health (2005b). *Supporting People with Long Term Conditions: An NHS and Social Carte Model to Support Local Innovation and Integration.* London: DH.

Department of Health (2006a). *Our Health, Our Care, Our Say.* London: DH.

Department of Health (2006b). *Working Together to Safeguard Children: A Guide to Interagency Working to Safeguard and Promote the Welfare of Children.* London: DH.

Department of Health (2006c). *Modernising Nursing Careers: Setting the Direction.* London: DH.

Department of Health (2008). *Delivering Health Closer to Home: Meeting the Challenge.* London: DH.

Department of Health (2009). *NHS 2010–2015 : from good to great. Preventative, people-centred, productive.* London: DH.

Finch, J. (2000). Inter-professional education and team working: a view from the educational provider. *British Medical Journal* 321: 1138–140.

Foucault, M. (2001). *Madness and Civilisation.* London: Routledge.

Goodman, B. & Clemow, R. (2008). *Nursing and Working with Other People.* Exeter: Learning Matters.

Gordon, F. & Walsh, C. (2005). *A framework for inter-professional capability: developing students of health and social care as collaborative workers. Journal of Integrated Care.* 13 (3): 26–33.

Handy, C. (1998). *Understanding Organizations.* Harmondsworh: Penguin.

Keunssberg, E. (1967). *Conference Report, Family Health Care: The Team.* London: Royal College of General Practitioners.

NIMHE / Department of Health (2004). *The Ten Essential Shared Capabilities.* London: NIMHE / DH.

Meads, G., Jones, I., Harrison, R., Forman, D. & Turner, W. (2009). How to sustain interprofessional learning and practice: messages for higher education and health and social care management. *Journal of Education and Work* 22 (1): 67–79.

Miers, M., Rickaby, C. & Pollard, K. (2008). *Making the Most of Inter-professional Learning Opportunities: Professionals' and students' experiences of inter-professional learning and working.* London: Higher Education Academy / Health Sciences and Practice.

Morrison & Jenkins (2007) Sustained effects of interprofessional shared learning on student attitudes to communication and team working depend on shared learning opportunities on clinical placement as well as in the classroom. *Medical Teacher* (29): 450–456.

OFSTED (2008). *Report into the Death of Baby P in the London Borough of Haringey.* London: OFSTED.

O'Hallaran, C., Hean, S., Humpheries, D., & Macleod0Clark, J. (2006). Developing common learning: the new generation of project undergraduate curriculum model. *Journal of Interprofessional Care* 20(1): 12–28.

Pollard, K., Rickaby, C. & Meirs., M (2008). *Evaluating Student Learning in an Inter professional Curriculum: The Relevance of Pre Qualifying Education for Future Professional Practice.* London: Higher Education Academy/Health Sciences and Practice.

Scull, A. (2007). *Madhouse: a Tragic Tale of Megalomania and Modern Medicine.* New Haven: Yale University Press.

Secretary of State for Health (2000). *The NHS Plan.* London: The Stationery Office.

Whittington, C. (2003). Collaboration and partnership in Context In. J. Weinstein, C. Whittington and T. Leiba (eds.) *Collaboration in Social Work Practice.* London: Jessica Kingsley.

World Health Organization (2006). *The world health report 2006 — working together for health.* Geneva: World Health Organization.

Chapter 6
The nurse-patient relationship

John McKinnon

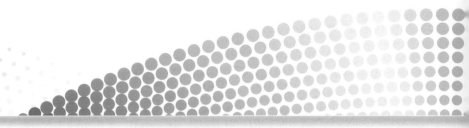

Introduction

In this chapter the nature of the nurse-patient relationship **and its value in health care will be discussed. The reflective logs of student nurses will be presented in order to illustrate the impact of** patient-centredness **on practice outcomes. Psychological and sociological frameworks together with current health care research across a range of practice areas will also be used to further demonstrate this. We will see that the nurse-patient relationship is an irreplaceable channel through which need can be individually assessed, and a package of care can be most effectively negotiated, delivered and evaluated. The meaning of partnership will be explored in a context of** empowerment **leading to arguments for patient leadership in care planning.**

Imagine a world in which one is required to disclose the most intimate details of one's private life to strangers. This may include divulging fears, hopes, pain, habits socially acceptable and not so socially acceptable. Imagine having to disrobe in front of strangers. Now imagine undergoing a treatment or clinical procedure which is based on best evidence, has an excellent success rate and is executed with expert precision but which is devoid of any meaningful human communication; no information, no words or glances of reassurance, no one to hear, acknowledge or listen to you.

The former scenario is not as extreme as it might appear. It is exactly what is expected of patients every day in health care systems around the globe. The latter situation is exactly how

the best health care experience would be without the nurse-patient **relationship**.

In today's tightly regulated health care system funding is targeted at services which are finely tuned to achieve tangible predictable outcomes. Length of hospital stays, waiting times, care pathways and levels of technical skill matched to profiles of tasks in clinical areas are all examples of this. However practice knowledge and skills central to nursing are neither visible, tangible nor easily measured. In such a climate of hard scientific values the importance of a nurse-patient relationship is easily underestimated by health care providers including some nurses themselves. Perpetual advancement in the technology of biomedical care and emphasis in practice on the skills to operate such technology coupled with acquisition of diagnostic and prescribing powers in nursing mean that the needs of **personhood** are easily eclipsed. This perspective reduces caring to little more than a production line process and contains a number of deficits (Benner *et al.*, 1996).

First, the patient is reduced to a set of problems, complaints and isolated organic disease states which need to be addressed (Evans, 2007). Second, care centres on preoccupation with issues other than the patient experience of health and illness and patient participation in their care is undermined together with the questions, opinions, fears, hopes and personal information they bring to assessment of need (Jones, 2007). Third, reactive pharmacological responses are privileged over proactive public health and social approaches to disease (Freund *et al.*, 2003). Finally and most crucially the professional carer is personally distanced from the one being cared for and consequently the fundamental state of humans as social beings is ignored (Malone, 2003).

The nurse-patient relationship is the missing component in this equation of caring. It describes the mutual trust and respect between patient and nurse which informs health care. The relationship stands distinct from that which exists in counselling practice although there are some overlapping principles. In counselling self-awareness, self-determination and empowerment through personal problem solving may be the sole end goals. This is not the case in nursing. In nursing the relationship with the patient permeates all care management and delivery and is attached to and enhances the acceptability of many other clinical and technical competencies. In this relationship developing patient self-determination and empowerment are the means as well as the end or care planning focused on promoting, restoring and sustaining health or helping towards a peaceful endlife experience (Benner and Wrubel, 1989). In addition the nurse-patient relationship involves family and trusted friends In care planning and carefully crafted advocacy; working across professional health and social care disciplines and collaborating with voluntary groups to optimize the human experience of health service (Gallup and O'Brien, 2003).

The relevance of attachment theory

Attachment theory bears witness to the centrality of the nurse-patient relationship. We are pre-programmed as prosocial at birth and throughout life we actively seek out the company of trusted others. This is particularly the case in times of stress and trauma when the challenges we face and the surroundings which house them are complex and unfamiliar to us, fragmenting our ability to cope and causing us to feel vulnerable. Engagement with other individuals whom we perceive as caring results in restored feelings of security, comfort and self-confidence. A failure to recruit human support results in further distress, insecurity, a lack of self-worth and even despair. This can lead to a lack of cooperation, anger, frustration and learned helplessness. Personal security, on the other hand, is a thinking and feeling state which promotes independence and buys time for us to regroup and plan to meet our needs (Belsky and Cassidy 1994).

This understanding of how people move and thrive in the world explains why the findings of a wide body of research into how patients perceive quality of care differ from that espoused by health care planners. There are more complaints from patients about poor personal communication including not being listened to than any other part of health care (Stickley and Freshwater, 2006). Shattell (2004) cites a range of studies in which patients reportedly felt dehumanized by a lack of eye contact but valued and restored by nurses who were willing to listen to them. Patients have been shown to be far less troubled by clumsily conducted procedures or tardiness in

responding to requests than by nurses who cannot remember their names or who fail to respect their individuality. Nurses who by their behaviour actively acknowledge the likes, dislikes and overall concerns of their patients are highly prized (Reiman 1986; Attree 2001). Williams (2001) underlines the importance of emotional and personal closeness at times of vulnerability such as bereavement or the period immediately before receiving a general anaesthetic.

If attachment theory explains the need for informed human relationships as part of health care, it also explains the skill and potential in such relationships. McQueen (2004) has described the ability to interpret the behaviour and feelings of others by effectively exercising empathy as emotional intelligence. Emotional intelligence is also characterized by self-monitoring behaviour which acknowledges prejudices and suspends value judgements. This is a social competence; finely tuned physical and emotional deportment to construct a working relationship and an environment in which the patient feels cared for. This provides a platform of trust on which health care can be most effectively negotiated, delivered and evaluated (Malloch, 2000).

This perspective on caring differs from one which gives pride of place to targets protocols and pathways. Humanity, the unexpected and the unpredictable are respected as the norm. The so-called 'routine' predictable episode of care is recognized as a piece of fiction or at least something which can only be identified with hindsight. This is unsurprising when the multiple contingencies and exit points of each context of human experience are considered. Sarah Cowley's study of public health nursing (1995) showed that practitioners frequently shift the focus of practice away from predetermined objectives to address more pressing needs which are hidden until the time of the episode of care. Cowley concluded that 'routine' was an inappropriate term which oversimplified the practice situation and devalued the skills necessary to move effectively within it.

The nurse continually works through a range of ad hoc assessment responses and practices to sustain patient comfort helping them to adapt in the face of change. This is a commonsense approach which is sensitive and reciprocal to the particulars of a situation which caused Berg and colleagues (2007:100) to speak of the nurse-patient relationship as being 'asymetrical and tied to time and context'. Pathways protocols and other guidelines are revealed as complementary rather than exclusive tools which are only as good as the expertise of those who use them.

The complex discursive nature of this process raises questions as to how it can be dismissed as a negligible aspect of health care.

The sociology of caring

Nursing is for the most part a female populated profession and this means that the appraisal of caring in nursing is a feminist issue. The traditional belief that caring is naturally synonymous with goodness in womanhood historically conducted in exchange for little or no payment exerts a substantial influence on the way professional practice in this domain is valued. Despite progress made by women in the secular workplace, the greater the correlation that can be made between their secular job description and the traditional role of caring, nurturing and subservience the easier it becomes to trivialize expertise as natural behaviour common to women.

This shapes the socialization of nursing to a position of deference believing managerial and medical expertise to be superior (Crowe, 2000). This position also works to oppose men in nursing developing their caring role and implies that their chief interest should somehow lean toward acute technical interventions or towards management. Traditional perspectives on women and caring mean that the nurse-patient relationship can be moved down the ladder of funding and planning priorities below technical roles.

In reality the reverse is true. The nurse-patient **relationship** is the tool which maximizes all other health care intervention. Caring is in itself an insufficiently simple and nebulous term with which to describe the multifaceted nature of nursing practice (Tarlier, 2004). The greater the investment in the expert personal delivery of health care through high levels of qualified nurses the more positive the outcomes including the extent of patient satisfaction will be. Conversely the poorer and more diluted the skillmix the poorer the standard of personal care will be (Carr-Hill *et al.*, 1992; Redfern, 1996). A careful examination of the construction of this relationship will illustrate how deceptively complex it is.

Constructing the nurse–patient relationship

There are number of features to the successful nurse-patient **relationship**. Some pervade all personal contact. Others are developed and achieved over time.

Engagement

Engagement is the demonstration of willingness to become involved; the evidence of a desire to pursue an understanding of the patient's situation as they see it (Berg *et al.*, 2007). **Engagement** lays the groundwork for trust and lends credibility to other skills which are actioned. **Engagement** is indicated by a variety of non-verbal behaviours which signal openness. Eye contact is essential. If this is absent it may render other non-verbal or verbal communication open to suspicion of insincerity. An open facial expression and non-threatening body position which visibly attend on the patient also provide evidence of active genuine interest. Relationships set in motion through **engagement** also provide familiarity in what can be an unfamiliar clinical environment. This is demonstrated in Case Study 6.1.

Case study 6.1: A familiar face by Kati Lucas, second year nursing student

Adam was a young man I met in my first year of study. He suffered a brain injury after falling off a balcony landing on a concrete surface. He had also gone on to develop epilepsy. He had been a very active young man but had now lost the ability to speak, walk, to use initiative and to perform any basic task. Seeing the small but significant progress he had made (following physiotherapy) in the few weeks from when he was admitted to the ward to when he was transferred to the rehabilitation unit inspired me.

Whenever I looked after him I understood the importance of eye contact and trying as hard as possible to communicate with him. Despite his compromised state he needed to know who I was and that I was 'there' for him.

Previously, Adam had made very little sign of self-awareness; he had given me a 'thumbs up' once and had smiled as I was passing through the bay. A year on when I was placed on the rehabilitation ward, Adam could laugh appropriately; he showed understanding and sometimes could interact with staff members he knew well through grunting. Other times he was very vacant and showed absolutely no sign of understanding or awareness, which I found hard to deal with. Sometimes I thought he was ignoring me, other times I didn't think he registered that I was there. Nevertheless I persisted in looking him in the eye and speaking with him as I would any other patient. The grief and anxiety being experienced by his family was written on their faces whenever they visited Adam but I encouraged them to do the same: keep looking at him and talking to him about familiar events. By liaising with the physiotherapists and occupational therapists I also recognized the value of reinforcing the exercises they had prescribed for him.

Adam made a startling recovery. It started off with very small progress; one day his father passed him a mobile phone and Adam was pressing buttons as if trying to write a text message. A few days later he spoke and said, 'Hello Dad' with a big smile. About a month later he recognized me and could say my name! I was so happy for him I could have cried and it made me reflect on how much I love this job and even though there are so many bad days associated with nursing there are some wonderful ones. The human spirit is robust. Where many people would have given up and sunk into depression Adam and his family remained upbeat. I like to think their outlook on life was kept high due to the excellent care and friendship they all received on the rehabilitation unit. I will never forget how he went from being quite comatose at times to suddenly finding the strength from somewhere to start talking.

Discussion points

- What does Kati's experience show about the importance of engaging with patients even when their level of consciousness is variable?
- Discuss the neuropsychological theory underpinning the recall and retention of long-term memory in the face of cerebral injury.
- How does Kati's experience distinguish the role of the nurse-patient relationship in rehabilitation following cerebral trauma from that of physiotherapy or other rehabilitative measures.

Patients, particularly those with long-term conditions value continuity (Berg *et al.*, 2006). Continuity is especially valuable when a patient's level of consciousness is variable and when memory is compromised as in the case of Kati Lucas' patient (Case Study 6.1). Long-term memory is not limited to a distinct structure in the brain but is stored within a relationship of personal meaning and context networked across cerebral structures. Memory networks are linked to the special sense cortices to trigger salient information retrieval. This arrangement makes compensation possible especially in the period of recovery following trauma (Cohen, 1993). The smell of red wine may trigger the memory of a mediterranean holiday. The sound of a favourite musical artist may stimulate memories of time spent with friends and loves ones and the sight of a familiar face may call to mind the encouragement received from that individual (Rose, 2006).

A sense of **personhood** recovered for someone by a nurse providing a environment of personal familiars is never more important than in a patient who is confused and disorientated. Working in tandem with rehabilitative specialists and maximizing the worth of their work through liaising with visiting relatives, Lucas assisted her patient to regain his place in the social world; something which could not have been achieved by physiotherapy or other rehabilitative measures alone.

Listening

'It is easy to take listening for granted and, through our own preconceptions, to fail to really listen'.
Stickley and Freshwater, 2006:14

My experience as a lecturer in undergraduate nursing studies tells me that of all the communication skills, listening is the most difficult to master. The tendency among many student listeners is to underestimate the potential for healing at work in listening alone. For many students listening exercises are the first real test of their ability to remain within the boundaries of competence. When problems of which they have no knowledge or experience are shared with them they panic and

the need to care for another 'by doing' drives them to 'leap in' with offers of help which they are not able to fulfill. Helping is about listening much more than doing.

Listening is also the crucial phase of a larger process in practice. Pathophysiological knowledge and skills of examination and diagnosis depend on listening to reach accurate findings. During history taking it is important to allow the patient to tell their story in their own way with intervention by the practitioner only to clarify detail (Epstein *et al.*, 2000). Poor listening results in an incomplete patient profile which may result in care which is poorly focused and insensitive to a patient's beliefs, values, allergy status or current medication.

McCormack (2003:204) argues that patient values beliefs and concerns are best understood when they are 'integrated into the biography of the individual'. When patients are allowed to explain their position through narrative the nurse is able to apprehend information in context and therefore understand the motives underpinning their behaviour. This is a person-centred method of listening in practice which helps ensure that concerns privileged by the patient are given primacy in assessment and allowed to shape care. The method contrasts with the findings of one study (Jones, 2007) in which admission was presented to patients as a bureaucratic onerous task which warranted an apology. The author describes the early establishment of a 'fixed relationship' (2007:218) with the nurse in the role of interviewer and the patient in the role of information giver. Moreover no time was allowed for patients' questions or opinions. Jones points out that his findings are supported across a wide body of literature.

The projected attitude of the listener is also important.

In any private relationship our view of a person is conditional on their behaviour towards us and towards others. In the nurse-patient relationship the nurse views the patient positively for the duration of care regardless of their behaviour outside the boundaries of that care. This is unconditional positive regard and it is based purely on the patient's status as another human being. Unconditional positive regard is what permits the nurse to provide care for someone whose political or religious position, moral and ethical reasoning might in another setting distance them from that one. It is listening without judging (Rogers, 1994). This is demonstrated in Case Study 6. 2 below.

Case Study 6.2: Unconditional positive regard

Leon

Leon is a 32 year old African Carribean man born in the UK. He has a large tattoo on the outer aspect of his right upper arm and a metal stud in his right eyebrow. His hair is short and tramlined. He smokes approximately 15 cigarettes per day. He is an unemployed painter/decorator/plasterer. His mother was a single parent and suffered from depression. She committed suicide six years ago. He was excluded from school several times and well known to local police at an early age. He was involved in a gang at age eleven and a drug dealer by the time he was 16 years old. He has served custodial sentences for carrying firearms and grievous bodily harm against women.

He has been admitted to hospital with an old stab wound which has become infected and a superimposed chest infection resulting in visible weightloss. He has no visitors and spends his time own his own sitting in bed or in a chair listening to his ipod. He speaks only when spoken to.

Within days his condition has responded to antibiotics and he can be discharged with advice to keep the wound clean and dry. He requests some help to stop smoking.

Discussion points

- What are this patient's rights to treatment and care?
- How might knowledge of Leon's past social history affect the thinking and/or behaviour of health care professionals who are looking after him?
- In addition to a smoking cessation referral what other community services might benefit Leon?
- Why and how might of placing his social history on one side affect Leon's thinking and behaviour and work to inform practice?

Under the 1986 World Health Organization Convention on Human Rights in Health Care (WHO, 1986) Leon is entitled to health care and to participate in that health care regardless of whether or not his behaviour meets with the approval of health professionals and society at large.

A superficial glance at this patient's history could lead health professionals to dismiss Leon as a violent and disruptive member of society and his history of violence against women could lead female members of staff to view him with caution; only approaching him when absolutely necessary. Leon's laconic presentation and his physical appearance may reinforce negative stereotyping. Consequently the nurse-patient relationship required to optimize care would be inhibited and remain undeveloped.

However there are clues in Leon's social history that suggest poor attachment which would explain poor communication skills particularly with those in authority along with low self-esteem. His mother suffered from long-term mental illness from when he was a child and there is no evidence of any other positive role models. Instead as in the case of many young men in his situation Leon has invested in unhealthy peer groups and associated negative behaviours to gain approval (Graham and Power, 2004). Owning Leon's perspective on his life history will assist the nursing team to place preconceived notions to one side and construct a more positive plan of care.

A public health nursing approach should seize this episode of care as an opportunity to offer positive life chances to Leon. In addition to smoke cessation referrals, a vulnerable adult referral to social services or to a community social exclusion project might serve to address his needs in a more holistic way.

Responding to Leon's request at this vulnerable time in his life may prove to be a turning point in his view of himself in relation to society placing his social exclusion in reverse. In achieving concordance with Leon, the nursing team will have acted in a socially informed way developing new skills in anti-oppressive practice.

The proactive properties of listentening

Listening has proactive properties in that it can stem anxieties and fears real and unfounded which might otherwise lead to damaging health behaviour or disease states. It has a healing power of its own by virtue of the value it imparts to the one being listened to (Stickley and Freshwater, 2006). This is observable in more than a personal feeling of self-esteem. For example a perceived feeling of comfort within the self fuels a powerful cortical affective component which provides pain relief by inhibiting impulses ascending the spinal cord (Gould and Thomas, 1999).

The skilled listener does not listen merely with their ears but recognizes the role of the face and the body. Listening therefore also involves self-awareness (Stickley and Freshwater, 2006). The eye contact open facial expression and body posture commenced at **engagement** are maintained here. In a Northern European culture sitting at right angles to the patient will present a non-hostile impression (Fig. 6.1). Other cultures may tolerate a sitting arrangement where nurse and patient are placed opposite each other (Egan, 2002).

Listening is about observing as well as hearing. The patients emotional and cognitive status are often betrayed by their body language. Mirroring the patient's changing body language can appear a disingenuous activity to the novice listener but once integrated into caring behaviour will reap benefits. **Empathy** is the goal of any caring listener. It is the ability to grasp the frame of reference of another. According to Kirk (2007:239) to exercise **empathy** is:

'to understand what it is like to be in someone else's position (what it is like to live that person's life) or, perhaps less ambitious, (ii) to understand what it is like to experience phenomena as someone else experiences them'.

When listeners mirror the body position of their patients they convey physical evidence of their **empathy.** Furthermore as emotions influence body movement observable in the patient by the nurse, so body movement of the nurse will inform his or her emotions. Adopting the body language of the patient throughout active listening will assist the nurse to **feel** the disposition of the patient (Immordino and Damasio, 2007).

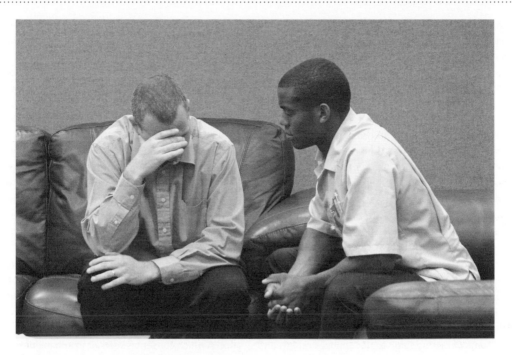

Fig. 6.1 Listening with the whole body.

When the listener finally speaks it should initially be to feed-back to the patient a summary of what has been said in order invite clarification or correction. This reaffirms to the story-teller the engaged empathic state of the listener (Shattell *et al.*, 2007).

Engagement and embodied listening prepare the way for the development of a working partnership which can result in empowerment.

Concordance

Concordance in health care is a partnership of equals on which care planning is negotiated. It is born from the recognition of patients as having the right to participate in their own care framed within the international convention on human rights in health care (WHO, 1986). Public criticism of the historical lack of accountability among health care professionals and a series of high profile cases of negligence have also played a part in the evolution of the concept.

Concordance replaces the concept of compliance in which the nurse assumes the role of expert. In the compliance culture 'sensible' patients follow the instructions of the nurse even at the cost of their own beliefs and values. 'Difficult' patients ignore question or attempt to negotiate their care. In a con-cordant culture the nurse earns trust as a skilled professional bringing evidence-based knowledge in practice to any encoun-ter. However the nurse understands that patients are also 'experts in their own lives' and bring socially contextualized

knowledge arising from the lived experience of health and ill-ness that is shaped by family relationships, housing, geograph-ical placement, employment and financial status (Russell *et al.*, 2003).

Case Study 6.3: Patient-centredness by Daniel Gray, first year nursing student

One 93 year old lady with a history of falls was with us for around 8 weeks. I noticed that as I allowed more time to get to know her it became easier to know what she wanted and needed. Likewise she seemed to be more comfortable with me. Not that I did anything special, I just talked with her, listened to her, and got to know her as a person rather than only approaching her when a certain intervention was due.

She was actually a very interesting lady, who had trav-elled to distant places and met people from different nations and tribes. She had endured a difficult and abusive upbring-ing as an unwanted child. Marriage had brought happiness and stability to her life but now she was a widow and alone. Her recent admission and planned transfer to a residential home meant permanent separation from her beloved cat. She was not always the most welcoming, sociable or coop-erative person on the ward. In fact she could be grumpy and unwilling to do things, but knowledge of her past and present circumstances enabled me to empathize with her situation and better equipped me to provide the care she needed.

For example, having got to know this patient better, I soon realized how she liked to be addressed and spoken to, and how she didn't like to be spoken to: a simple thing but one that made a big difference to her and to our relationship. During mobilization I was able to help her productively and in a way that she was comfortable with. I learned that when moving her, what was vital was time, patience and listening to how she wanted to be supported; safeguarding and encouraging her movements. Rather than rushing her about and doing most of the moving for her, she benefited by getting a better chance to actually mobilize within her limits, and by doing things her way. Because of this I was able to help maintain and improve her mobility and maximize her independence.

Other things such as placing extra pillows around her for support to prevent her knocking herself as she slept, and cutting up some of her food due to her limited strength and dexterity, all came from having a better knowledge of the patient either through observation or conversation.

Nurses can expect too much from patients; forgetting that everybody is different. They can expect patients to follow a longstanding routine that has worked well for them even though it isn't really what the patient wants. Then when the patient doesn't comply, nurses become irritated and less willing to help. When there's a lot of work to be done it's understandably difficult, but there is a need to treat each patient as an individual.

Discussion points

- How does Daniel's experience show that patient-centredness is a prerequisite to concordance?
- How is a patient-centred approach constructed?
- What support for concordance is found in social psychology?
- How can the paternalistic and concordant perspectives on consent be distinguished?

Daniel Gray's experience (Case Study 6.3) illustrates how **patientcentredness** is a prerequisite to **concordance.** On first impressions Gray's patient is uncooperative and temperamental. A **paternalistic** approach to care might view the way to positive outcomes blocked by this old woman's lack of compliance with a mobilization programme. However his personal interest in his patient and his place in her biography provide Gray with insight into the interpretation she places on her hospital admission, the concerns which arise from this interpretation and the behaviour this shapes. Gray molds and negotiates

care on the basis of his patient's view of her needs and 'limitations'. **Concordance** is achieved and sustained resulting in a positive health outcome.

There is nothing particularly remarkable about this outcome. Patients' values and beliefs arising from religious cultural and subcultural folklore both influence and are influenced by their view of health and health care experiences (Henley and Schott, 1999). Ignoring the need to factor in respect for belief diversity into care threatens to disable practice and increase patient vulnerability (Cioffi, 2006). Unlike compliance, **concordance** is consistent with contemporary psychological perspectives on reasoned action. Our behaviour is motivated much more by what matters to us than by established fact and certainly more than by what we have been told to do by others (Armitage and Connor, 2000). Consequently positive health outcomes are are more likely when a care plan takes account of a patient's anxieties and sentiments, practical needs, ethical and religious beliefs (McKinnon,2007).

Consent is at the heart of concordance and unlike compliance in which consent is seen as an end incident, concordance sees consent as a process where sensitivity is shown to time, place and patient perspective. At key stages in this process exploration of the harm and benefits of each care option mean patient choice is appropriately informed by evidence (DH, 2001a).

Since the international ratification of patients rights, listening to and acting on patients concerns as part of a concordat has become a statutory requirement for practicing nurses around the world. For example the Nursing and Midwidery Council of the United Kingdom (NMC, 2008:2) highlights the need to 'make the care of people your first concern, treating them as individuals and respecting their dignity'. Under the section on collaboration with patients clause one states:

'You must listen to the people in your care and respond to their concerns and preferences'.

Clause three states:

'You must recognize and respect the contribution that people make to their own care and wellbeing'.

These approaches to practice cannot therefore be viewed as optional or conditional upon context. However while concordance is an egalitarian relationship it is also a commutative one.

Concordance is not the same as **consumerism.** Consumerism implies that there are no limits to the demands patients may make on practitioners. **Concordance** means that patients have responsibilities as well as rights. This is the beginning of empowerment because it encourages patients to act on their own behalf (Hook, 2006). Interestingly in Berg *et al.*'s observational study (2007:103) concordance thrived in part because patients took responsibility for the care 'they believed they needed'. Examples of Concordance are given in Case Study 6.4.

Case Study 6.4: Examples of concordance

Joe

Joe arrives in the evening to commence the latest phase of his chemotherapy for recently diagnosed leukaemia but informs his nurse at the last minute that he wishes to discontinue the treatment as he cannot face the accompanying malaise and vomiting any longer. In the course of conversation the nurse learns that Joe is exhausted following a particularly trying day in which his car had broken down and he has had to assume care of his two children. The nurse explores the possibility with Joe that his decision to discontinue chemotherapy might be a result of his exhaustion and discouraged frame of mind and that following a night's rest he might feel differently. Following consultation with Joe's physician it is agreed that treatment should be deferred to the following afternoon.

Stephen

Following a rigorous diet and exercise programme Stephen has lost 10 kilograms and his triglycerides have shown some improvement. However with an imminent family celebration approaching when food is a central part of the festivities Stephen confides in his nurse practitioner that he is losing heart. It is agreed that on the day of the family party Stephen can refrain from his diet programme but take small portions reverting to his diet the following day.

If **patientcentredness** and **concordance** are important in nursing those with acute and chronic disease they are essential in the broader field of public health where interdisciplinary collaborative working with disadvantaged groups is integral to practice and lifestyle change is the end goal of care planning. For example Daiski's study of the homeless (2007) shows how a lack of service user partnership results in services which are irrelevant to need or out of reach to those who need them most.

However well intentioned, the services in question were not shaped around the concerns of homeless people as individuals which included the stigma associated with receiving benefit, the threat of worsening health and the fear of dying alone and friendless. Also in initiatives aimed at smoking cessation, smokers are unlikely to quit smoking without personal support which recognizes the role of the habit as a source of relief from stress and works to find realistic life alternatives (Naidoo et al., 2004).

Failure to form service user partnerships with clients and client groups which inform public health practice can serve to marginalize further the very people whose needs nurses are aiming to meet (Wilson and Neville, 2008).

Beyond concordance

Empowerment is the provision of resources to enable and skill individuals communities and groups to improve their quality

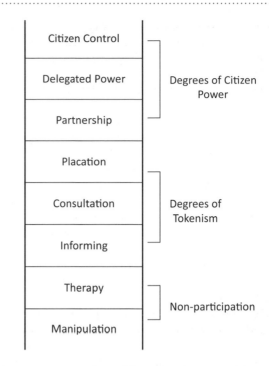

Fig. 6.2 Arnstein's Ladder of Citizen Participation. Reproduced with permission Arnstein S. R. (1969).

of life on their terms. It is about helping people to help themselves (Case Studies 6.5 and 6.6). As early as 1969 Sherry Arnstein (1969) argued for the place of citizen participation in shaping their environment. Her ladder of participation is an effective model (Fig. 6.2) in showing how professed **empowerment** can range from tokenism; the mere passage of information and soliciting of opinion, to real leadership and power. Paternalism has been deeply ingrained in professional life. Partnership as represented by **concordance** rests uneasily between measures of placation and genuine shared control depending on the culture in which practice takes place. It would be naive to think that the cultural shift necessary to house patient participation is complete.

Recent studies (Millard et al., 2006; Oudshoorn et al., 2007) portray nurses as reluctant to share their knowledge with patients often only involving them in decision making when they find it expedient or when compelled by circumstances to do so. A level of power beyond the partnership of concordance is warranted in which patients have leadership in healthcare. Many who suffer from chronic disease have developed expertise in their condition which can be shared with others including many health professionals. Harnessing the 'expert patient' (DH, 2001b) means building teaching and patient support programmes which are service user led. Valuing the rich lived experience of patients also means that with appropriate training and remuneration expert patients may comment assist and lead on health care planning and professional recruitment (Laverack, 2005). Examples of Empowerment are given in Case Study 6.5.

Case Study 6.5: Examples of empowerment

Getting by with a little help from her friends

A highly popular post-natal support group is in progress in a housing estate characterized by poor housing, high unemployment and crime. The only local shop is a newsagent. Dawn, a single mother with two young children, tells her public health nurse that she is tired of having to pay a taxi exorbitant fares in order to access fresh produce at a branch of a major supermarket chain 3 miles away. The public health nurse organizes a meeting between Dawn and some of her friends, the local branch of the Womens Institute, town councillors and social services.

The Womens Institute agree to permit the use of their hall to house a food cooperative for parts of three days a week. Dawn and some friends agree to staff the cooperative. One of the town councillors agrees to introduce Dawn to local suppliers of fruit and vegetables who have been rejected by national retailers because the produce does not tolerate transport over many miles. One of Dawn's friends Linda has the agreement of her partner Phil to use his van after work to collect produce from suppliers. The public health nurse successfully bids for monies from the PCT directorate to fund basic bookkeeping training for Dawn.

Discussion points

In what ways is the public health initiative described here superior to the opening of a small local fruit and vegetable shop by a retailer?

- For Dawn?
- For Dawn's friends and the community at large?
- For the public health nursing team?

In the course of developing a food cooperative, Dawn and her friends are far more than the passive consumers of a new business. They have taken charge of a source of public health improvement in their local community. In the course of doing this they have developed new skills, improved their self-esteem and social mobility. For the public health nursing team resources are used in a tailored, targeted and more cost effective way. The nurses become facilitators of health rather than providers.

Case Study 6.6: Out with the fags and in with a new career

Maggie has just stopped smoking after fifteen years of being a smoker. She achieved this with individual support from her public health nursing team and several weeks on nicotine patches. When the public health lead sets up a local support group she asks Maggie to speak to the members of the group about her experiences and shortly after Maggie takes responsibility for co-leadership of the group. The PCT supply her with a mobile phone to receive calls from other smokers seeking personal support. Funding is allocated to sponsor Maggie on a short part time counselling course. A few months later Maggie is encouraged to apply for a service user representative role with the PCT and when she is successful advises the executive on strategy. Following further training Maggie now sits on the interview panel at a nearby univeristy interviewing applicants for a public health nursing degree programme.

Discussion points

- Why does Maggie in the role of support group leader carry more credibility than a public health nurse in the eyes of local smokers who would like to give up?
- What are the other health benefits of service user representation for Maggie?

Maggie's knowledge of the local community and their knowledge of her as an ex-smoker means that she carries a form of credibility that is unique to being part of a peer group. Local smokers will trust her judgement and count her empathy as more genuine and reliable than the most expert public health nurse. Furthermore Maggie carries none of the authoritarian trappings associated with professonals which can prove intimidating to some service users who perceive that they are adversely judged by society. The role service user representative means that Maggie is enabled with new skills of negotiation and the new 'heard' status of her advice promotes her self-esteem and confidence which in turn improves her the quality of her life choices and chances. These are health gains which complement and extend beyond those of stopping smoking.

The time factor

There are occasions when extra time spent on the personal aspect of patient care will prove essential and attempts to dismiss this as impractical will prove a false economy in care planning. There are other situations in which the pace and intensity of treatment make development of specific relationships between nurses and patients unlikely. In the light of this, contemporary research is helpful and suggests that refuting patient-centredness and a lack of willingness to engage with patients has far more to do with task orientation and personal prejudice than with lack of time (McCabe and Timmins, 2006).

Catherine McCabe's study (2004) of patients' experiences of care showed **patient-centredness** as a different way of being and framing communication and intervention rather than a more time consuming exercise. Shattell (2004) showed that preoccupation with tasks caused nurses to exaggerate the amount of time taken to develop relationships with patients. Kirk (2007) makes the distinction between intimate clinical relationships and interactions portraying the nurse as one sufficiently skilled to place herself in an immediate helping position with a vulnerable patient who does not know her.

These arguments help dispel the notion that there is no time in modern health care for **patient-centredness**. On the contrary patients are demeaned by anything less. An absence of **patient-centredness** also demeans nursing practice reducing it to a set of subservient tasks rather than an evidence based knowing which helps the patient interpret their needs in the context of sickness and health.

Conclusion

'The ability to be flexible and adaptable without losing sight of purpose, to be able to work with human individuality rather that against it, is what we are striving to develop in the nurse of 2000 and beyond' Dearmun (1992:28).

Ann Dearmun's words seem timelier now than when they were written if only to show the perennial value and power in the nurse-patient relationship. The relationship sustains the patient and informs the nurse seeking to provide appropriate care through **engagement** listening and **concordance**. Concordance is served by **patient-centredness.** Furthermore the relationship empowers patients to move beyond being mere recipients of care to becoming sharers and leaders in care planning for themselves and others.

Summary

The nurse patient relationship provides a channel through which all need is assessed and health care negotiated and delivered in a way which respects personhood. Caring is an insufficiently simple and nebulous term with which to describe the dynamics of the nurse-patient relationship. Engagement is the means by which the nurse evidences willingness to become involved in the patient's situation and is exhibited in appropriate eye contact, facial expression and body language. Listening is the most important part of assessing and helping and has a healing power of its own. Concordance is an equal partnership between nurse and patient arising from engaged embodied listening. Empowerment is the provision of resources to enable and skill individuals communities and groups to improve their quality of life on their terms. Nurse-patient relationships do not require more time but are a different way of framing care.

 Online Resource Centre

For more information on the nurse patient relationship visit the Online Resource Centre —
http://www.oxfordtextbooks.co.uk/orc/linsley/

References

Armitage, C.J., & Conner, M. (2000). Social cognition models and health behaviour: A structured review. *Journal of Psychology and Health*, 15 (2):173–189.

Arnstein, S. (1969) A Ladder of Citizen Participation. *Journal of the American Institute of Planners.* 35(4):216–224.

Attree, M. (2001). Patients' and relatives experiences and perspectives of 'good' and 'Not so Good' quality care. *Journal of Advanced Nursing*, 33(4): 456–466.

Belsky, J., Cassidy, J., (1994). *Attachment: Theory and Practice.* In: Rutter, M. and Hay, D., (Eds) *Development through Life: a Handbook for Clinicians.* Oxford: Blackwell Science: 373–402.

Benner, P., & Wrubel, J.(1989). *The Primacy of Caring: Stress and Coping in Health and Illness.* Menlo Park:Addison Wesley.

Benner, P.,Tanner,C.A. & Chesla, C.A. (1996). *Expertise in Nursing Practice, Caring, Clinical Judgement and Ethics.* New York: Springer.

Berg, L., Skott, C., & Danielson, E. (2006). An interpretive phenomenological method for illuminating the meaning of caring relationship. *Scandinavian Journal of Caring Science.* 20(1): 42–50.

Berg L., Skott C., & Danielson E. (2007). Caring relationship in a context: Fieldwork in a medical ward. *International Journal of Nursing Practice*; 13(2): 100–106.

Carr-Hill R., Higgins M., Dixon P., Gibbs I., Griffiths M., McCaughan D. & Wright K. (1992). *Skill Mix and the Effectiveness of Nursing Care: A Report to the Department of Health.* University of York: Centre for Health Economics.

Cioffi J. (2006). Culturally diverse patient–nurse interactions on acute care wards. *International Journal of Nursing Practice* 12(6): 319–325.

Cohen, R.A., (1993*). The Mutual Constraint of Memory and Attention.* In: Cohen. (ed.) The Neuropsychology of Attention. London: Plenum Press 381–392.

Cowley,S. (1995). In Health Visiting,a routine visit is one that has passed. *Journal of Advanced Nursing.* 22,(2):276–284.

Crowe, M. (2000). The nurse-patient relationship: a consideration of its discursive context. *Journal of Advanced Nursing,* 31(4): 962–967.

Daiski, I. (2007). Perspectives of homeless people on their health and health needs priorities. *Journal of Advanced Nursing.* 58(3): 273–281.

Dearmun, A. (1992). Reflections of a Lecturer-Practitioner. *Paediatric Nursing* 5, (1): 28.

Department of Health (2001a). *Good Practice in Consent.* London: The Stationery Office.

Department of Health (2001b). *The Expert Patient: a new approach to chronic disease management for the 21st century.* London: The Stationery Office.

Egan, G. (2002). The *Skilled Helper— a problem management approach to helping.* Seventh Edition. Pacific Grove: Brookes Cole.

Epstein, O., Perkin G.D., de Bono, D.P. & Cookson, J. (2000). *Clinical Examination.* (2nd ed.) London: Mosby.

Evans, A, M. (2007) Transference in the nurse-patient relationship. *Journal of Psychiatric and Mental Health Nursing* 14 (2):189195.

Freund, P.E.S., McGuire, M.B. & Podhurst, L.S. (2003). *Health, Illness and the Social Body: A Critical Sociology.* (2nd ed.) *New Jersey:* Prentice Hall.

Gallup R. & O'Brien L. (2003). Re-establishing psychodynamic theory as foundational knowledge for psychiatric/mental health nursing. *Issues in Mental Health Nursing* 24(2): 213–227.

Gould, D., & Thomas, V.N. (1998). *Pain mechanisms: The neurophysiology and neuropsychology of pain perception.* In: Thomas, V.N., (1998) *Pain, its nature and management.* London: Bailliere Tindall: 1–19.

Graham, H.,& Power, C. (2004). Childhood Disadvantage and Adult Health: A Lifecourse Framework. London: Health Development Agency.

Henley, A. & Schott, J. (1999). Culture, Religion and Patient Care in a Multi-ethnic Society. London: Age Concern UK.

Hook, M.L. (2006). Partnering with patients — a concept ready for action. *Journal of Advanced Nursing* 56(2), 133–143.

Immordino, M.H.,& Damasio, A. (2007). We Feel, Therefore We Learn: The Relevance of Affective and Social Neuroscience to Education. *Mind, Brain and Education. 1(1):3–10.*

Jones, A. (2007). Admitting hospital patients: a qualitative study of an everyday nursing task. *Nursing Inquiry*; 14(3): 212–223.

Kirk, T.W. (2007). Beyond empathy: clinical intimacy in nursing practice. *Nursing Philosophy.* 8(4):233–243.

Laverack, G. (2005). *Public Health: Power, Empowerment and Professional Practice.* Basingstoke: Palgrave Macmillan.

Malloch, K. (2000). Nurse-patient Relationships: Essential Skills for Expert Nursing Practice. *Creative Nursing. 6(4):12–13.*

Malone R.E. (2003). Distal nursing. *Social Science and Medicine* 56 (11): 2317–2326.

McCabe, C. (2004). Nurse–patient communication: an exploration of patients' experiences. *Journal of Clinical Nursing* 13(1): 41–49.

McCabe, C., & Timmins, F. (2006). *Communication Skills for Nursing Practice.* Basingstoke: Palgrave Macmillan.

McCormack, B. (2003). A conceptual framework for person-centred practice with older people. *International Journal of Nursing Practice.* 9(3): 202–209.

McKinnon, J. (2007). *Patient Centred Planning and Concordance.* In: McKinnon, J., (Ed.) *Towards Prescribing Practice.* Chichester: Wiley: 35–58.

McQueen, A.C.H. (2004). Emotional Intelligence in Nursing Work. *Journal of Advanced Nursing.* 47 (1) 101–108.

Millard, L., Hallett, C. & Luker, K. (2006). Nurse–patient interaction and decision-making in care: patient involvement in community nursing. *Journal of Advanced Nursing.* 55 (2), 142–150.

Nursing and Midwifery Council (2008). *The Code: Standards of Conduct Performance and Ethics for Nurses and Midwives.* London: NMC.

Naidoo, B., Quigley, R., Taylor, L. & Warm, D. (2004). *Smoking and public health: a review of reviews of interventions to increase smoking cessation, reduce smoking initiation and prevent further uptake of smoking.* London: Health Development Agency.

Oudshoorn, A., Ward-Griffin, C., McWilliam, C. (2007). Client–nurse relationships in home-based palliative care: a critical analysis of power relations. *Journal of Clinical Nursing* 16(8):1435–1443.

Redfern, S. (1996). Individualised patient care: a framework for guidelines. *Nursing Times* 92(5): 33–36.

Reiman, D. (1986). Non Caring and caring in the clinical setting *Top Clinical Nursing* 8(1):30–36.

Rogers, C. (1994). *Freedom to Learn.* Third Edition. London: Macmillan.

Rose, D. (2006). *Consciousness, Philosophical, Psychological and Neural Theories.* Oxford:Oxford University Press.

Russell, S., Daly, J., Hughes, E. & Hogg, C. (2003). Nurses and 'difficult' patients: negotiating non-compliance. *Journal of Advanced Nursing* 43(3): 281–287.

Shattell, M. (2004). Nurse–patient interaction: a review of the literature. Journal of Clinical Nursing 13 (6):714–722..

Shattell, M, M., Starr, S.S., & Thomas, S.P., (2007). Take my hand, help me out: Mental health service recipients' experience of the therapeutic relationship. *International Journal of Mental Health Nursing.* 16 (4): 274–284.

Stickley, T., & Freshwater, D. (2006). The Art of Listening in the Therapeutic Relationship. *Mental Health Practice.* 9(5):12–18.

Tarlier, D.S. (2004). Beyond caring: the moral and ethical bases of responsive nurse–patient relationships. *Nursing Philosophy.* 5(3): 230–241.

Williams, A. (2001). A study of practising nurses' perceptions and experiences of intimacy within the nurse-patient relationship. *Journal of Advanced Nursing; 35*(2):188–196.

Wilson, D., Neville, S. (2008). Nursing their way not our way: Working with vulnerable and marginalised populations *Contemporary Nurse.* 27(2): 165.

World Health Organization (1986). Resolution of the Convention of Human Rights. Ottawa, Canada: WHO.

Chapter 7
Accessing and using information in clinical practice

Sonia Budgen

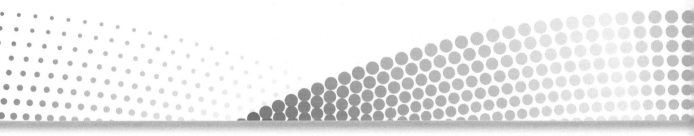

Introduction

As health care becomes more knowledge intensive, nurses are challenged to effectively manage clinical information and keep abreast of professional knowledge. The demands upon nurses to use computer technology in care delivery are increasing. National policy, and in particular Connecting for Health (CfH), dictates that nurses embrace and actively integrate such initiatives within their clinical practice. This chapter explores the impact of electronic communication on health care, health care professionals and the role of the nurse in accessing and using information. The chapter ends with a look at some of the overriding issues when accessing and using information, including issues of security, confidentiality and information governance.

Case Study 7.1: *Using technology to improve health*

With a combined age of 193, Rose Sanders and Violet Gyves are not the most likely computer game fans, but the pair have become hooked on playing with their Nintendo Wii console. The grandmothers love to duck and weave in front of the television screen as they try out their skills on Wii Boxing, a game which requires them to simulate punching an opponent.

Mrs Sanders and Mrs Gyves were introduced to the Wii by managers at Greensleeves Nursing Home in Crawley, West Sussex, to help improve their fitness and flexibility.

They became so enamoured with it that, together with their fellow residents, they raised £500 with a raffle and cake sale to buy two consoles and a selection of games.

Mrs Sanders, 98, who used to fly in Spitfires during her time in the WAF, said: 'It's great fun. It makes a change from Coronation Street, doesn't it?'

Mrs Gyves, 95, a fan of British boxer Henry Cooper, said: 'We were absolutely ecstatic to get the Wiis.

Rose and I love playing the boxing game — it's a great way to keep fit and it doesn't hurt to take out some aggression now and again.'

Care home manager Trevor Bartley said the Wiis had already 'worked wonders' with the residents, who are all women, helping them to sharpen their minds and get some exercise.

Source: http://www.telegraph.co.uk/connected/main.jhtml?xml=/connected/2008/07/11/nwii111.xml

Who would ever think that technology could be used for the benefit of physical fitness? This is just one example of how technology can be used to improve and maintain good health.

An overview of the UK National Programmes for Information Technology and eHealth

The UK National Programmes for Information Technology supports the NHS to deliver better, safer care to patients, by bringing in new computer systems and services usually by a Local Service Provider (LSP). The key to these reforms is the transition towards an increasingly joined up electronic healthcare system and collection and use of data. This will enable health and social care staff to communicate effectively and provide a seamless support for the patient. 'eHealth' will play a large part in enabling health care to be more effectively available to those who require it (Baker et al. 2002). eHealth refers to the whole scope of information technology (IT) usage in health and health care, including electronic patient records, health care decision support systems and the use of short message service (SMS) (see information box — below).

Box 7.1 New systems and services being introduced into the NPfIT (other countries will be implementing similar functionality)

Choose and book
This is a national electronic referral service which gives patients a choice of place, date and time for their first outpatient appointment in a hospital or clinic.

My health online (Wales)
This has a similar functionality as choose and book (see website —
http://www.wales.nhs.uk/IHC/page.cfm?pid=33598&orgid=77)

The Electronic Prescription Service (EPS)
This will enable prescribers — such as GPs and practice nurses—to send prescriptions electronically to a dispenser (such as a pharmacy) of the patient's choice. This will make the prescribing and dispensing process safer and more convenient for patients and staff. It allows prescribers in GP practices to generate and transmit electronic prescriptions.

Healthspace
This is a secure website where patients can store their personal health information online, such as height, weight and blood pressure.

N3
The national network, provides fast, broadband networking services to the NHS, offering reliability and value for money. The high speed network makes it possible to deliver the reforms and new services needed to improve patient care.

The NHS Care Records Service (NHS CRS)
This is a secure service that links patient information from different parts of the NHS electronically, so that authorized NHS staff and patients have the information they need to make care decisions. There are two elements to the NHS Care Records Service: detailed records (held locally) and the Summary Care Record (held nationally). The NHS Care Records Service will enables each person's detailed records to be securely shared between different parts of the local NHS, such as the GP surgery and hospital.

Picture Archiving and Communications System (PACS)
This enables images such as x-rays and scans to be stored electronically and viewed on screens, creating a near filmless process and improved diagnosis methods. Doctors and other health professionals can access and compare images at the touch of a button.

NHS Connecting for Health
This service came into operation on 1 April 2005 and is an agency of the Department of Health. It supports the NHS to deliver better, safer care to patients, by bringing in new computer systems and services — (http://www.connectingforhealth.nhs.uk/)

Nurses are becoming more acquainted with **eHealth** and are positive about its benefits in health care (RCN, 2006b). Used appropriately, the tools and services which contribute to eHealth provide better, more efficient health care services for all. eHealth covers the interaction between patients and health service providers, institution-to-institution transmission of data, or peer-to-peer communication between patients and/or health professionals. Examples include health information networks, electronic health records, telemedicine services, wearable and portable systems which communicate, health portals, and many other information and communications technology —ICT-based — tools assisting disease prevention, diagnosis, treatment, health monitoring and lifestyle management. Although there is a foundation of nursing knowledge, medical science and technology advances require a lifelong learning process for a clinical practice nurse. To keep pace with expanding amounts of evidence and knowledge, nurses must know how to access the knowledge that they need in order to practise.

The primary design behind these systems is based on how information and data is gathered, stored, and used in an entire institution or service rather than in terms of a specific process. For example, when a medication order is placed, the system will have access to all information about the patient including diagnosis, age, gender, weight, and allergies as well as the medications currently being taken. The order and patient information will be matched against knowledge, such as what drugs are incompatible for simultaneous use with the prescribed drug, the correctness of the dosage of the drug, and the appropriateness of the drug for this patient. The system will deliver warnings at the time the medication is ordered to allow difficulties to be dealt with at the time of order entry. The same information will be available to the dietician in planning the patient's diet as well as the nurse doing care and discharge planning. Additionally, access to the current knowledge base about a given condition in the form of practice guidelines will be easily accessible. Practice guidelines will be accessed from a computer and kept up to date by professionals whose job is to synthesize research and produce these guidelines. This new systems will not only save time but will also reduce errors caused by the necessity for multiple data entry and the previous inability of professionals to have at their fingertips all the patient data and information.

Electronic records of this kind also make it easier to schedule appointments for patients, keep track of follow-ups, and ensure patients' general practitioners are informed of the results of their referrals. When it comes to preventive healthcare, eHealth tools can help achieve much higher coverage, for example, ensuring that children receive the full programme of vaccinations at the correct ages. Thanks to these improvements, health care providers can better address increasing demand for health care, and cover the costs of new, advanced treatments.

In turn, eHealth systems provide patients with better information — on treatments, on their condition, and on improved standards of living — and make it simpler for health care professionals to access and share information, both general and patient-specific. The use of electronic patient records allows doctors to see much more of a person's medical history than do paper files, which typically only include information on treatment in a single surgery or hospital. A patient's condition can be monitored remotely, either freeing up a hospital bed which would have been required with previous monitoring equipment, or providing a better standard of care for the patient. Online tools can help patients to understand their conditions better and make it easier for them to find and talk to fellow sufferers, for example through online support groups.

Widespread implementation of e-Health will enable more 'patient-friendly' health care services to be developed. This will offer health care providers a chance to become more flexible and better able to address the differing needs of individual patients. Whilst today patients have to go to the doctor (or the doctor come to them), online and mobile tools are already opening up the possibility of remote diagnosis. Similar tools can also enable health professionals who travel to see patients to provide more sophisticated treatments. eHealth services promise to raise the quality of care in remoter and rural areas, thanks to modern communications infrastructure.

However, a recent RCN project (Baker, *et al.,* 2008) looking at the professional issues experienced by nurses working in an electronic environment found that there is a huge gap between the eHealth future as envisaged by policy leaders and the current experience of frontline nurses. One of the main reasons for computer and information systems failing to support nursing practice is that they are frequently developed with limited input from nurses. This has done nothing to promote ownership and user involvement amongst nurses, so often regarded as the key components to successful systems implementation (Linsley and Hurley, 2005). Clinical engagement (Budgen, 2005) is necessary to ensure professional issues are addressed within the implementation of eHealth. Part of the despondency felt by nurses towards the use of computers and information technology, is that it is perceived that the information they gather seldom relates to their practice (Barker, *et al.,* 2008). The ability to adapt an information system to meet the needs of all its users whilst delivering the essential information to support the nurse in practice must be one of the fundamental aspects of health information technology. Ideally, the nurse should be able to engage with these systems of information as a process of their work and develop their own interpretations of the information provided in order to construct their own meaning of that information for use in clinical practice.

A nurse, like all other health care professionals, is primarily a knowledge worker. To practice effectively, nursing must be supported in this role. Synder-Halpern, *et al.,* (2001) described nurses as data gathers, information users, knowledge builders and knowledge users. The nurse collects clinical data, structures these data, and transforms them into information that is interpreted with the nurse's speciality information and used in clinical decision-making When clinical data are collected and used to create knowledge, the nurse functions as a knowledge builder. In the knowledge user role, the nurse combines her speciality knowledge with the clinical data as part of both information use and knowledge building. These functions are supported, but not replaced, within the clinical area by information technology.

The only truly unique feature of nursing is the 24-hour care that it provides. This demands that nurses have more involvement with their patients and inevitably need information that other disciplines do not — information that is specific to the practice and management of nursing care. Because nurses provide most of the care given in hospitals and in the community it is essential that they develop the skills of information technology in order to become part of this movement. Nurses understand how patients or their clients progress through health care, and will become the main users of any clinical system implemented into health care settings. Nurses in all practice areas (home, long-term care etc) need to synthesize many pieces of information using creativity and intuition and going beyond medical analysis done by physicians. Nurses synthesize knowledge by evaluating the information they have on hand at the point of decision-making. This knowledge may be gained through using technology, communicating with a colleague, or speaking with the patient, family, or other significant social support person.

The nurse must become 'savvy' in the operational aspects of health care. With projected advances in technology, nursing science, biological sciences and genetic science, nurses need the ability to synthesize more information with more depth. They must evaluate complex and sometimes ambiguous patient care scenarios in different provider settings and with interdisciplinary teams to ensure safe, excellent care. What is needed is a nurse strategic leader with in-depth knowledge about core health care processes to be supported by technology for the software to be designed, tested and implemented for any IT tool to be a success. These 'leaders' must be experienced nurses who have an understanding of technology, strategic visioning and organizational finesse. They are not just at managerial level, but are increasingly likely to be those who deliver services, those who have regular and direct contact with communities and who understand the needs of these individuals.

Exposure to workshops and working with the **clinical informatics** departments are the most beneficial ways of improving understanding in the design of software and ensuring these systems meet the needs of nurses at the coal face. Nurses will have to champion the use in computers to demonstrate how effective and crucial they are in the 'business' of nursing to provide clinical data for benchmarking and audit. In order to achieve these benefits, they must be underpinned by standardized infrastructure to ensure interoperability of systems (Ozbolt, 2004) and thus seamless communication. These standards are called **data standards**, which are a set of rules ensuring each clinical term or phrase used has a single definition (Wallis, 2007).

Clinical decision support software

The ability to adapt a computer system to meet the needs of all its users in practice must be one of the fundamental aspects of health information technology. Ideally, the nurse should be able to engage with computers as part of their work and develop their own interpretations of the information provided by computers to order to construct their own

meaning of that information for use in clinical practice. To this end computers should be seen as an integral part of and not something separate to, clinical practice if they are to make a worthwhile contribution to the work of those that use them.

Where computer systems have been developed with the nurse in mind they have tended to incorporate an element of decision support. The development of computerized decision support systems has stressed the need for clinical practice standardization as a means of providing baseline information to evaluate practice processes and patient outcomes.

A good example of **clinical decision support software (CDSS)** is that used by NHS Direct/NHS 24. It provides a set of questions to a problem which is being addressed. The health professional will check with the client they are advising and depending on their answer will either prompt further questions or supply the health professional with other possibilities. It is a very structured form of decision support and, when nurses use this tool they must ensure that it remains as a tool and not a dictate for care. Another example of this is the **NHS Clinical Knowledge Summaries** (formerly 'PRODIGY') which is more interactive; the health professional is looking for information or up to date guidelines on a particular disease/condition. Information sheets can be printed off for the client.

Such systems can only advise nurses based on the knowledge that they contain. Nurses who come to rely exclusively on the advice of such systems may not be able to discriminate when the computer decision support software may not be applicable and they should seek other knowledge resources. Clinical practice standardization also underscores an assumption that clinical practice variation represents resistance to change when it may actually reflect legitimate variation based on the nurse's use of professional artistry in new and uncertain clinical practice situations (Linsley and Hurley, 2005).

Activity box

A recent report (Dowding, *et al.*, 2007) explores how new technologies are used to inform nurse decision-making in practice and the potential effects this may have on the process of care and patient outcomes. The findings highlighted a lack of robust evidence to support the introduction of CDSS for nursing practice and a recommendation to evaluate new technologies.

Read Dowding, D., *et al.* (2007) and give consideration to its findings. Clearly, while many aspects of information systems can help and inform the practice of nurses, standardized clinical practice is not one that reflects the requirements of either nurses or those that they care for.

Information governance

Information Governance (IG) concerns the way information is used i.e. — it ensures the necessary safeguards for, and appropriate use of patient and personal information. Currently paper-based patient records are transferred from one health care professional to another (General Practitioners are the exception) which is not always secure. As a consequence, one of the main benefits and improvements of these implementations is that patient information is secure and accessible by health care professionals that have authorized access (DH, 2002). In England this is called **role-based access (RBAC)** which in addition, requires a **legitimate relationship (LR)** with the patient that the health care professional wishes to access other UK countries will have a similar structure.

Case Study 7.2: Helen Wilkinson

16 June 2005: Columns 495–502 The United Kingdom Parliament

Helen works as a practice manager. She has worked for the NHS for twenty years, therefore she commands an excellent understanding of how the NHS functions. Helen discovered that the University College London Hospitals trust had sent computer records of every hospital medical treatment she had ever received to a private company, McKesson, which holds a mass of NHS records. Those records are then passed on, as Helen's were, to computer systems used by the NHS. Helen's records thus became available to several NHS bodies.

Helen asked to see her records under the **Data Protection Act 1998,** as she is fully entitled to do. She discovered when she examined them there was a serious mistake. She was effectively and mistakenly registered as an alcoholic. Helen, concerned about the many people who have access to even the correct parts of her record, and the even larger number who may have access to it as the NHS computerization programme proceeds, requested this error be removed from the NHS system altogether.

NHS patients have the right to object to data about them being held in a form that identifies them, but only when that causes or is likely to cause substantial or unwarranted damage or distress. It is not clear if those data are held by a number of NHS bodies, as in this case, who decides whether damage or distress is caused or is likely to be caused.

As there was no straightforward process to address this issue Helen took drastic action and withdrew from the NHS as a patient altogether. This would ensure her records, including the mistaken identity of her as an alcoholic, could be removed from the NHS computer system. In summary this patient has had to withdraw from the NHS to protect her privacy.

For full report access: http://www.theyworkforyou.com/debates/?id=2005-06-16b.495.0

The incident reported here is due to 'user error'; when a user of the system has accessed the incorrect record and entered the information. This 'error' can be traced back to the originator but is never deleted. This is called an **audit trail**. For systems to be safe and display accurate information users must ensure **data quality**. Data quality is important in any information system: high quality information is vital to safe and effective patient care and for this purpose 100% accuracy 100% of the time must be the goal (DH, 2004).

Discussion points

- How do health professionals manage errors when they occur (that are know to them)? If you make a mistake in patients' notes what is your current way of addressing this?
- Think about implications to the patient. Is it right that this particular patient was allowed to have their records deleted from their care record? What would happen if the patient is admitted as an emergency? How are their records stored?

When an error occurs in a **hard copy**, the health professional will strike a line through it and write the correct information. This amendment is always signed and dated. In a computer system **everything** is recorded and nothing is deleted. It would be possible to strike through particular information (a line through the text) and this would still be available to be read by users who have appropriate access. This can be tracked via audit by the user identification (ID) logged in at the time. Alternatively the error can be 'soft deleted' which means the information is hidden within the database and it not seen on the display i.e. the information will be stored and accessed only in exceptional circumstances by designated roles.

Patients that are treated in emergency care settings will automatically be electronically traced on admission and a new record of care will be commenced. Locally defined policies will be in place if patients do not wish to have an electronic healthcare record.

Nursing Practice box

A patient visits the GP with a problem of a sexual nature. This problem is entered into the patient's electronic notes and is successfully treated.

Years later a senior receptionist at the practice meets this patient above socially. The receptionist wants to find out more about this person. The receptionist unethically and illegally accessed this patient record, which is held on a national NHS computer database and ferrets out private and confidential details, without the consent of this patient or the patient knowing of this breach of privacy.

Within an electronic system it would be impossible for any member of staff to access the patient record unless they have a legitimate relationship with the patient and their role profile allows them to open and view this information. If health care professionals' access patient records that they do not have legitimate relationships with i.e. their next door neighbour or a personal friend they will be accessing clinical information unlawfully. This would be traced via regular audits of the system.

Is the example above any different to how clinicians' access notes currently (i.e. paper based)? How many times have you seen health and social care professionals look through patient notes and wondered if they should be privy to that part of a patient's clinical history? It is so easy to do and no record of this access is documented.

Activity box

Look up the term **Caldicott Guardian**. Find out why this is important to the health care organizations. Are you able to identify the Caldicott Guardian for your organization?

All clinical staffs are bound by the Caldicott Principles which are:

1. Justify the purpose(s) of using confidential information
   Every proposed use or transfer of patient-identifiable information within or from an organization should be clearly defined and scrutinized, with continuing uses regularly reviewed, by an appropriate guardian.

2. Do not use patient-identifiable information unless it is absolutely necessary
   Patient-identifiable information items should not be included unless it is essential for the specified purpose(s) of that flow. The need for patients to be identified should be considered at each stage of satisfying the purpose(s).

3. Use the minimum necessary patient-identifiable information that is required
   Where use of the patient-identifiable is considered to be essential, the inclusion of each individual item of information should be considered and justified so that the minimum amount of identifiable information is transferred or accessible as is necessary for a given function to be carried out.

4. Access to patient-identifiable information should be on a strict need-to-know basis
   Only those individuals who need access to patient-identifiable information should have access to it, and they should only have access to the information items that they need to see. This may mean introducing access controls or splitting

information flows where one information flow is used for several purposes.

5. Everyone with access to patient-identifiable information should be aware of their responsibilities
   Action should be taken to ensure that those handling patient-identifiable information — both clinical and non-clinical staff — are made fully aware of their responsibilities and obligations to respect patient confidentiality.

6. Understand and comply with the law
   Every use of patient-identifiable information must be lawful. Someone in each organization handling patient information should be responsible for ensuring that the organization complies with the legal requirements.

Caldicott Guardians are senior staff in the NHS and social services appointed to protect patient information.

Information on the Caldicott Guardians can be found at: — http://www.dh.gov.uk/en/Publicationsandstatistics/Publications/PublicationsPolicyAndGuidance/DH_062722

Confidentiality

What is confidentiality?

As a registered nurse, midwife or specialist community public health nurse you must protect confidential information and use it only for the purpose for which it was given (NMC, 2008a)

A duty of confidence arises in a professional relationship where one person (the confider) makes a disclosure of essentially 'private' information to the professional in the expectation that the information will remain confidential. The basic rule is that the information will not be passed to a third party without the express permission of the confider.

Activity box

The RCN has guidance on confidentiality. Use search facility on the RCN home page with keyword 'confidentiality' for further information.

The overall objective is to enable the NHS to share information with all those necessary to provide good care to patients while meeting patients' rights and needs for confidentiality (NHSIA, 2002). This will be achieved by:

1. Sharing patient-identifiable health records for health and social care

2. Giving people the information they need to know to do their job in caring for the patient.

A recent project — the **Shared Record Professional Guidance Project** aimed to resolve developing issues within a shared electronic record environment and to issue a set of guidelines (see http://www.rcgp.org.uk/news_and_events/news_room/news_2009/srpg_shared_record_professiona.aspx) that considered the governance, medico-legal and patient safety consequences of a shared record.

To address information of a sensitive nature a **computer information systems** (CIS) will require functionality such as a **sealed envelope** (England). The level of access the user has will determine a: if the user observes the sealed envelope within the electronic patient record and b: whether it can be 'opened' and viewed. Conversely, health professionals can limit the amount of information a patient can see by a **clinical seal**, which could be used in mental health for example.

Box 7.2 Sealed envelopes (CfH 2006a)

The NHS Care Records Service will enable users to limit access to sensitive information within patient records. A patient will be able to request that specific sensitive information within their clinical record is accessible only with their consent. This is sometimes referred to as a patient 'sealed envelope'. A clinician will also be able to withhold certain types of information from patients in a clinician 'sealed envelope' . 'Sealed envelope' and 'sealing' are metaphors; no information within the patient record is expected to be physically sealed or moved as a result of sealing. Information on 'sealed envelopes' can be found at: **http://www.connectingforhealth.nhs.uk/systemsandservices/infogov/confidentiality/sealedpaper.pdf**

Currently there is much debate about issues concerning confidentiality and sealed envelopes. These issues are about the operational and practical implications that occur and the best way they can be managed. It is not a reflection on the ability of an IT system — it is the human interaction and interpretation that requires careful thought. Therefore the nurse will need to ensure training and understanding has taken place to explain and guide the patient in this area.

Box 7.3 Questions regarding patient and clinical information

There is an excellent resource on the **Connecting for Health** website: 'The NHS care record service — a guide for the nursing community' (2006b) which answers thirty nine questions regarding patient and clinical information. It can be downloaded at: **http://information.connectingforhealth.nhs.uk/prod_images/pdfs/29486.pdf**

Information ethics within health care

Information ethics broadly examines issues that relate to ownership, privacy, security, community and access to confidential records. In a society increasingly defined as an 'information society' dilemmas regarding all aspects of **information management** are becoming increasingly important, more so with the challenges information technology introduces. Reliance on professional codes of practice to guide the user ensures these issues are kept to a minimum, however situations arise where there is no 'best practice' guide and often it is up to the individual to ensure protection and security are paramount.

Box 7.4 Data security

The reputation of the NHS to securely hold information has been severely thwarted during 2008 with various NHS Trusts loosing confidential patient information usually in the form of USB memory sticks or laptops.

The theft of a USB drive at an NHS Hospital Trust in 2007 has shown the need to keep portable devices secure. The trust policy stated that 'confidential data should be stored on 128-bit encrypted USB sticks, with "if found" labels on them, and be used solely on Trust computers'. However, according to an F1 doctor at the Trust in a letter to the British Medical Journal; out of 50 junior doctors 36 stored patient data electronically, 20 using a USB stick, 3 a floppy disk and 13 a hospital computer hard drive. None of the USB sticks has 128-bit encryption, and only three had password protection.

Is the scenario above any different to medical staff transporting patient notes in the boot of their car? What about the tracking of patient notes? How are patient notes tracked in your organization?

Why do you think Specialist nurses would need to keep a database of their patients? Should they be allowed to have their own database or should it be 'owned' by the trust?

Patient information should be kept on NHS premises and should be tracked via the medical records department. Many health care organizations have implemented electronic tracking of patient notes so that they can be found quickly. Eventually all NHS patient information will be electronic and will enable staff to access the record from any designated location and record patient care activity.

Specialist nurses need to record the care and advice they give to their patients. Many specialist nurses do not have the ability to record clinical information electronically and use Access databases. Some may have USB memory sticks. This is an ethical dilemma which is being addressed in NHS Trusts. All patient information that has been captured by the NHS is the property and responsibility of the NHS. Specialist nurses may use the information from their databases to provide clinical outcomes of their activity.

A common occurrence is to access a system when a user has logged in and not logged out. It has been known for a particular member of staff to log in 'for the day'. This is not good practice as there is no audit trail and can implicate staff in violation of data protection. However, information ethics is still embryonic as the use of internet and software develops. New situations are presenting every day and the nurse should seek advice from their Information Governance department if in doubt.

Training

Training is very important for effective use of IT systems. It supports change and improvements in clinical and working practice in order to deliver the full benefits of the technology. Training not only addresses how to use the technology but includes appropriate scenarios, information management techniques and rationale. Issues with training are invariably underestimated and commonplace in the implementation of IT systems (Jones, *et al.,* 2002); many examples include, no protected time, lack of tailoring to the needs of the individual, training given too early (or there is a delay in implementation and the user requires a 'refresher' before 'go live'). Therefore, nurses need to ensure they are competent users of systems in order to record the care they give. To prepare the health care workforce for this particular change many hospitals and health care environments have encouraged the enrolment of staff to the **European Computer Driving Licence (ECDL)**, which provides an understanding of key principles and policies relating to health care information systems and the practical skills required (see www.ecdl.nhs.uk).

Mobile working

The ability of the NHS to absorb and effectively utilize advances in mobile technology is becoming more apparent, especially with the move to bring care closer to people's homes (DH, 2007b). Nurses will need to access records and information from many locations. Therefore, mobile working can be described as 'working on the go' — accessing and recording data and information about the client wherever the

professional happens to be; supporting the government to deliver high quality and safe care to patients in settings that are more convenient for them (DH, 2007a).

Box 7.5 Mobile technology

Telemedicine

This is the use of ICT, such as a video conferencing link, to enable a doctor in one place to examine a patient who is in another place, perhaps miles away.

Telenursing

This is where a nurse uses a link to a patient's television set at home to monitor medication or provide advice and support.

Telehealth

This is the preferred overarching term as it is seen to be more inclusive/multidisciplinary in scope and focuses on health rather than disease and illness.

Store and forward telehealth

This is where information is captured and stored, then sent to a specialist at another location.

Real time telehealth

This a live link between clinicians that allows real time interaction to take place. This often involves teleconfering, either using dedicated equipment or, increasingly, webcams and personal computers.

Remote monitoring

This is where sensors can be used to capture and transmit data. This technology may be used for home based dialysis or heart monitoring and may allow patients to be treated at home instead of at the hospital.

Telecare

This refers to the remote delivery of care, ie using sensors to detect when frail or elderly people fall in their own homes or wander into an unsafe environment.

The mobile health worker — North Lincolnshire Community Nurses get mobile

Community nurses in North Lincolnshire are to get wireless rugged laptops in one of the largest deployments yet of mobile technology to staff working outside hospitals. BT Health will

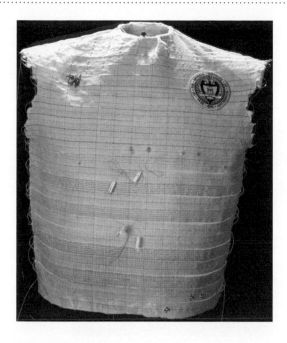

Fig. 7.1 New systems of working introduced as part of Connecting for Health.

supply up to 400 community staff with wireless connected, semi-rugged Panasonic Toughbooks.

The wireless linked laptops, which include a smart card reader, will provide staff with secure access to clinical records, email and support systems and data when working in the community or in a patient's home.

The Smartcard reader will enable the trust to use the mobile service in conjunction with NPfIT identification smartcards, required to access the NHS spine and applications such as the Personal Demographic Service and Care Records Service. BT calls the service Mobile Health Worker — a managed service tailored to the particular NHS customer that covers the devices they choose, a managed, secure end-to-end service, a managed service desk and mobile express GPRS access.

District Nurse Kathy Drayton, who works for North Lincolnshire said: 'Many of the patients seen in their own homes have complex needs — and being able to access their medical records during the visit means you can make more informed decisions about planning care and treatment'.

Accessed at: http://www.ehiprimarycare.com/news/3500/north_lincs_community_nurses_get_mobile

Wearable systems

Taking monitoring a stage further there are a vast array of 'wearable systems' available which allow physiological measurement and monitoring. This particular model — the wearable mother board—has three main types of sensors; bioelectric

(ECG and EMG), movement (chest sensors to provide tide volume and respiratory rate) and temperature.

Activity box

- Can the wearable motherboard be worn on a client you have or are caring for?
- What type of problems do you think might be encountered with the wearing of this?
- Are there any safety issues?
- What are the benefits?

Discussion points

The type of problems encountered could be personal cleaning, requiring assistance to remove and replace these garments, educating the user. Safety of the client will be improved (to prevent falls or anticipate an exacerbation of a chronic illness). Benefits would include tracking longer-term changes in patients with long-term conditions, managing the client in their own environment rather than hospital.

Robots

Another way of monitoring clients is by robots.

The value of the therapeutic relationship between the nurse and patient is as important as the clinical relationship. As technology advancements reframe the definition of presence, whether virtual or in person, the patient remains at the center of care. Nurses bring legitimacy to however presence is defined. Patient's needs are the basis by which both virtual and presence relationship can be equally considered as caring. Patient's needs are the basis by which both the virtual and presence relationship can be equally considered as caring. Nurses of the future will value both virtual and presence-based caring. Generational issues of nurses need to taken into consideration. Both new and experienced nurses must be able to respond to different patients' needs while working in such virtual environments as telenursing and e-intensive care units (The American Organizations of Nurse Executives, 2009).

Issues relating to consent

Consent is defined as 'a patient's agreement for a health professional to provide care' (DH, 2001). There is also further guidance in clause three of the NMC code of conduct and the RCN website. What does consent mean in the context of routine nursing?

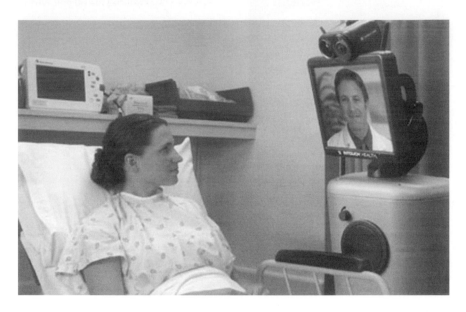

Fig. 7.2 The interaction between patient and doctor using robot technology. © 2010 In Touch Technologies, Inc.

Nursing Practice box

Improving consent skills

- Consent not only applies to surgical procedures and invasive techniques — consent must be obtained from a legally competent client before examinations, treatments or care is delivered.
- Ensure consent is part of a process in a pathway of care, and that it has been obtained.
- When obtaining consent consider the following criteria to ensure it is legal: that the client has the capacity, sufficient information to make a decision and that the consent is voluntary

---

Consent types

Informed Consent is an ongoing agreement by a person to receive treatment, undergo procedures or participate in research, after risks, benefits and alternatives have been adequately explained (RCN, 2006a).

There are two types of informed consent: (HPC, 2006)

- **Implied consent** — if identifiable information is being used to care for a client then implied consent is taken e.g. client holds out arm for blood pressure to be taken.

- **Express Consent** — when a health professional is given specific permission to do something.

Activity box

The RCN has issued guidance on consent, especially to young people. See link http://www.rcn.org.uk/__data/assets/pdf_file/0006/178971/003256.pdf

---

Nursing Practice box

- A patient refuses treatment that is in his or her best interest — what do you do?
- When is it justifiable to act without obtaining consent?

If treatment is refused, the issue is whether the patient is competent to refuse and is aware of the consequences — i.e. that death could occur — then legally the patient can refuse treatment.

Acting to save a life in a medical emergency is an occasion when it is acceptable to act without the consent of the patient.

When consent is obtained it must be recorded and easily accessible for viewing.

The importance of clinical information management

Organizations routinely capture vast quantities of data at macro and micro levels. The ability of decision makers to extract meaningful information in a timely and accurate manner provides a competitive advantage to any service. This is called **business intelligence**, which can be further broken down to **nursing intelligence** and therefore it is important for the nurse to become competent in processing information; especially within the particular service care is delivered (micro level). Nurses should know for example, what the incidence of **methicillin resistant staphylococcus aureus** (MRSA) within their unit compared to the national incidence, or what percentage of their caseload have a Body Mass Index (BMI) greater than 27.

Nurses should also be able to demonstrate an understanding of how patient needs and high quality clinical outcomes can be met in the most cost effective way possible e.g.: using the right product for the right purpose. Currently there has been discussion on how this is possible — current information systems do not provide this rich activity **data** because this has not been a high priority target. Specialist nurses have been collecting data on their care for a number of years but this has been subjective in nature, and not consistent. However, understanding and interpreting information is a skill that is now required of all nurses and the challenge that then follows is what and how do you address these issues raised.

Box 7.6 Nursing indicators

How do nurses measure the effectiveness of their care? What quality **nursing indicators** are currently used to demonstrate the nursing intervention?

Casey (2006) states there are two assumptions:

- Monitoring the quality and effectiveness of what we do and making necessary improvements in practice are core activities for all practising nurses
- General measures of quality and performance include the nursing contribution. The focus of specific measure of nursing quality should be those aspects of care and patient experiences that are affected by the judgements and decision of nurses.

Health care quality is not an easy thing to measure. Direct measures such as risk adjusted outcomes of individual patients require costly and time consuming data collection — unless electronic records are in use and capture this data.

Cost effectiveness is now central to health care reforms with a whole raft of policies introduced to drive up value for money, e.g.;

- Payment by results,
- Payment by outcomes,
- Practice based commissioning.

Nurses will have to prove to commissioners of care that they provide cost effective services. This will be accomplished by accurate, timely coding of clinical activity performed and is pivotal to providers' financial stability. Inaccurate coding loses vital revenue and could mean downsizing or closure (Newbold, 2006) of services.

Currently the DH is looking at ways to reward nurses fro scoring highly in a proposed system that will measure safety, effectiveness and compassion in nursing. The report (Griffiths, *et al.*, 2008) looks at how elements of nursing will be measured.

Healthcare Commission's investigation into Maidstone and Tunbridge Wells NHS Trust (CHAI, 2007)

The Healthcare Commission carried out this investigation to look into outbreaks of **Clostridium difficile** at the Maidstone and Tunbridge Wells NHS Trust. One of main findings was that 'the Trust has no effective system for surveillance of **C. difficile**'. System failures included the lack of local, consistent data capture of the patient journey throughout the trust. Under 'findings of fact' it said:

- Little progress had been made in terms of awareness, identifying the cause and reducing the rates.
- The trust was not compliant in meeting fully the requirements of the mandatory reporting scheme for **C. difficile**.
- Discrepancies in data submitted to CHAI regarding the number of patients with **C. difficile.**
- Before 2006 information submitted was out of date, did not include basic information and did not trigger actions.

Information systems have a crucial part to play in healthcare; the above example demonstrates a whole information system failure with regard to patient activity with severe consequences. Without aligned information systems (i.e. systems that **support** health care) and interpretation it is very difficult to see any trends in performance. The implementation of **CIS** will provide data capture on many of these criteria above, but health professionals including nurses must ensure that systems match the current and future needs of health care.

This is achieved by analysing the work flow and data capture which is then transformed to an electronic system.

Nurse specialists cover a whole range of activities including administration which is difficult to capture in current systems. Therefore it is difficult to make the outcomes of practice visible and demonstrate the outcomes of these roles (O'Dowd 2007).

Box 7.7 Using personal digital assistants (PDAs)

A user-friendly auditing system is helping specialist nurses demonstrate the value of the important work they do.

Clinical nurse specialists (Cancer) at Royal Berkshire NHS Foundation Trust have developed an effective system to measure, audit and appraise their activity using a **personal digital assistant (PDA).** They record activity which is saved and then docked **(store and forward)** with the team's computer.

Whilst is it good that nurses are able to demonstrate their activity and outcomes, think about the time it takes them. Care or activity is recorded elsewhere in a system and then re-recorded in their database. This is known as double entry. What would be the best way to do this? Think about the current way the care you provide is recorded — how could this be collected without double entry?

The vision is to capture data once and use it many times. Therefore if the screen you are completing does not capture a particular item (more important for the specialist) it will not be recorded and therefore cannot be used for reporting and predicting outcomes.

Record keeping

Poor record keeping and documentation remains one of the most common reasons for being removed from the NMC register (NMC, 2007). Being able to record care electronically will provide an opportunity to improve the recording of nursing care, providing nurses are involved in the design of these systems. There is a helpful section from the NMC website on advice sheets which provide information on the standard of professional conduct required of nurses and midwives in the exercise of their professional accountability and practice.

See http://www.nmc-uk.org/aSection.aspx?SectionID=11

Concerns have been highlighted regarding the time away from a patient when entering care onto an electronic record. There can be many reasons for this, not just because it is a computer. For example, there may not be enough computers available (Levy and Casey, 2004; 2005), or the network is slow and takes much longer to move from screen to screen than anticipated. These problems are not about the actual

---

Box 7.8 HORUS

Go to the **Connecting for Health** Website and look for the Nursing Clinical Lead who can be contacted with questions and queries. http://www.connectingforhealth.nhs.uk/engagement/clinical/ncls/nurses

A helpful acronym recommended by **NHS Connecting for Health** for record keeping (CfH, 2005) is the HORUS model:

H held securely and confidentially

O obtained fairly and efficiently

R recorded accurately and reliably

U used effectively and ethically

S shared appropriately and lawfully

---

programme running on the computer but more about the operational preparation before 'go live', which is why electronic implementations become complex and difficult to master, and why nurses will need to 'champion' this tool. With the event of mobile working this will become less of a problem. However, nurses must acknowledge that a little extra time spent on careful data entry will provide them with a valuable resource to demonstrate their effectiveness.

Box 7.9 Lessons learnt from the Shipman case

Harold Shipman, a GP caused death to patients by overdosing them with opiates and later falsified the electronic records to cover his tracks. If the contents of the patients' records had been visible to patients or their carers the chances of this going undetected would have been minimal. Dr Hannan who has taken over the very same practice where Shipman previously worked has offered his patients complete access to their own electronic medical record to restore confidence in their GP. Although in the initial stages, patients are able to request repeat prescriptions book appointments and view blood results. Not surprisingly, lessons learned from this project are influencing the implementation of the summary care record.

Freedom of information

The Freedom of Information Act 2000 and **Freedom of Information (Scotland) Act 2002** grants anyone rights of access to information that is not covered by the **Data Protection Act 1998**, i.e. information which does not contain person's identifiable details. See **http://www.nmc-uk.org/aFrameDisplay.aspx?DocumentID=4803**

Communicating with clients using email and the internet

To facilitate the **public health** agenda communicating via email with clients is a new way of working and should be capitalized on. Clinicians will be able to remind their clients about goals and objectives to reach targets or just provide monitoring advise.

Dean (2008) proposed the following:

- Along with the increase in internet usage, the popularity of email as a means of communication has also risen, and health care providers are beginning to experiment with its potential.

- NHS Direct has an email service that will respond to queries about specific health conditions, treatments or NHS services (www.nhsdirect.nhs.uk).

While research on using email in clinical practice is mainly from the US, evidence suggests that patients would welcome it as a means of communication with practitioners (Sittig, *et al.*, 2001).

Implications for practice

- As the popularity of the internet and email grows, patients may increasingly expect to use it as a means of communicating with practitioners.

- Using email has implications for confidentiality, resources and accountability; these need to be carefully considered when designing email services for health care settings.

- Patients may benefit from the convenience and accessibility of email, which may ultimately empower then to be more responsible for their own health.

- A range of methods for communicating with health care professionals must always be available to meet the needs of patients who lack access to computers, computer skills or general literacy.

- Training may be beneficial before communicating with patients by email to develop a writing style that is clear, easy to read, informative and empathetic.

Summary

The ultimate aim of health information technology is to create information systems that are integrated with one another and also to provide a universal, birth-to-death health care record. This system would not only allow a person to be treated anywhere in the country using this record, but it would also

incorporate knowledge based systems as both factual databases and decision support tools.

The demands upon nurses to use computer and information technology in care delivery are increasing. National policy, and in particular **Connecting for Health**, dictates that nurse embrace and actively integrate such initiatives within their clinical practice. This requires nurses to become more informed and participatory in utilizing information technology for the betterment of the profession and the patients that they care for.

 # Online Resource Centre

For more information on recording patient information visit the Online Resource Centre — http://www.oxfordtextbooks.co.uk/orc/linsley/

References

Baker, B. Edwards, B. Lane, D. Sibson, L. Bryson, M. & Nolan, S. (2002). *Definition of eHealth*. [cited 25 March 2006]. Adapted from Gott, M (1993) Telehealth & Telemedicine in the Electronic Home. Available from: http://www.ehealthnurses.org.uk/ehealthgrp.html

Baker, B., Clark, J., Hunter, E., Currell, R., Andrewes, C., Edwards, B., & Vincent, C., (2007). *An investigation of the emergent professional issues experienced by nurses when working in an eHealth environment. A collaborative project between the Information in Nursing Forum at the Royal College of Nursing and the School of Health & Social Care*, Bournemouth: Bournemouth University.

Ballard, E. (1997). Important considerations about nursing intelligence and information systems. *Studies in Health Technology Information* 46:44-9.

Budgen, S. (2005). Is there an agreed definition of Clinical Engagement? *Royal College of Nursing Information Group Newsletter*. Spring:.2.

Clark, J. (2003). (ed.) *Naming Nursing*. Proceedings of the first ACENDIO Ireland/UK conference held in September 2003 in Swansea, Wales, UK. Germany: Verlag Han Huber, Bern, 35.

Cockcroft, L., (2007). Grandmothers hooked on Nintendo Wii boxing. *Daily Telegraph*. [cited 1 August 2008]. Available from: http://www.telegraph.co.uk/connected/main.jhtml?xml=/connected/2008/07/11/nwii111.xml

Commission for Healthcare Audit and Inspection (2007). *Investigation into the outbreaks of Clostridium difficile at Maidstone and Tunbridge Wells NHS Trust*. London: CHAI

Connecting for Health (2006a). *'Sealed Envelopes' briefing paper: 'Selective Alerting' Approach*. London DH

Connecting for Health (2006b). *The NHS care record service — a guide for the nursing community*. London: DH.

Dean, A. (2008). Communicating with patients using email and the internet. *Nursing Times*; 104(7): 29-30.

Department of Health (2000). *The NHS Plan: a plan for investment; a plan for reform*. London: DH.

Department of Health (2001). *HSC 2001/023: Good practice in consent: achieving the NHS Plan commitment to patient-centred consent practice*. London: DH

Department of Health (2002). *Delivering 21st Century IT Support for the NHS*. London: DH.

Department of Health (2004). A Strategy for Information Quality Assurance. [cited 3 August 2008]. Accessed @ http://www.dh.gov.uk/en/Publicationsandstatistics/Publications/PublicationsPolicyAndGuidance/DH_4125508

Department of Health (2006a). *Our Health, Our Care, Our Say: A New Direction in Community Services*. London: The Stationery Office.

Department of Health (2006b).*The Expert Patients Programme*. [cited 1 August 2008]. Accessed @ http://www.dh.gov.uk/en/Aboutus/MinistersandDepartmentLeaders/ChiefMedicalOfficer/ProgressOnPolicy/ProgressBrowsableDocument/DH_4102757

Department of Health (2006b). *The Caldicott Guardian Manual*. London: DH.

Department of Health (2007a). *Our NHS, Our Future. NHS Next Stage Review. Interim Report*. London: DH.

Department of Health (2007b). *Shifting Care Closer to Home*. London: DH.

Department of Health (2007c). *Consultation on a review of PCT's Professional Executive Committees (PECs)*. London DH.

Dowding, D., Foster, R., Lattimer, V., Mitchell, N., Owens, R. & Randell, R. (2007). How do nurses use new technologies to inform decision making? In: *The 2007 International Nursing Research Conference, Dundee, UK 01 - 04 May 2007*. Middlesex, UK: RCN Publishing.

Griffiths, P., Jones, S., Maben, J., Murrells, T. (2008). *State of the Art Metrics for Nursing: A Rapid Appraisal*. London: National Nursing Research Unit, Kings College.

Health Professions Council (2008). *Confidentiality — Guidance for Registrants*. London: HPC.

Jones, A., Hart, A., Henwood, F. & Gerhardt, C. (2002). *The Use of Electronic Patient Records (EPRs) in the Maternity Services: professional and Public Acceptability*. [cited 23.01.05]. Available from: <www.inam.brighton.ac.uk/eprproject.htm>

Levy, S. & Casey, A. (2004). *Speaking Up. Nurses and NHS IT Developments*. [cited 17.06.04]. Available from: http://www.rcn.org.uk/downloads/research/ nurses-it-devs-survey.doc

Levy, S. & Casey, A. (2005). *A year on …. Nurses and NHS IT Developments*. [cited 12.07.05]. Available from: http://www.rcn.org.uk/downloads/press/nurses-it-devs-survey2005.doc

Linsley, P. & Hurley, J. (2003). *Web learning in post registration nurse education: application and theory. A practical experience of combining humanistic, educational and technological considerations. Information Technology in Nursing*, 15 (4): 16-19.

National Health Service Information Authority (2002). *Caring for Information — Model for the future*. London: DH.

Newbold, D. (2006). Caring about the Costs. *Nursing Standard* 20(29):24-25.

Nursing and Midwifery Council (2007). *Professional conduct committee and the conduct and competence committee (Audit 2005/06)*, London: NMC.

Nursing and Midwifery Council (2008a). *The Code of Conduct*. London: NMC.

Nursing and Midwifery Council (2008b). *Confidentiality Advice Sheet*. London:. NMC.

O'Dowd, A. (2007). Social taboo or specialism? *Cancer Nursing Practice* 6 (1):14-15.

Ozbolt, J. G. (2004). Nursing Terminology summit conference promote data standards. *Computers, Informatics, Nursing* 22(1):44-49.

Royal College of General Practitioners (2009). *Final report of the Shared Record Professional Guidance project*. London: The RCGP Health Informatics Group/Connecting for Health.

Royal College of Nursing (1999). *Future NHS Staffing*. Select Committee on Health. [online]. Houses of Commons [cited 29 March 2006] Available from: http://www.publications.parliament.uk/pa/cm199899/cmselect/cmhealth/38/8121016.htm

Royal College of Nursing (2006a). *Informed Consent in Health and Social Care Research*. London: RCN.

Royal College of Nursing (2006b). *Putting Information at the Heart of Nursing Care*. London: RCN.

Sittig, D.F., King, S., Hazlehurst, B. (2001). *A survey of patient provider email communication: what do patients think?* International Journal of Medical Information. 61: 71-80.

Snyder-Halpern, R., Corcoran-Perry, S. & Narayan, S. (2001). Developing clinical practice environments supporting the knowledge work of nurses. *Computers in Nursing*. 19(1): 17-26.

Wallis, A. (2007). Clinical Data Standards and Nursing. *Nursing Management* 14(2):26–28.

Chapter 8

The importance of nursing to public health: the political and policy context

Abigail Masterson

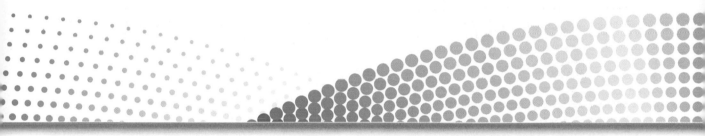

Introduction

The nursing workforce is the largest group of health professionals employed by the NHS and so nursing has a vital contribution to make to the public health and should be of great interest to politicians and policy makers. However nurses and nursing have historically been rather invisible in many key health policy debates and many nurses are uncomfortable with the idea of engaging in policy analysis and indeed politics, seeing these activities as a distraction from their core purpose of care delivery (Maslin-Prothero and Masterson, 2002). This chapter outlines the political drivers and overarching policy related to the public health agenda. It will begin by exploring how public health policy has historically been formulated in the UK. It will examine the link between nursing and public health policy and argue that all nurses should be interested in politics and policymaking because of their impact on both the profession itself and the nature of practice.

Why nurses need to be interested in politics and policy making

Currently in the UK, as in many parts of the world, nurses lack autonomy, accountability and control over their working environments and the scope of their practice (Maslin-Prothero and Masterson, 2002). For over twenty years there has been international recognition that nursing and nurses should become more involved in policy debates (WHO, 1987). A recent relaunch of the 2000 International Council of Nurses position statement emphasizes that:

'... nurses have an important contribution to make in health services planning and decision-making, and in development of appropriate and effective health policy. They can and should contribute to public policy related to preparation of health workers, care delivery systems, health care financing, ethics in health care and determinants of health. Nurses must accept their responsibilities in health services policy and decision-making, including their responsibility for relevant professional development. Professional nursing organizations have a responsibility to promote and advocate the participation of nursing in local, national and international health decision-making and policy development bodies and committees. They also have a responsibility to help ensure nurse leaders have adequate preparation to enable them to fully assume policymaking roles'.

ICN, 2008:1

The development of the NHS: an idiosyncratic but critically informed whistle-stop tour

The establishment of the NHS itself provides a useful focus for understanding politics and policymaking. Although the NHS was formally established on 5 of July 1948, the NHS and indeed the Welfare State itself was actually the result of a slow process of evolution dating back until at least the sixteenth century and is fundamentally connected to the experience and consequences of war and the needs and consequences of capitalism.

Since the **Poor Law of 1597**, English Parliaments have recognized a mandatory responsibility on the State to assist the old, the sick, the incapable, and, when absolutely necessary, the able-bodied. The **1601 Poor Law Act** in England created a collectivist, national system, paid for by levying local rates (or property taxes) and which, amongst other things, included the establishment of poorhouses (workhouses) with infirmaries for those who were old or ill and poor. Over the next two centuries the system came under increasing pressure as a consequence of the industrial revolution which involved huge movements of people into the towns and cities. However, the poor law system was increasingly seen to be too costly and was widely perceived as encouraging the underlying problems i.e. encouraging people into poverty and making them dependent on handouts. Over time therefore the purpose of the poorhouse changed from that of a support to a deterrent or threat.

The **Poor Law Amendment Act of 1834** created a national body (the Poor Law Commission) to oversee the operation of the poor law system. This Act is very important in terms of understanding current apparent inequities and different approaches to health and social care as it coined the principle of 'less eligibility' and the notion of deserving and undeserving

poor. So already over 100 years before the formal inception of the NHS there was substantial and increasing state involvement in the provision of health and social care.

The early twentieth century saw the State taking even more responsibility for the provision of health care. During the early 1930s, the Labour-led London County Council demonstrated the advantages of a purely public service by rationalizing hospital care, providing common staffing standards, funding back-up laboratories and generating the infrastructure of what emerged as a mini NHS before the war. This experiment provided a blueprint for Labour's post-war health policy, operating under the direct gaze of Westminster and Whitehall.

Capitalism in the late nineteenth and early twentieth century needed large numbers of fit workers concentrated near factories. The Industrial Revolution and the growth of the towns and cities required by capitalism had created a number of serious social and health problems. A number of measures were brought in to alleviate the conditions of ordinary people such as the Public Health Acts of 1872 and 1875 which set up Health Authorities throughout England and brought in a range of measures related to sewerage and drains, water supply, housing and disease.

Why was war important?

During the Boer War (1899-1902) the medical condition of the working class recruits was a cause of grave concern. Four out of ten young men offering themselves as recruits to the British army had to be rejected (even against the extremely minimal medical test), because their bodies weren't up to the job. They had bad teeth, weak hearts, poor sight and hearing, physical deformities of all kinds. Most obviously, they were too short: in 1901, the infantry had to reduce the minimum height for recruits from 5ft 3ins to 5ft. This increased attempts to improve the nation's health.

From 1907 medical tests and free treatment were provided nationally for school pupils. In 1911 the government introduced the **National Insurance Act** that provided insurance for workers in time of sickness. This National Health Insurance scheme, the brainchild of Lloyd George, lasted from 1912 until 1948, combining what we would now classify as social security benefits and a rudimentary health service. It offered basic GP care and sickness benefits in return for a tri-partite contribution, covering all workers earning less than a specified minimum annual income — but not their families and dependants.

In World War 1 (1914–1918) as a consequence of the tremendous sacrifices made and concern about shifting political movements and ideologies in other parts of Europe as well as the increasing strength of the Labour Party in the UK there was significant investment in social reform. It also had an impact on the 'battle' for state registration in nursing as the war illustrated the administrative importance of some nationally recognized standard in grading staff and matching skills to needs.

During the Second World War (1939–1945) the public hospitals (former workhouse infirmaries) and the Voluntary Hospitals (e.g. St Bartholomew's, St Thomas' in London) were joined together in the Emergency Medical Service. The Ministry of Health thus assumed 'central' control over and took responsibility for finance of the entire hospital service for the first time. The Second World War also brought people from different social classes in much closer contact with each other thus highlighting class inequalities and increasing a societal commitment to social justice, social change and increasing equity in life chances and opportunities. Before the end of The Second World War the government announced its intention to develop a national hospital service and followed this up by the publication of the Beveridge Report in 1942 which recommended the establishment of a centrally organized and funded totally comprehensive health service.

The NHS and the legacy of negotiation and bargaining

The NHS is a uniquely UK initiative closely tied to our social history. Interestingly in view of the current tense relationship between the British Medical Association and the Government and concern over GPs in particular, one of the original arguments for setting up a state-run health service was that, as government employees, GPs would be liable to stricter official controls. The medical profession conversely have long been opposed to State control and wary of the financial consequences. GPs were only enticed into the 1911 *National Insurance Act* arrangements because the government agreed that payment would be based on the number of patients on a doctors list rather than a fixed salary and the exclusion of higher income groups to enable the continuation of lucrative private practice.

In the 1940s the decision taken by the wartime coalition government to establish the NHS was largely welcomed by the general public but its final structure was the product of considerable bargaining, negotiation and compromize between competing political and professional interests. Aneurin Bevan (usually known as Nye Bevan) the Minister of Health responsible for the formation of the NHS, famously claimed to have 'stuffed consultants' mouths with gold', splitting the medical profession and giving himself the leverage to create the health service he envisaged. The resulting 1948 structure therefore was based on historical structures such as an 'independent' GP service and consequently maintained (or even enhanced) the autonomy of the medical profession. Needless to say the nursing profession had little effect on the decisions made.

> **Box 8.1** Key moments in the history of heath care
>
> • Aneurin Bevan's National Health Service Act
>
> Aneurin Bevan's *National Health Service Act* passed through parliament and became law in November, 1946. Bevan told the 1946 Royal College of Nursing Conference:
>
> 'When I had your invitation to come and address you this evening I accepted with alacrity because I realized from the very start that, no matter how distant my relationship with the doctors might become, I had to be most friendly with the nurses, if I was ever to get our health service going properly'.
>
> • NHS Founding Day
>
> The NHS Founding Day was July 5th 1948. Hospitals previously run by voluntary foundations and local government, 1550 in total, were nationalized. National control was established through the creation of a set of health authorities financed partly from national insurance but mostly from general taxation.

Globalization

As outlined above, policies have traditionally been seen to be the products of politics at the level of the nation state. However globalization and the evermore interconnectedness of the world requires a re-conceptualization of policy to include the practice of a range of supranational actors and the ways in which supranational organizations shape national policy. We will now explore this in more detail looking at nursing and nurses as a focus.

Globalization: a threat to professional self-regulation?

Nursing in the UK is a self-regulated profession. Currently, the nature and function of the profession of nursing, is ostensibly controlled by the nation state through the state sanctioned regulator — the Nursing and Midwifery Council (NMC) — which sets standards of conduct and competence for its registrants in order to protect the public. However we will explore how this control is in fact limited and constrained by supranational actors such as the European Union (EU) and other political changes such as devolution.

The relationship between the state and nursing in the UK is close, both because the profession is regulated through statute and therefore any major changes to the profession have to be approved by parliament, and because the majority of nurses work in state provided and funded health services. The government departments of health in the four countries of the UK offer guidance concerning the nature and scope of practice in their services both through nursing specific policy documents such as **Modernizing Nursing Careers (2006)** and through National Service Frameworks which, in addition to identifying the standards of service provision the public can expect, also identify the role and competencies of the professionals involved in delivering these. Indeed, even in non-state provided or funded services such as private nursing homes the government stipulates the nursing roles and staffing structures required.

Nursing in the UK has been a statutorily regulated profession since 1919. The NMC is the regulatory body. Its purpose is to establish and improve standards of nursing care in order to serve and protect the public. The NMC is elected and funded by the profession. It maintains a register of qualified nurses; sets standards for education, practice and conduct; provides advice on professional standards; and considers allegations of misconduct or unfitness to practice due to ill health. NMC registration is required to work in the UK as a registered nurse.

Despite this apparent control over nursing by its professional body and the nation state the EU has already had a significant impact on the essence, structure and function of nursing in the UK; and the European institutions are increasingly displacing national institutions as the principal loci of policy change. Although the EU does not usually intend to make health policy in practice other policies, such as the commitment to freedom of movement and smooth functioning of the internal market, can have a significant impact on health policy and even the role and function of nurses and nursing as we will now explore.

Shaping preparation for practice

Most EU countries only offer a general nursing qualification whereas the UK registers four distinct types of nurses:

- Adult (general),
- Child,
- Mental health,
- Learning disability.

In 1977 two EEC directives with significance for nursing were agreed by the Member States. The first (77/452/EEC) was concerned with the mutual recognition of diplomas, certificates and other evidence of the formal qualifications for a range of professions including nurses responsible for general care. This was to facilitate the movement of professionals within the European Community (EC), 'freedom of movement'

as noted above, being one of the basic rights of individuals living in the EC. The second (77/453/EEC) specifically concerned the minimum standards of professional training of nurses responsible for general care. This directive stipulated that courses of preparation must comprise 4,600 hours of practical and theoretical instruction, identified the subjects to be studied, and the type of clinical instruction required; and was enacted in the UK through a Statutory Instrument, **The Nurses, Midwives and Health Visitors Rules 1983**.

General nurses who have completed programmes of study that meet the EU requirements can automatically register in any EU country of their choice. So for example, a nurse who completes an appropriate programme of study in Spain can opt to register in the UK rather than in Spain. Registration in the country of employment is however essential for employment in that country i.e. a nurse trained in the UK who wishes to work in Spain must register in Spain.

Courses in general care nursing in the UK meet with EEC requirements and have done since 1977 (EEC 2003).

However, the UK also registers direct entry qualifications in mental health nursing, children's nursing and learning disability nursing. In many other EU countries such qualifications, if available at all, can only be taken after completing a course of study and registering as a general care nurse. Consequently these qualifications are perceived to be 'specialist' qualifications and are not recognized by the EU. Therefore UK nurses holding these qualifications are prevented from registering in other EU countries without undergoing additional education in general care nursing.

This has led to a perception that the UK is out of step with other European countries in the way that it educates its nursing workforce and concern that UK nurses, other than those who have undertaken a general pre-registration programme, are disadvantaged when it comes to seeking employment in the European Community. For example an EC report celebrates the fact that the number of such 'specialist' nurses is declining as their existence is seen to be a barrier to the labour mobility desired (EC, 2000). These perceptions and concerns have resulted in the NMC being pressured by the EU to reconsider the structure of its professional register and the future of its qualifications in mental health, children's and learning disability nursing.

Mutual recognition of qualifications

In 2000, the Lisbon European Council set as a target that the EU should become the most competitive and dynamic knowledge based society in the world by the year 2010. Quality education and training, optimal use of human resources and developing flexible labour markets are seen to be key in achieving the Lisbon objective. Consequently EC Directives covering nursing are intended to ensure that training and qualifications comply with agreed minimum standards throughout the EU so that regulators in the member states such as the NMC can have confidence in giving automatic recognition to the qualifications held by migrants from other Member States and systems for mutual recognition of qualifications are intended to facilitate the movement of nurses across the EU. However despite all sorts of 'harmonization' initiatives, across Europe there remain considerable differences in the numbers of nurses per head of population and their function, autonomy and scope of practice.

Moving towards a global model of nursing

We shall now consider some supranational organizations: The World Health Organization and the International Council of Nurses and their impact on nursing in the UK.

The World Health Organization

The World Health Organization (WHO) was founded in 1948 and is a specialized agency of the United Nations with responsibility for international health matters and public health. The **WHO Declaration of Alma-Ata 1978** stipulated that nursing services should focus on health rather disease (see Chapters 1 and 3). It is increasingly clear that spending more of our attention and resources to promoting and maintaining health for individuals, families and communities should result in a healthier population and less need for illness care. Nurses have been at the forefront in advocating for, developing and applying new methods to maintain and promote health and prevent illness. The shift to primary health care, health promotion and disease prevention creates opportunities for unique and independent roles for nurses, and at the same time raises a number of issues regarding the scope of nursing practice.

The WHO nursing unit maintains a database of best practice projects and actively works to assist nurses internationally to share a common understanding of the essential nature of nursing and a collective practice development agenda. Through this work the WHO can be seen to encourage policy transfer and ultimately policy convergence. Because of the great disparity in health resources across the globe and the huge variation in education, function, and status of nurses internationally, much of the WHO nursing unit work is targeted at raising standards of nursing education and practice in countries where these are perceived to be underdeveloped. Countries such as the United States of America (USA) and the UK supply most of the 'best practice' examples which are then promoted by the WHO in the less developed health systems. Thus the WHO can be seen as a tool of globalization that the UK uses to export its vision of nursing.

International Council of Nurses

The International Council of Nurses (ICN) was founded in 1899 by nurses from England, the USA and Germany and is now a federation of 122 national nurses' associations. Its mission is to represent nursing worldwide, advancing the profession and influencing health policy. The ICN accounts for the bulk of internationally focused regulatory activity and since the 1980s it has published a succession of documents promoting its position on regulation. Such documents reflect and even cite examples from UK regulatory policy as examples of good practice. In 1999 the establishment of international competencies for general nursing applicable to multi-country licensure was identified as a key focus of ICN activity. As the competencies proposed appear to mirror those already demanded in the developed world the ICN is at least in part contributing to the development of a global nursing workforce which arguably is likely to be of most assistance to the developed countries.

Throughout their careers nurses develop expertise through education, experience, research and the development of skills in response to the context of their work setting. Because nurses provide the coordination and care for many different kinds of clients, from neonates to entire communities, many different kinds of expertise develop. While there may be some common understanding of what the core of nursing, is the spreading out from that core finds nurses at different places in their own professional development and understanding of the depth and breath of nursing practice. For example, as nursing expands into areas traditionally viewed as medical services. This creates a need for a definition of scope of nursing practice that is sufficiently broad and flexible to enable appropriate expansion of nursing practice, and at the same time provide a reasonable degree of direction on the boundaries of the discipline.

Recruitment policy

Health expenditures across the globe are increasing faster than population growth and faster than inflation. Cost-effective health care means ensuring the right service is efficiently provided at the right time, in the right place, by the most appropriate and least expensive mix of health care providers. Health human resource planning, which addresses this last point, has become a key focus for improving cost-effectiveness. The concentration on the role of all health care providers by governments and other stakeholder groups must be able to decide what they do, why they do it, why it is important for this to be done and why they should do it rather than somebody else.

The UK has long depended on overseas trained nurses, particularly from its former colonies, to staff the NHS however the numbers involved are rapidly increasing and a third of nurses in central London are now from overseas. Over the last decade registrations from developed nations such as Australia, New Zealand and the USA have fallen but have significantly increased from developing nations such as the Philippines, India and Ghana. Similar numbers of UK registered nurses apply for registration in developed countries as are accepted by the NMC from the same countries however very few UK registered nurses apply for registration in developing countries.

The international recruitment of nurses regularly captures much media attention in the mainstream press and concerns have been expressed about the impact of the UK government's policy on the health systems of developing countries and the need for **ethical recruitment**.

Technology

The increase in access to the internet has opened up relatively cheap access to nursing and health knowledge from any country in the world (see Chapter 7). The internet is however dominated by the English language and western nursing values. The majority of the information it contains in the form of online journals, literature from nursing associations and even contributions to professionally orientated chat rooms derives from the USA, UK and Australia.

In the future it should become possible using interactive communication technologies for clinical images to be beamed across the globe for interpretation in another country. This would potentially allow nurses to diagnose and make treatment decisions at a distance and in turn enable nurses to have instant access to specialists across the globe. Such transnational clinical activity would raise further issues for the future of nation specific professional regulation. For example, to adequately protect the public, should the nurses involved also be registered to practice in the country from which the images are being sent and where the decision will be applied.

Devolution

The 1997 Labour Party election manifesto pledged to introduce a devolved form of government for Wales, Scotland and Northern Ireland. In 1998 this promise was realized with the creation of an elected parliament in Scotland, an elected assembly in Wales and an elected assembly in Northern Ireland. Prior to devolution differences in health policy across the four countries had been minimal; devolution has provided new freedoms and opportunities to pursue and develop their own health policy. Devolution has created distinct differences between the health services of England, Scotland, Wales and Northern Ireland, particularly in their organization and management.

Although the broad aims for health services across the four countries of the UK are similar i.e. the need to streamline the acute sector, provide more care in community settings and make more preventative interventions, particularly for individuals with long-term conditions, these aims are being pursued in different ways. Policy and services and therefore roles of health professionals, such as nurses and midwives are becoming increasingly distinct which may ultimately pose challenges for UK nurse mobility and work and career opportunities particularly in border areas (Maslin-Prothero, *et al.,* 2008).

Current policy issues for public health nursing

High quality care for all — 'The Darzi Report'

In June 2008, after a series of consultations and the publication of an interim report, Lord Darzi launched **High quality care for all: NHS next stage review final report** (Darzi, 2008), outlining his vision and recommendations for next steps for the NHS. He set out a vision for an NHS that is clinically effective, personal and safe for all, and which:

- Helps people stay healthy,
- Has quality at its heart, gets the basics right every time, and gives the public information about the standard of quality achieved,
- Works in partnership with its staff enabling them to lead and manage the organizations in which they work,
- Integrates health and social care,
- Works within a constitution setting out rights and responsibilities.

Quality in this context spans: patient safety; patient experience and effectiveness of care and as Darzi noted:

'Nurses will always be at the heart of shaping patient experience and delivering care'
Darzi 2008:17

Transforming Community Services

More than 90% of all contacts with the NHS already take place outside the hospital (DH, 2008). GPs and practice nurses are providing an increasing range of services including blood tests and minor surgery. Developments in technology are allowing more and more treatments and services to be delivered outside of hospitals or other health care environments (HM Government, 2009).

Transforming Community Services (TCS) is a radical change programme for the delivery of primary health care services in order to meet the aspirations of the **NHS Next Stage Review** (DH, 2009e). It includes a number of initiatives designed to help staff provide high quality evidence-based care, and achieve positive outcomes for the community they serve. It suggests that community nurses should be able to assess, diagnose and treat and that they are therefore likely to require advanced level knowledge and skills in physical assessment and pharmacology. Similarly the development of new assistant practitioner roles is advocated and it is recognized that to fully realize this transformation a radical shift in the competence and capabilities of the current and future nursing and midwifery workforce is required (DH, 2009f).

Promoting health

The progress on health inequalities over the last ten years has been summed up as 'much achieved; more to do' (DH, 2009d). In England there has been a general improvement in health outcome overall with improvements in a number of critical areas such as declining mortality rates in targeted killers (cancers, all circulatory diseases and suicides), increased life expectancy, now at its highest ever level and reduced infant mortality, now at its lowest ever level. However in some areas persistent challenges remain such as rising rates of diabetes and new challenges have emerged such as rising rates of Chlamydia.

Similarly for the determinants of health, although improvements have been made in some important areas such as a reduction in the number of people who smoke and the quality of housing stock and so on, increasing levels of obesity in adults and children is a growing concern. In addition within this overall positive picture, health inequalities are often present and there are huge geographical inequalities across the country (Health Improvement Analytical Team — Monitoring Unit 2009). Health inequalities are not only apparent between people of different socio-economic groups — they exist between different genders, different ethnic groups, and the elderly and people suffering from mental health problems or learning disabilities also have worst health than the rest of the population (Secretary of State for Health 2009).

One of the key commitments given in the *Next Stage Review* final report is a commitment to health promotion and helping people stay healthy (Darzi 2008). Primary Care Trusts (PCTs) are expected to commission comprehensive well being services, and opportunistic health promotion interventions in primary and secondary care are also advocated (Secretary of State for Health 2009). The valuable health promoting role of nurses and midwives in all settings and services has been regularly emphasized (DH, 2007a; HM Government, 2004).

Patients as partners

The NHS Constitution sets out rights and responsibilities for staff and health service users (DH, 2009b). The NHS is not yet truly patient centred but must become more so. Personal care plans and personalized budgets will allow patients much greater involvement in their care and extended choice of the most appropriate type of treatment as well as when and where they are treated (HM Government, 2009).

The quality and productivity challenge

Over the next five years the NHS will be moving from a position of growth to one of consolidation (DH, 2009a; Flory, 2009). The quality and productivity challenge requires a fundamental change in the way that services are delivered and innovation to improve productivity and quality outcomes. In practice this will require attention to reduce inappropriate clinical variation e.g. different rehabilitation and mobilization plans for two patients with the same health needs undergoing the same elective surgical procedure and supporting the development of evidence-based and cost effective care. It is also likely to necessitate pathway redesign and moving more care into the community.

In terms of nursing, there will be significant pressures to improve productivity by developing new ways of working, creating new assistant and advanced practice roles and increasing the flexibility and adaptability of the nursing workforce in general.

Discussion point

When you were on your last clinical placement did you observe any opportunities to redesign services or pathways to improve patient experience?

From April 2010, PCTs and Trusts will be required to produce annual quality accounts and report publicly on their quality performance (DH, 2009c). Accurate, timely, meaningful and comparable measures or metrics of quality related to nursing and midwifery will therefore be required. Nurses and midwives working at all levels and across different settings will need to be able to measure and act on patient experience.

Alongside these general policy drivers which will have an impact on nursing and midwifery there are also a number of nursing specific policy directives which are of particular importance. For example from 2012 the minimum award for pre-registration nursing programmes in the UK has been approved by the Nursing and Midwifery Council as nursing registration with a degree and with a mandatory **preceptorship** period to follow initial registration (NMC 2008).

An important workstream, led by the Chief Nursing Officer England is **Modernizing Nursing Careers** (DH, — CNO'S Directorate, 2006). The document outlines the programme of work and emphasizes the vital contribution of nurses and nursing to achieving the health care reform programme. It forecasts:

- Care taking place in and outside hospital with the workforce moving between,
- Nurses starting their career in the community,
- A career framework that allows nursing to 'grow its own' with multiple entry points for those taking up nursing as a second career or as mature entrants,
- Plurality of provision offering alternative employers and employment models including NHS Foundation Trusts, self employment and social enterprises,
- A flexible principle based curriculum that is built around patient pathways, with a strong academic foundation and interdisciplinary learning,
- A framework that supports movement between career pathways, practice, management and education, and that values and rewards different career types,
- A better balance of generalists and specialists to provide integrated networks of urgent, specialist and continuing care,
- Careers built around patient pathways using competence as the currency for greater movement and flexibility,
- A career structure with increased number of assistants working as part of multidisciplinary teams,
- Standardization of advanced level skills,
- Patient pathway based careers focusing on nursing roles rather than titles,
- Nursing roles defined according to patient need — to provide intervention that is timely, accurate and swift,
- Nursing teams to become more self-directed and professionally accountable,
- Nurses leading, coordinating and commissioning care, as well as giving care, to bring about change measured by health gain and health outcomes,
- Care based on evidence and critical thinking and assisted by new technology.

In a further report (DH, 2007b) ten key roles for nurses are outlined to support service transformation and change through the development of nursing and midwifery practice. Nurses will be expected to:

- Order diagnostic investigations such as pathology tests and X-rays,

- Make and receive referrals direct, say, to a therapist or pain consultant,
- Admit and discharge patients for specified conditions and within agreed protocols,
- Manage patient caseloads, say for diabetes or rheumatology,
- Run clinics, say, for ophthalmology or dermatology,
- Prescribe medicines and treatments,
- Carry out a wide range of resuscitation procedures including defibrillation,
- Perform minor surgery and outpatient procedures,
- Triage patients using the latest IT to the most appropriate health professional,
- Take a lead in the way local health services are organized and in the way that they are run.

In a similar vein, *Facing the future* (DH, 2007c) called for health visitors to head up multi-skilled teams and to focus on the most complex cases and most vulnerable children enabling general nurses and nursery nurses to deliver the more straightforward elements of support.

Summary

Nurses are central to public health. The rapid review of current health policy above has indicated that health organizations will only be able to deliver world-class health care if nurses are fully engaged and nursing skills are fully utilized. Nurses will need to seize the health promotion opportunities present in every patient encounter. Advanced clinical skills will increasingly need to be a core element of many nurses practice. Nurses will need to be equipped to take on leadership roles in many areas of care, leading multi-professional teams and coordinating and commissioning care as well as delivering it. Nurses in all settings will need to take responsibility for delivering evidence-based care, improving services and being accountable for ensuring that patients enjoy a high quality experience. Increasingly nursing roles will cross organizational boundaries and careers will be developed around patient pathways. Many nurses will need to take on advanced roles and exercise a high degree of influence across local health economies.

Nurses have been said to be '...notoriously bad at being political' (Casey 1996:1), not only regarding their role and place in existing health care structures but also about other issues and areas which effect health. However nurses need to understand and engage with the policy process in order to maximize their contribution to public health.

Online Resource Centre

For more information on the political and policy context visit the Online Resource Centre — http://www.oxfordtextbooks.co.uk/orc/linsley/

Further reading

Aiken, L.H., Buchan, J., Sochalski,, J., Nichols, B. & Powell, M. (2004). Trends in International Nurse Migration. *Health Affairs*, 23(3): 69-77.

Batata, A. S. (2005). International nurse recruitment and NHS vacancies: a cross-sectional analysis. *Globalization and Health* 2005: 1:7.

Buchan, J., Parkin, T., & Sochalski, J. (2003). *International Nurse Mobility: Trends and Policy Implications*. Edinburgh: Queen Margaret University College.

Campbell, M.L. (2006). Nurses in international health care: migrants or commodities? *Health (London)* 10(3): 361-7.

Crook, C. (2001). Globalization and its critics. *The Economist* Sept 29: 3-5.

Department of Health (2004). *Code of practice for NHS employers involved in the recruitment of healthcare professionals*. London: DH (NB replaced the 2001 version).

Giddens, A. (2000). The globalising of modernity. In D. Held & A. McGrew (Eds) *The global transformations reader: an introduction to the globaliza tion debate*. Cambridge: Polity Press 92-98.

Gough, P., Maslin-Prothero, S. & Masterson, A. (1994). *Nursing and social policy: care_in context*. Oxford: Butterworth Heinemann.

Kings Fund (2004). *London Calling?* London: King's Fund.

Masterson, A. (1998). Discourse analysis: a tool for change. In Smith, P. *Nursing Research — setting new agendas*, London: Edward Arnold.

Masterson, A. (2002). Commentary: Issues of qualification assessment for nurses in a global market. *Nurse Education Today* 22(1): 57-59.

Masterson, A. (2004). Closer European integration: a threat to self regulation. *Nursing Management* 11(3): 14-19.

Masterson, A. & Cameron, A. (2002). The influence of professional and statutory bodies on decision-making. In A. Young & M. Cooke (eds.). *Managing and implementing decisions in health care*. London: Bailliere Tindall 27-45.

Reinicke, W. (1998). Globalization and public policy: an analytical framework. In W. Reinicke (ed.) *Global public policy*. Brookings Institution Press 52-74.

References

Casey N. (1996). Editorial. *Nursing Standard* Oct 2, 11(2): 1.

Darzi, A.(2008). *High Quality Care for All, NHS next stage review final report. London:* DH.

Department of Health (2007a). *Choosing Health Progress Report*. London: DH.

Department of Health (2007b). *Developing key roles for nurses and midwives - a guide for managers*. London: DH.

Department of Health (2007c). *Facing the future: A review of the role of health visitors*. London: DH.

Department of Health (2008). *NHS next stage review: Our vision for primary and community care*. London: DH.

Department of Health (2009a). *Creating an innovative culture. Guidance for strategic health authorities (SHAs): new duty to promote innovation*. London: DH.

Department of Health (2009b). *NHS Constitution*. London: DH.

Department of Health (2009c). *Quality reporting in 2008-09 Annual Reports and Accounts: A consultation for NHS foundation trusts and NHS organizations in East of England*. London: DH.

Department of Health (2009d). *Tackling Health Inequalities: 10 Years On. A review of developments in tackling health inequalities in England over the last 10 years*. London: DH.

Department of Health (2009e). *Transforming Community Services: Ambition, Action, Achievement Transforming Services for Acute Care Closer to Home*. London: DH.

Department of Health (2009f). *Transforming Community Services: Enabling new patterns of provision*. London: DH.

Department of Health — CNO'S Directorate (2006). *Modernising nursing careers setting the direction*. London: DH.

Flory, D. (2009). *The Quarter*. London: DH, Quarter 1 2009/10.

Health Improvement Analytical Team — Monitoring Unit (2009). *Health Profile of England 2008*. London: DH.

HM Government (2004). *Choosing health. Making healthy choices easier*. London: HM Government, Cm 6374.

HM Government (2009). *Working Together — Public Services on your side*. London: Her Majesty's Stationery Office.

International Council of Nurses (2008). *Participation of Nurses in Health Services Decision-making. Policy Development Position Paper*. Geneva: ICN. http://www.icn.ch/PS_D04_ParticipationDecisionMaking.pdf last accessed 26/04/09.

Maslin-Prothero S. & Masterson A. (2002). Power, Politics and Nursing in the United Kingdom. *Policy, Politics & Nursing Practice*. 3 (2): 108-117.

Maslin-Prothero, S; Jones, K. & Masterson, A. (2008). Four parts or one whole: the National Health Service (NHS) post devolution. *Journal of Nursing Management* 16: ,662-672.

Nursing and Midwifery Council (2008). *Confirmed principles to support a new framework for pre-registration nursing education*. London: NMC.

Secretary of State for Health (2009). *The Government's Response to the Health Select Committee Report on Health Inequalities*. London: TSO, Cm 7621.

The European Parliament and the Council of the European Union (2001).

Directive 2001/19/EC of the European Parliament and of the Council of 14 May 2001 amending Council Directives 89/48/EEC and 92/51/EEC on the general system for the recognition of professional qualifications and Council Directives 77/452/EEC, 77/453/EEC, 78/686/EEC, 78/687/EEC, 78/1026/EEC, 78/1027/EEC, 80/154/EEC, 80/155/EEC, 85/384/EEC, 85/432/EEC, 85/433/EEC and 93/16/EEC concerning the professions of nurse responsible for general care, dental practitioner, veterinary surgeon, midwife, architect, pharmacist and doctor. Strasburg: European Parliament.

The European Parliament and the Council of the European Union (2003). The European Qualifications (Health Care Professions) Regulations 2003. Strasburg: European Parliament.

World Health Organization (1987). *Leadership in nursing for Health for All: A challenge and Strategy for Action*. Tokyo Japan: WHO 7-11.

Part 3

Key skills for nurses delivering the new public health agenda

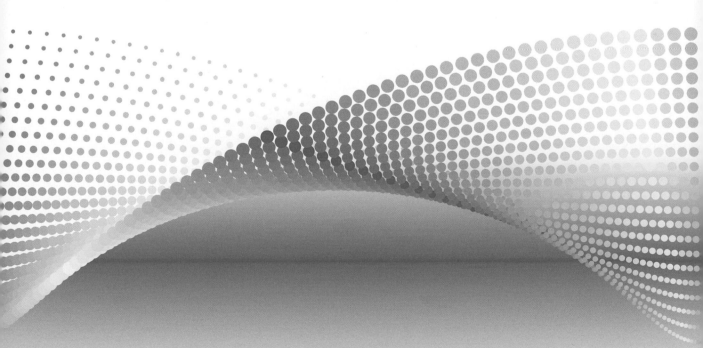

Chapter 9

Health needs assessment: caring for the individual and the population

Maria Joyce, Tracy Pilcher and Dianne Ramm

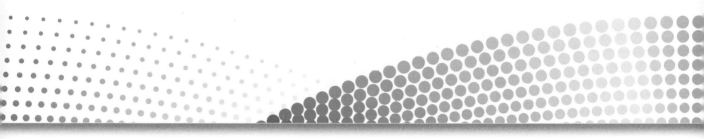

Content

Introduction

A full understanding of individual and community needs must be acquired to achieve a level of service that satisfactorily meets the needs of the public (DH, 2007). In order to provide effective health care, health needs assessment can occur at a population or individual level. At an individual level it can occur through the process of history taking and physical assessment, which will ensure that the individual's health needs are assessed, and at a community level tools such as health needs assessment (HNA) can support the assessment of health needs of the wider community. This chapter will start by looking at the process of assessment of an individual patient, and will explore the key skills required by the nurse in Section One. It will then move on to address health needs assessment at a wider level through the exploration of the health needs assessment at a community population level in Section Two (pages 113 onwards).

Section One: Conducting a nursing assessment of an individual patient

Individual nursing assessment

The aim of a general nursing assessment is to identify the individual health and social care needs of the patient (Peate, 2007). It is the first stage of the nursing process, in which the nurse and patient work together to solve problems and make decisions in a holistic, individualized way, thus avoiding a **task-orientated approach** (Peate, 2007). Patient assessment is a complex activity, in which the nurse utilizes a range of inter-personal and communication skills in order to establish a therapeutic dialogue with the patient, gently probing for further information when necessary, and signalling the need to move on when the conversation in one area is exhausted.

Principles of taking a history

Bickley (2007) refers to the health history as a conversation with a purpose. Whilst undertaking a health history, the practitioner is seen to draw on many of the interpersonal skills that they have developed and used in everyday practice, but with unique and important differences. Within the everyday world of the health care practitioner the conversation is centred upon their own needs and preferences. However, in the professional world the conversation is focused on improving the health and well-being of the patient. This conversation has three purposes; to gather information, to offer information, and to establish a supportive and trusting relationship (Bickley, 2007).

The skills usually associated with interviewing are therefore of equal relevance and importance in the context of assessment (Peate, 2007). The assessment process should not be reduced to a 'tick box' exercise, in which the patient is subject to repetitive questioning, with the nurse merely recording the 'answers'. An experienced assessor will discreetly record responses as the discussion progresses, either electronically or in handwriting, but will not slavishly adhere to a particular format, or list of questions, as this would represent a ritualistic and service-led, rather than patient-centred approach (Walsh and Ford, 1992).

When approaching the patient, Cox (2004) suggests that the nurse should put the patient at ease by adopting a friendly and confident manner, and should always greet the patient using their formal title such as 'Good morning Mrs Green' until the patient has given the practitioner the permission to use a less formal title. She goes on to suggest that when first greeting the patient the nurse should shake the patient's hand, or hold the patients hand. Listening carefully and not interrupting the patient help to demonstrate respect (Peate, 2007). The assessment should be conducted in a professional, non-judgemental manner, using language that the patient readily understands, free from jargon and medical terminology (Bach and Grant, 2009: NMC, 2009). This aids communication, the aim being to facilitate a rapport in which sensitive topics can be raised '...in an atmosphere of trust and confidentiality' (Pierce, et al., 2001:594).

Principles of assessment

According to Baid (2006), inspection is the first phase of the physical assessment, which starts the moment contact is made. As the patient walks into the room the nurse is using his/her assessment skills to begin to build up a picture of the patient. By using their assessment skills the nurse is able to observe for signs such as the patients posture, gait, whether they are able to move freely, or whether they are demonstrating signs of pain. Listening to the patient speaking will reveal important information about the patients' neurological and respiratory function. Baid (2006) suggests that during the initial inspection of the patient, the nurse should pay attention to the overall appearance of the patient, including their mood, alertness, behaviour, signs of pain, distress or confusion. If a neurological impairment is suspected the nurse should then go onto to undertake a fuller assessment using a tool such as the **Glasgow Coma Score (GCS)**.

In the community setting, several visits to the home environment or clinic may be required before a patient feels comfortable enough to discuss personal or potentially embarrassing issues causing them concern, which may adversely affect their health and well-being. Although this process may appear time consuming, the nurse can establish valuable relationships with patients and carers during this period, which enables the development of a more individualized plan of care (Pritchard, 1999).

Nursing problems may raise complex issues for the patient in relation to the acceptability of treatment options and consequently, there is no one 'correct answer'. Time taken during the assessment process will promote a greater insight and understanding of the person's daily life, routines and preferences, enabling the nurse to suggest timely and individualized support and care, in tune with a patient's circumstances. For example, a middle-aged lady with venous ulceration of her lower limb may be advised to elevate the limb and rest. However, she may also be the main carer for her frail, elderly husband who has severe dementia. When there are a variety of possible options available, it will take time to learn about the family, their perceptions and attitudes towards, for example, respite/day care or help in the home, in order to assist them appropriately (Bryans and McIntosh, 1996).

Interventions or services which may be welcomed and appropriate at one juncture may not be deemed acceptable at another. As the quality of the data obtained is dependent on the therapeutic relationship which gradually develops between the patient and the nurse, assessment is best viewed as an ongoing process. This 'continuous nature' of community nursing assessment has been acknowledged previously in the literature (Bryans and McIntosh, 1996:28). The information gathered during assessment will include subjective experiences or phenomena experienced by the patient, (Walker, 2004) in addition to measurable, objective data.

Completion of the assessment tool or form per se, does not represent the conclusion of the assessment. Once the data is collected and incorporated together with any relevant nursing observations and the results of medical tests/investigations, the nurse will review this complex, (and sometimes conflicting), information in its entirety, and make '...professional knowledge and experienced based interpretations' (Rose, 1994:29). This is the stage within the nursing process where the nursing diagnosis is made (Peate, 2007).

Principles of decision-making

It is then possible for the nurse to work collaboratively with the patient to prioritize the issues identified and together agree a plan of care to meet the patient's health and social care needs. Prioritization is important as the patient may have been attempting to cope with a particular problem for a long time, but has chosen to seek assistance at this specific point e.g. the need to address severe urinary urgency prior to taking a once-in-a-lifetime holiday. It is helpful, therefore, to establish what has triggered the referral, and to consider this first, as the patient's motivation to improve their health will then be at the optimum level.

The nurse will draw on the contemporary evidence base, sharing this information with the patient (Sackett, et al., 1996), thereby enabling them to make informed choices and decisions about the care that they will receive. This may include the provision of specific nursing interventions, health promotion advice, and/or the individual's referral options — the nurse using his/her knowledge and experience of local services and organizations where appropriate, to aid in this process.

Decision-making may take place over an extended period: it is therefore both challenging and stimulating and can only meet the patients' needs when the patient and their family remain at the centre of their care.

It is essential to give patients the information they require, at the correct level, in order for them to take control of the decision-making process, a particularly important concept when they are considering making changes in their behaviour designed to improve their health (Rollnick, et al., 2000). This is consistent with the aims of the **Expert Patient Programme**, (DH, 2006), which acknowledges that patients know the most about their own multiple pathologies and individual coping strategies.

The importance of the assessment process is therefore evident, as nurses assume increasing autonomy in relation to their professional roles in prevention, diagnosis and treatment.

Effectiveness

In 1999, the Audit Commission investigated the effectiveness of the care provided in relation to two major community nursing issues, continence care and leg ulcer management. The report concluded that '...comprehensive and accurate assessment is a major determinant of successful patient care' (Audit Commission, 1999:3). Thus, nurses who are appropriately educated and competent to perform advanced level assessments, working together with their medical colleagues to diagnose and to initiate appropriate treatments, can therefore substantially improve health and social care outcomes for patients.

More recently, community nurses are responding to demographic changes and the increasing numbers of people living longer, many of those with long-term conditions by developing advanced skills in physical assessment, associated with the concept of 'case management' (Baid, et al., 2009). This educational preparation enables the skilled and experienced community nurse to identify and respond rapidly to any deterioration in their patients, reducing unnecessary hospital admissions and maintaining patients where they most often wish to be — within their own homes.

Specialist assessment or referral

Throughout the assessment process, the nurse seeks to identify areas where a specialist assessment may be appropriate, that is, a positive response to a particular question will 'trigger' the need to perform a further, more specific assessment or initiate onward referral. Whether the nurse personally conducts these additional assessments, or alternatively, refers the patient, with their permission, to a specialist practitioner, will depend on the nurse's level of educational preparation, competency and also on local policy. However, it is essential that the nurse is aware of the significance of these specific 'trigger' areas, including how and when to refer for specialist support and advice.

Nursing Practice box

Where a patient suggests that they are not adhering to specific health promotion messages, for example, in relation to dietary intake, the nurse can offer reassurance that he/she will be non-judgmental and deal sensitively with the issues discussed. It is helpful to emphasize that it is much easier to provide options and choices designed to meet their needs where the patient provides accurate information. Both parties are 'on the same side' in this, having an interest in maintaining and improving the health of the patient (Rollnick, et al., 2000:57). This mutual aim can therefore, be openly acknowledged.

It is easy to be tempted to give health education advice during the assessment, especially if given an apparent cue by the patient e.g. 'I know I should stop smoking...' or 'I've heard I should drink cranberry juice'. However, it is inadvisable to do this until the assessment is complete, as not only is it extremely time consuming (so the assessment will overrun) but more importantly, the priorities for care may prove rather different when the full picture is known.

The assessment format and nursing models

Historically, many general assessment tools used in the community have been based on the Roper, Logan and Tierney model for nursing (Roper, *et al.*, 1996). This model has been used as a valuable framework for care delivery in many clinical care contexts, used also for teaching and learning in order to promote a holistic approach (Holland, 2004).

This model may be particularly suited to the community health care setting, due to its emphasis on the need to identify potential problems, maintain health and prevent disease. It therefore explicitly recognizes the role of the nurse as a teacher in public health (Holland, 2004).

The model recognizes many factors influencing the way that we choose, or are able to live, our daily lives. These are identified as biological, psychological, sociocultural, environmental and politico-economic (Roper, *et al.*, 1996). Within this model, the person's individuality forms the basis for this conceptualization of nursing, with twelve areas being described as 'Activities of Living' (ALs):

- Maintaining a safe environment,
- Communicating,
- Breathing,
- Eating and drinking,
- Eliminating,
- Personal cleansing and dressing,
- Controlling body temperature,
- Mobilizing,
- Working and playing,
- Expressing sexuality,
- Sleeping,
- Dying.

Roper, *et al.*, 1996

The ALs are influenced by the degree of dependence or independence the patient exhibits in carrying out these functions and also, where the person is on the lifespan. The nurse's role is to establish where the patient has a problem or potential problem, in performing one or more of these activities, and needs support in some way, whether or not this is currently provided. Thus, the ALs within the model may be used to provide a framework for the general assessment process, although their interrelatedness is explicitly recognized (Roper, *et al.*, 1996).

In recent times, the 'headings' used for the general assessment documentation have become increasingly 'user-friendly' with ALs not immediately relevant in all cases e.g. dying, being omitted. Specific concepts, perceived as being of vital importance in their own right, such as 'spiritual needs' and 'pain' may have been substituted in some assessment tools for local use.

As integrated community nursing teams increasingly access patient records electronically, there may be a move towards the standardization of general assessment templates in the future. However, the tool selected merely needs to facilitate the accurate recording of the comprehensive information obtained via the assessment process in a systematic, logical manner, for later retrieval and analysis. It is helpful if the format chosen incorporates areas for the documentation of free text, as this provides the opportunity for the nurse to individualize the information to that specific patient, and to their unique circumstances.

The formats used will doubtless continue to develop, with different terminology being utilized to suit local needs and preferences. However, it is helpful to keep in mind the model's fundamental concept of the independence/dependence continuum (Roper, *et al.*, 1996), together with the influences directly impacting on each area described earlier, in order to avoid the potential risk of adopting a rather one-dimensional, reductive approach to patient assessment.

Other models for nursing e.g. Orem's model for self-care (Orem. 1995) may be successfully employed to enhance the patient experience and promote the required holistic, patient-centred approach described (Peate, 2007).

The section relating to assessment of a patient in the community environment, which follows, is designed to provide useful insights into the initial assessment process for undergraduate student nurses, to aid them in developing their own skills in general nursing assessment. It is not designed to be exhaustive, as each individual assessment process will be unique. Any attempt to identify each and every likely permutation would risk 'spelling out so much it overwhelms' (Benner, 2001:242), rather than representing a useful starting point.

The following assessment process would be used in instances where a patient is referred to the community nursing team for the initial assessment of, for example, a patient with multiple sclerosis who has developed pressure damage to a heel, or a gentleman who has an indwelling urinary catheter for bladder cancer, discharged home for palliative care. However, the principles of holistic assessment described will be applicable to a variety of health care settings.

The assessment process: setting the scene

The assessment will begin with the introductions, the nurse 'setting the scene' for the assessment by ensuring the patient's physical comfort and privacy (Bach and Grant, 2009; DH, 2001a). Patient identification information will be taken, and their preferred style of address established.

It is helpful to explain that the aim is to establish what is currently happening for them, from their own perspective and give an indication of how long this will take. The patient's expectations regarding the outcome of the assessment process can also be explored at this point, as these may or may not be realistic and achievable.

The patient should be given the opportunity to decide who, if anyone, they wish to be present whilst the assessment takes place. The nurse may help further by suggesting some of the more personal topic areas that will be considered, and allowing the patient to reflect for a few moments, preferably on their own, in order for them to make a decision, free of pressure or coercion.

The nurse should be aware that everyone's relationships are unique —a person described as 'a neighbour' may be the patient's most close confidante and friend, sharing all the ups and downs of their everyday lives. The patient may therefore value their neighbour's presence. Alternatively, neighbours may be on nodding terms only, perhaps just taking in one another's post. It is essential therefore, not to make assumptions about the perceived closeness of a relationship.

Similarly, all families are different and subject to their own internal histories and changing dynamic. Where one mother may strongly express her wish to have her son or daughter present during the assessment, another may be appalled by the idea.

It is good practice to seek verbal consent for the assessment and formally record that this has been obtained, (or the opportunity for an assessment declined), whether or not the documentation used specifically requests this. A summary of these discussions and the agreed outcome should appear in the patient records, in line with best practice on seeking consent (DH, 2009) and record keeping (NMC, 2009).

Where there are barriers to communication, the patient's individual needs should be considered to optimize the quality of the information obtained (NMC, 2008a). For a patient with mild dementia, this may involve arranging the assessment when the patient's main carer is available and at a time of day when they are most likely to be most lucid and orientated.

If the nurse and patient are experiencing problems in understanding one another, an interpreter acceptable to the patient should be provided, to enable the patient to actively participate

in their assessment (Bach and Grant, 2009). If a patient uses sign language, such as **Makaton**, again an interpreter will be needed (DH, 2001a). Specialist speech and language therapists may also be able to provide assistance (DH, 2001a).

Additionally, there should be a discussion around the confidentiality of the information disclosed, including who will have access to it, under what circumstances, and detailing the information governance issues surrounding its storage and transmission, including the exceptions to the usual legal requirements e.g. where abuse is alleged or the law requires it (NMC, 2009).

Nursing observations including the vital signs

Examination of the vital signs refers to measuring the blood pressure, heart rate, respiratory rate and temperature. Other observations, including urinalysis, height and weight, are usually taken and recorded during the initial assessment process in order to identify any abnormalities and establish a baseline for future reference. Performing a baseline physical assessment and being able to differentiate normal from abnormal findings is one of the most important roles for contemporary health care practitioners (Baid, 2006; West, 2006: Docherty, 2002). Performing an accurate and timely baseline assessment will ensure practitioners are aware of when the patient's condition changes. Where any reading or measurement is outside normal limits this fact, together with any action taken, should be documented in the nursing notes (Hutson and Millar, 2009).

As discussed previously, nursing observation is a continuous process and is not restricted to the taking of physiological measurements. It involves monitoring the person's appearance, assessing their movement from the moment they walk in for any signs of limitations, and their demeanour, including facial expression and non-verbal communication for the presence of pain or distress, anxiety or agitation. The monitoring associated with nursing observations necessarily involves 'being there' with, and for the patient, which in itself is a valuable source of comfort (Burrows and Baillie, 2009).

Once the assessment is complete, the nurse should ensure that they record their findings in an accurate and precise manner into the patient's health care record.

The documentation used for assessment may include a list of acceptable abbreviations, approved via local clinical governance procedures. Abbreviations used frequently in nursing practice often relate to vital signs and may include BP (Blood Pressure), T (Temperature), P (Pulse) and R (Respirations). The use of abbreviations should however, be kept to an absolute minimum within health care records (NMC, 2009).

The interpretation of the significance of the clinical findings will result in either the recognition of the abnormality by the

---

Box 9.1 Setting the scene: summary

- Introduction,
- Confirm patient's expectation of assessment,
- Does the patient wish to have someone present?
- Seek and record verbal consent for the assessment,
- Recognize and respond to patient's individual communication needs,
- Discuss confidential nature of assessment and records made.

health care practitioner or the development of a differential diagnosis, depending on the role and skills and competencies of the individual undertaking the examination (Baid, 2006). Whilst some health care practitioners role will be focused on the identification of abnormal findings, and then referral to other members of the health care team. Health care practitioners working in autonomous roles will have the necessary knowledge base and professional responsibility to act independently on their physical assessment findings.

Allergies

Assessment forms generally prompt the nurse to enquire about any allergies or allergic responses the patient might have had in the past, whether related to food, sticking plasters, animal dander or medications prescribed or purchased over the counter (OTC). Patients may state that they have an allergy, when this may more accurately be described as an intolerance or sensitivity, but nevertheless this should be recorded, as their response may worsen with repeated exposure to the allergen/antigen.

The patient should be asked what happens when they eat that particular food or take/are given the medication. Where the patient suggests that this reaction is potentially serious, and 'shock' or 'anaphylaxis' have been experienced in the past, the nurse should not only record the information, but also ensure that it is communicated to the wider health care team.

Medications

All current medications, including those prescribed or purchased over the counter (OTC), including dietary supplements, herbal and any complementary medicines should be recorded. Bickley (2007) suggests that a drug history includes information about the drug name, dose, route and frequency of medications. It is essential to identify what the patient is actually taking and cross-reference this against their current medical and nursing prescriptions to identify any discrepancies.

The prescription of four or more medications (polypharmacy) is a particular risk factor in the development of drug interactions in older people. Polypharmacy develops over time, often with medications being added to counter side effects caused by others, or specific medication not being discontinued when no longer required (DH, 2001b).

It is helpful to ask the patient to see their medication and to review this together. In this way, it is easier to assess whether the patient has developed some form of logical system to prompt them to take each medication at the appropriate time, or alternatively, whether they could be helped to achieve this. Patients may use a box with individual compartments (purchased from the pharmacist) or utilize a simple tick list which means that, should they be unsure, they can check when their last dose was taken and when the next is due.

Practices such as opening capsules or grinding tablets up may be volunteered, so the nurse can identify the need for medications that are easier to swallow. Where patients administer their own insulin or other medication, any issues or concerns the patient has in relation to storage, injection technique and disposal can be revisited and addressed.

Patients may accumulate excess stock of a particular drug because they have stopped taking it or experienced side effects, which they have not reported. The reasons why particular medications proved unsuitable or unacceptable should be discussed, as the patient may have legitimate concerns or, alternatively, inaccurate health beliefs about a particular medication, which could usefully be explored.

Where contraindications to the prescribed medicine are discovered or where the medicine is deemed, following assessment, to be no longer suitable, the nurse must contact the prescriber without delay (NMC, 2008b).

Although time consuming, the nurses' role in providing skilled and effective communication about medications is appreciated and valued by patients, increasing their knowledge and compliance (Keleher, *et al.,* 2009).

> ### Box 9.2 Nursing observations: summary
>
> - Record vital signs (blood pressure, heart rate, respiratory rate and temperature),
> - Record baseline observations (including urinalysis, height and weight),
> - Note general appearance,
> - Establish if patient has allergies and if appropriate communicate it to the wider health care team,
> - Review medications both prescribed and those purchased over the counter:
>   - Note the drug name, dose, route and frequency of medications,
>   - Identify any issues with adherence,
>   - Identify any issues with self administration,
>   - Identify any side effects or contraindicators. If appropriate communicate with the prescriber.

Medical and surgical history

Assessment formats often include a check list, detailing the main long-term conditions, to enable the nurse to place a tick besides any which are medically confirmed e.g. cancer, cerebrovascular disease, neurological disease, osteo/rheumatoid arthritis, renal, dermatological and endocrine disorders. It is helpful to establish whether the patient has regular contact with health care professionals and the amount and frequency of hospital admissions within the last 12 months. It is necessary to establish whether there is a family history of particular conditions or illnesses which may be relevant to the patient's current health and well-being (Peate, 2007). The purpose of the family history is to learn about the health status of the patient's blood relatives and immediate family, the presence of diseases with hereditary tendencies, and sources of physical, emotional, or economic support or stress within the family structure (Wilkins *et al.*, 2000).

Any surgical operations should be noted, particularly where they may have relevance to the presenting problem(s) and any complications which may have arisen. The patient's understanding of their current problem(s), (the reason for this assessment), should be recorded, as this may provide clues regarding their insight into the problem/condition, their coping strategies and their motivation to consider changes in their health related behaviour in the future.

Price *et al.* (2000) suggest that it is good practice to start with a broad or open question, to give the patient the opportunity to put problems into his or her own words. For example 'In what way do you feel worse today?' The answer that the patient gives is described as the 'presenting complaint'. The presenting complaint should only be a few words, such as headache or laceration to the shin. Price *et al.* (2000) identify that if there is more than one presenting complaint these should be listed in turn.

The complaints can be ordered by time, which emphasizes the pattern of symptoms and by severity. Price *et al.* (2000) suggest that it is useful to make this list during the first time that the practitioner hears the patient's account, and this list should be confirmed with the patient, before the practitioner moves on to ask more closed types of questions. If an important symptom is not present then this 'negative finding' should also be recorded and communicated.

> **Box 9.3** Medical and surgical history: summary
>
> - History of long-term conditions,
> - Family history,
> - History of surgical operations,
> - The patient's current problem(s), and the reason for this assessment,
> - Presenting complaint:
>   - time,
>   - severity,

Social history

The nurse will ascertain who the patient lives with, any dependents, whether they have a partner, and gain an understanding of their immediate relationships and extended family networks, particularly where relatives have caring responsibilities. Any difficulties experienced in, for example, their relative or friend providing, or the patient accepting, this care should also be identified.

The tenure regarding accommodation should be documented, for example whether the patient lives in their own home, council or housing association property, or rents from a private landlord. The patient may be receiving residential or nursing care in a care home or alternatively, be currently homeless or temporarily living in a hostel. It is useful to record the particular type of accommodation as this may be useful in considering potential access or mobility problems e.g. bungalow or ground floor level flat, three storey house with stairs or care home with lifts to all floors.

> **Box 9.4** Social history: summary
>
> - Family relationships,
> - Social relationships,
> - Carers,
> - Accommodation.
>
>   Ability to maintain independence in everyday living (see Activities of Daily Living)

Physical examination

Undertaking a comprehensive health history and the subsequent examination of the patient is a developing role for health care practitioners working in a variety of different roles and practice settings. The level of physical examination performed will, therefore depend on locally agreed policy/protocols, the educational preparation required to undertake this role and that person's individual skills and competencies.

The information gathered during the health history will allow the appropriately trained health care practitioner to decide which body systems to examine, as well as the extent of the investigations. A focused examination will be carried out if the health history suggests that only a specific area of the body requires examination. Alternatively, some clinical situations may require the health care practitioner to undertake a more indepth examination.

Patients may view the physical elements of the assessment with some anxiety, as the process of examining the patient may make the patient feel vulnerable, as they are physically exposed and apprehensive about possible pain (Bickley, 2007). It is important that the health care practitioner is aware of this, and undertakes the examination in a manner which minimizes these feelings.

The activities of daily living
Maintaining a safe environment

This activity of living may include the financial welfare of the patient, for example their ability to provide for their family, to heat the house and pay the bills following a change in circumstances as a consequence of long-term illness. Community nurses are uniquely placed to identify eligible people who may not be claiming their full benefit entitlements (Hoskins and Smith, 2002).

Additional areas for consideration may include the identification of potential hazards within the home — a lack of aids, such as grab rails and ramps to promote safe movement or the presence of high kerbs, steps or the absence of a downstairs bathroom or toilet facilities to promote health and hygiene. It is helpful to know whether the patient has, and uses, a body-worn alarm which may be triggered to summon help in the event of a fall in their home or garden.

Where moving and handling is identified as problematic, or representing a risk to the patient or their carers, a moving and handling risk assessment should be completed (Johnson, 2005). Referral for an occupational therapy assessment may be considered, to promote independent living. This inter-professional collaboration ensures that the patient is provided with the appropriate community equipment such as profiling beds, hoists, transfer boards and slide sheets.

Additionally, an occupational therapist may be able to arrange for adaptations to the patient's home, such as ramps, grab rails and stair lifts to promote their mobility and reduce the risk of trips and falls. It is necessary to establish therefore, whether these measures have been considered previously and declined, or whether the need is more recent and as yet, unexplored.

Communicating

This section relates to communication via speech, and potential barriers including language, but also to the senses of hearing and sight. Any impairment and the aids used by the patient to assist them in communicating, such as hearing aids or glasses for reading, together with the effectiveness of these, should be recorded. If the patient is registered as blind, or partially sighted, this should be noted.

This area also includes cognition — whether the patient has a learning difficulty or dementia, for example and how this affects their daily life. Any particular, individualized methods for communicating should be documented, such as signing e.g. Makaton, cards incorporating symbols or pictures, the use of high technology aids.

Breathing

Breathing is essential for life itself, facilitating the exchange of oxygen for carbon dioxide and helping to maintain homeostasis. It follows, therefore that any difficulties in breathing may impact upon the individual's ability to maintain their independence in everyday living.

During assessment, it may become evident that the patient is experiencing problems with breathing. How severe is this? Does the patient have difficulty in breathing, on speaking or only on physical exertion? Is the colour of their skin pink and healthy and well-perfused with blood, or are their lips and extremities cyanosed? Are there any sounds associated with the patient's breathing, such as an audible wheeze on inspiration or expiration? Does the patient appear to be in pain or discomfort on breathing and is this positional? These questions can be answered by the nurse observing the patient during the early stages of the assessment.

If the patient has a diagnosed medical problem affecting their breathing, it is necessary to establish who they have seen previously, their diagnosis and current prescribed care. The conversation though should not merely focus on what the patient's medical team has established, as that will be available in the medical records. The nurse needs to investigate instead, the effect their problem has on the patient's quality of life and what specific activities the patient cannot now perform without assistance. Where oxygen is provided for home use, it is necessary to ensure that the prescription is fulfilling the patient's needs and that there are no problems with accessing and using vital equipment, such as nasal cannulae and/or masks.

In addition to recording breaths per minute, the depth and regularity of their breaths, and whether the accessory muscles of respiration are employed, are also important observations (Hutson and Millar, 2009). Where there is cause for concern, including a new problem, or deterioration in a known condition, such as an increasingly productive cough, the nurse should seek medical assistance urgently.

Where the patient had not thought about their breathing until mentioned by the nurse, or alternatively, their breathing is normal for them, the nurse can continue with the assessment.

It is useful to ask about smoking in relation to breathing and to record current smoking habits and patterns and to record this e.g. ex-smoker, non-smoker, smokes more than ten cigarettes per day. Where patients have attempted to stop smoking unsuccessfully in the past, the methods tried, including medication and any support accessed, either formal or informal, should be recorded. This will facilitate future discussions, for example, about smoking cessation, to be meaningful and individualized.

Eating and drinking

The nurse should identify the patient's nutritional intake and any factors that may affect the patient's ability to eat and drink, including their cultural and religious dietary observations (Staniland and Gascoigne, 2009), any history of eating disorders, malabsorption and/or problems with teeth, gums or dentures.

It is useful also to ascertain the patient's understanding in relation to a healthy diet, and not to use rhetorical questions, as these may both provide information and suggest the anticipated response, for example: 'You know all about 'five a day'? This sort of questioning will result in the accumulation of inaccurate data, which fail to reflect the patient experience and are therefore, not meaningful.

If a patient is experiencing problems with shopping and cooking, the nurse should note this, as there may be options for the patient to consider, including the delivery of frozen, pre-prepared meals.

Patient perceptions around diet are important, as patients with diabetes mellitus may believe, for example, that they need to buy foods specifically labelled 'diabetic', which are expensive and unnecessary. It is useful to explain to the patient that the discussion will focus on what is happening for them now, from their perspective, so that they know not to expect interpretation of the information during the assessment. In this context, it follows that there are no 'wrong answers', and the patient may be consequently reassured.

It is essential to establish whether the patient has recently gained or lost weight and, if so, whether this was intentional. Any change in appetite should also be identified. Their current weight and height should be recorded and their Body Mass Index (BMI) calculated, bearing in mind that a low body mass in old age is associated with an increased risk of morbidity and mortality (McCormack, 1997). For more detail on how to measure BMI, see Chapter 15, Tackling Obesity.

Nurses have a vital role to play in identifying people at risk of malnourishment and to then act on these findings (Marsh, 2009). Nutritional screening tools, such as the **Malnutrition Universal Screening Tool (MUST)** (Todorovic, *et al.*, 2003) are increasingly used during assessment to identify both obese and underweight adults, whether the initial contact is in the community or hospital setting.

Any artificial feeding such as supplements or the use of enteral feeding e.g. via Percutaneous Endoscopic Gastrostomy (PEG) should be documented, together with the current regime. It is useful to establish who administers the feed and ensure that they are confident in this and to record details of the dietician and the pharmacist providing support.

Where a patient has experienced a stroke, it is essential to enquire about any difficulties with swallowing, whether they are able to empty their mouth completely after eating and whether they received a specialist assessment e.g. from a physiotherapist or speech and language specialist. It is always helpful to establish the previous involvement of health care professionals (in any area of care), to promote continuity for the patient and minimize the duplication of services.

Where the patient has received, or is receiving chemotherapy, they may experience mouth ulceration or oral thrush. There will be occasions when oral care is of paramount importance — e.g. in terminal care or for patients who experience nausea and vomiting.

It is appropriate to ask about alcohol intake in order to establish whether the patient feels they already have an alcohol dependency, or may be at risk of developing a problem, in order that this may be pursued, and referral for specialist help offered.

Eliminating

This activity of daily living has the capacity to cause embarrassment, because it involves discussion of parts of the body and bodily processes which are usually deemed private, kept hidden and may also be perceived as not nice or dirty (Roe and May, 1999). The topic should therefore be explored with sensitivity and may be signposted beforehand, for example, by saying: 'I need to ask you about your routines in relation to your bladder and bowels now —is that ok?'

The purpose of this initial assessment is to establish whether or not the patient experiences any problems, so questions such as 'Do you have any difficulties with your waterworks/opening your bowels?' might prove helpful.

Where patients describe experiencing 'constipation' or 'diarrhoea', the meaning the patient attributes to this should be explored in detail. There may be differences between the definition that the patient uses, to that understood by the medical and nursing professions, leading to the potential for confusion in diagnosis. For example, faecal incontinence can be caused by severe impaction (i.e. constipation) with overflow (Nazarko, 2002). Should the term 'diarrhoea' be used by the patient and accepted without question, the opportunity to establish the correct diagnosis, educate the patient and prevent recurrence may be missed.

The use of the **Bristol Stool Form Scale** (Walker, 2009) is valuable, both in providing a useful frame of reference, and also, by its existence, serving to normalize a potentially embarrassing situation. It effectively legitimizes this discussion, assisting the patient to understand that such conversations are usual practice within the context of a nursing assessment.

The term 'incontinence' should be avoided as this has negative associations and may also be considered a taboo subject (Norton, 1996: Morris, 1999). Substituting euphemisms for incontinence are similarly unhelpful. 'Have you had any accidents?' can genuinely be misconstrued by the patient as meaning trips and falls. Instead, patients may feel more able to volunteer the information that they 'don't always get there in time', so this form of discussion, led by the nurse, may elicit factual information, perhaps for the first time.

Where patients experience involuntary leakage from their bladder or bowel, this should trigger referral for further assessment aimed at the identification of the cause(s) and exacerbatory factors (Button et al., 1999: DH. 2000).

Where patients have already experienced difficulties and have been assessed by a Specialist Nurse, Physiotherapist, Urologist/Urogynaecologist/Colorectal surgeon for their continence or urology care, this should be documented. Any aids used to promote independence and maintain continence, including the use of commodes, raised toilet seats, grab rails and urinals (including the type) should be noted.

Appliances used to manage a pre-existing problem should also be recorded, including stoma appliances, urinary catheters (whether indwelling, supra-pubic, urethral, intermittent or stricture therapy), sheath systems and incontinence pads and whether these are purchased privately or provided by the NHS. Where a patient suggests that an indwelling urinary catheter is used purely for incontinence, it is best practice to discuss whether alternative forms of management have been tried, and to establish when their continence needs will be reassessed (DH, 2003).

Personal cleansing and dressing (including skin integrity)

This area involves an exploration of any difficulties the patient experiences in maintaining their hair, skin, teeth and nails to their own standard of personal cleanliness. There are many influences upon a person's attitudes towards their own cleanliness, including culture and religious beliefs. What is essential in assessment, is establishing whether the patient is currently independent in this care, and has a support system in place that they find acceptable (e.g. arranged privately or via social services) or whether any problems have not been previously addressed.

Where a patient has a known dermatological condition, such as eczema or psoriasis, the nurse needs to establish how this affects the patient's daily life, the clothing they choose to wear, treatments and any strategies the patient uses to reduce exacerbations. Any difficulty in maintaining healthy feet, including care of the toenails, should be noted and any podiatry involvement.

If a patient has a wound of any kind, including ulceration of the lower limb, surgical wounds, or those sustained following trauma, this requires the completion of a further, specialized wound assessment, which may also include maintaining a photographic record, in line with local policy. Where individual health care organizations have agreed referral criteria for

access to tissue viability specialist nurses, these should be followed to ensure consistent practice and optimize patient outcomes.

Where patients are experiencing pain associated with a wound, formal assessment including the use of a pain scale designed to elicit information about pain intensity is recommended (Bowers and Barrett, 2009).

All patients seen within their own homes should have a risk assessment performed by a nurse who is competent in recognizing the risk factors that contribute to the development of pressure ulcers and who can initiate and maintain correct and suitable preventative measures (NICE, 2003). The assessments or risk should be ongoing throughout the patient's episode of care, to include the visual inspection of the skin as frequently as the patient's condition requires.

Although risk assessment tools designed to identify patient at increased risk of pressure damage are often utilized during the assessment process e.g. Waterlow score (Waterlow, 1985), there is some debate about their predictive ability, and therefore the results obtained by their use should not replace clinical judgement (NICE, 2003).

Patients who are at risk of developing pressure damage include older people, pregnant women, those who are seriously ill, have impaired mobility (or who are completely immobile) and those wearing a prosthesis, plaster cast or body brace. Additionally, people who have neurological or nutritional compromise, are obese or have poor posture are at increased risk (RCN and NICE, 2005).

An individual's potential for developing ulcers may be further exacerbated by certain medications and the presence of moisture against the skin (NICE, 2003). The extrinsic risk factors to ulceration include pressure, friction and shear forces, which should, therefore, be identified during assessment, and eliminated or reduced (NICE, 2003).

Controlling body temperature

In health, an adult is independent in regulating their own body temperature, and is often unaware of the thermoregulatory systems in operation. However, in very young children these systems are immature, and in the elderly they may be less efficient, or alternatively, the potential for coping may be affected. This exposes these particular groups to the risks associated with extremes in temperature (Walker 2004).

The risk of hypothermia rises sharply in the winter months with the elderly being particularly vulnerable to the effects of poor housing, malnutrition and insufficient heat for their homes (Walker 2004). Reduced activity and physical fitness, the presence of long-term conditions and dementia or confusional states may all contribute to an inability to respond appropriately to changes in temperature (Herbert and Rowswell, 1992).

The nurse therefore needs to assess the patient's ability to cope with extremes of temperature and to establish whether they are particularly at risk. It is helpful to establish the patient's attitudes and beliefs about spending money on heating (Herbert and Rowswell, 1992) as this will influence their behaviour. Further areas for discussion include whether the patient has considered the benefits and grants they may be entitled to claim, for instance to provide loft and cavity wall insulation, whether they receive their annual vaccination against 'flu, establishing their level of social contact and their knowledge of the voluntary sector's contribution in providing advice about keeping warm in winter.

Mobilizing

This area focuses on whether or not a patient can walk unaided. Having knowledge of the patient's presenting complaint(s) and visiting them in their own home will provide clues such as the presence of a stair lift or grab rails. However, it is important to use open questions, such as: 'Tell me how you manage to get about with your hip as it is', in order to gain the patient's perspective. This may provide a more accurate picture, for example by eliciting the reason why they choose not to use a particular aid, rather than just the fact that they were once issued with one.

Where wheelchairs or walking aids, such as sticks or frames are used, it is useful to identify when they were provided, and whether their mobility has improved or deteriorated since. Referral for a specialist reassessment of their mobility may then be considered.

It is useful to explore how the patient's illness or condition is affecting the patient's lifestyle and what social activities, if any, it limits. Where immobility prevents the patient attending day centres or shopping, there may be sources of alternative transport available, including local provision of specialized taxi services for the elderly or specifically for wheelchair users. Additionally, the nurse can ensure that the patient is aware of local and national mobility schemes, providing access to car parking, some with a reserved space guaranteed and the use of a wheelchair or mobility scooter included.

Working and playing

Work is a meaningful, regular activity for which a person has a responsibility, indicating their status, purpose and providing a sense of achievement. It is not necessarily paid, but involves a measure of personal organization, social contact and daily structure (Whittam, 2004). In the context of this model, 'play' refers to activities which are pursued away from the work environment, such as sporting interests, hobbies and holidays.

During assessment, it is helpful to establish what the patient would normally do in relation to work and leisure activities and to assess whether these activities have been adversely affected. This is significant because patients may be at risk of adopting adverse recreational habits, such as poor diet and the increased risk of alcohol and recreational drugs where opportunities are restricted, for example when someone loses their employment due to ill health injury, redundancy or retirement (Whittam, 2004). Patients may also be at risk of psychological stress, anxiety and/or depression as they seek to cope with a new, and possibly enforced, situation.

Expressing sexuality

Historically, sexual expression may have been a neglected area during nursing assessment with nurses exhibiting ageist attitudes (Brogan, 1996). Elderly people in health and illness have a right to holistic care, and therefore to have their needs in relation to the expression of sexuality acknowledged (Webb, 1992).This is particularly so in relation to urology/continence where for example, indwelling urinary catheters may be used without due consideration of a person's sexual needs (Wilde, 2003).

In framing questions, sensitivity and tact are required. During the initial assessment, it is helpful to limit questions to those which may provide valuable information in relation to the presenting condition(s) and associated problems, as the relevance of this enquiry is readily apparent e.g. 'Does your indwelling catheter affect your sexual relationship at all?' The patient is then provided with an opportunity to discuss any issues or concerns. In this example, the subsequent discussion may be very fruitful, as alternative forms of bladder management, such as intermittent self-catheterization (ISC) may then be explored (Doherty, 2006).

Sexuality should perhaps be viewed in its wider context during a general nursing assessment, that is, to include sexual health, self esteem and the wider issues relating to body image, such as those which may be experienced post mastectomy or following amputation of a limb.

Sleeping

Sleep is rather akin to breathing in the healthy person—it is taken for granted until a problem manifests. The ability to sleep may be affected by a patient's health problems, including acute or chronic pain, stress, depression and/or anxiety (Jenkins, 2004).

On assessment it is helpful to identify the person's usual sleep habits and whether they employ specific strategies to aid them to sleep well, for example, by making sure the room is completely quiet and dark, reading a book or having a specific drink before bedtime.

It is necessary to establish whether the patient relies on medication and whether this is prescribed or OTC. The usual amount of hour's sleep can be recorded, which is of particular significance where this is disturbed by their needs in relation to another AL, for instance the need to empty the bladder during the night, or difficulty in breathing.

It is helpful to ask the patient to reflect on what was happening for them a around the time the problem started e.g. early morning waking, as this may help them to make associations between life events, or the commencement of new medication, and the onset of their symptoms.

Dying

As suggested earlier, the final act of living — that of dying — may be omitted from the assessment process, being deemed inappropriate in the majority of patient care episodes. However, Roberts (2004) suggests that this may deny the patient their opportunity to discuss any fears and real concerns in relation to dying, whatever their presenting illness or condition.

Where patients do have a terminal illness and commence the dying trajectory, palliative care aims to alleviate distressing symptoms and concentrate on enhancing the patient's quality of life. The nurse will therefore discuss the patient's care needs, including their preferences and choices, aiming to assist them as they move along the independence/dependence continuum. It is vital to establish whether the patient already has the support of the local Macmillan/palliative care team, Marie Curie nurses etc. and whether agreed management or clinical treatment plans and personal/preference plans are in place in line with the **Gold Standards Framework (GSF)** (National Gold Standards Framework Centre, 2006).

Towards the very end of a patient's life, that is, within the final forty-eight to seventy-two hours, the patient's multidisciplinary team may utilize the Liverpool Care Pathway (LVP), an integrated care pathway which provides guidance on, for instance, anticipatory prescribing, discontinuation of inappropriate interventions and comfort measures (NHS, 2009).

Spirituality has perhaps been viewed as relevant only in relation to suffering and the experience dying (Peate, 2007) when in reality, a sense of meaning is important to all of us throughout our lives. A patient's religious and/or spiritual belief systems may therefore be explored at any time during the assessment process. When faced with illness, our spiritual beliefs, including our purpose in life, and our hopes for the future can be threatened (Peate, 2007). Our needs in this area may consequently come to the fore.

If the subject of pain and/or discomfort is not discussed elsewhere in the assessment process, it should perhaps be explicitly raised to ensure that the patient has the opportunity to discuss any issues and concerns. Patients may experience physical, emotional and/or spiritual pain (Burrows and Baillie, 2009). During assessment a patient may, for example, share details of a recent personal bereavement, and this may affect their functioning in all aspects of their life, forming the focus around which the assessment pivots.

Summary of Section One: conducting an individual patient assessment

This chapter has so far considered individual patient assessment as a skilled process requiring considerable communication and collaboration between the patient and the nurse to be effective. Assessment represents therefore '...an inherently social, dynamic and interactive process' (Bryans and McIntosh, 2000:1245) in which both the patient and the nurse play an integral and vital part.

Having considered the comprehensive and holistic assessment of an individual patient, this chapter will now focus on the issues of importance in conducting an assessment of the health needs of a defined population.

Section Two: Health needs assessment of populations

Introduction

In the introduction to this chapter, we referred to the White paper **Our health, our care, our say** (DH, 2006). This paper set out a plan to improve the health and well-being of the population. The focus of this paper was on prevention of ill health and early intervention, patient choice, tackling inequalities and improving services with more support for people with long-term needs.

The paper recognized that whilst there has been progress in improving the health of some of the population, where patients live still has a major impact on health and the health care patients can expect to receive. It identified that health inequalities remained across social class, income groups and across different area of the country.

Provision of services to improve health are supported by effective health needs assessment which looks specifically at the health needs of the individual and communities (DH, 2000: DH, 2004), leading to more effective use of finances that will bring about real changes and improvement in public health. To identify these variations in an attempt to close the health gap, it is necessary to assess populations for their health status and the influences to their individual and collective health and well-being. This can be facilitated by undertaking health needs assessment.

So what is 'health needs assessment'?

Definition

Health Needs Assessment (HNA) is a process of identifying health needs either at individual level or community level to allow the planning and provision of services to improve health. Health needs assessment has been defined as:

'a systematic method for reviewing the health issues facing a population, leading to agreed priorities and resource allocation that will improve health and reduce inequalities'
HDA, 2005:3

Objective

Health needs assessment looks at a variety of features within a community group or population that are relevant to the health of that community. These may be needs that relate to physical illness and ill health. They may relate to housing, work or environmental concerns or even to issues arising relating to education provision.

These features can have a significant impact on individual health and well-being and are widely known as the determinants of health. They are illustrated in layers in the diagram by Dahlgren and Whitehead (1991) (see Chapter 14) with the individual at the centre and the influencing layers moving outward through to the wider societal influences.

The feature they have in common is that they all have the ability to impact on health at some level, in the present or in the future. They have been described as:

'those factors which must be addressed in order to improve the health of the population'
Billings. 2002:115

What is the purpose of 'Health Needs Assessment'?

Provision of resources

Health needs assessment has an essential role in supporting effective provision of resources, both physical and financial to appropriately identified communities. This means that resources are allocated to communities that need them most, and equally importantly, can receive the greatest benefit from these resources. These resources may be allocated geographically to the most socially deprived communities in line with data taken from deprivation indices (ID, 2000: IMD, 2004) but will still need a more exact form of planning to determine the type of actual service provision that is most appropriate and most acceptable at the point of delivery to patients.

Policy support

Health needs assessment has a much needed role in underpinning the shift of focus in health care provision from cure to prevention. It can identify where the health problems are most prevalent allowing early intervention through screening and health promotion to take place. Through this identification and targeted intervention, it supports the effective allocation of resources for improving individual health and lengthening life span. This makes the process meaningful for the community and it is reassuring for them to know that the process of HNA is being undertaken to measure health and identify health needs with the purpose of improving individual and/or community health. The interventions that come about following the process of HNA also ensure value for money for the public; the intervention has been planned to meet identified need, tailored to a specific community to bring about improvement in health.

Tool for gathering data

It has been recognized that there are insufficient mechanisms for PCTs and local authorities to gather reliable information relating to their populations despite being required to target these groups for health interventions (Wanless, 2004). Government policy, in addition to focusing on prevention rather than cure, is also driving a move from hospital to community based care amidst an environment of finite resources for the provision of health care. This necessitates the assessment of the health needs of individuals and communities through the use of a practical tool to gather information. This tool can be the method of health needs assessment. The information gathered through HNA, after analysis, will allow services to be commissioned to bring about beneficial changes to individual and population health.

Strengthening workforce

Recent key documents in health policy, have highlighted the need for a public health focused workforce, that is skilled, flexible and well resourced to underpin the move from acute hospital based care to care that is provided in the community (DH, 2004; DH, 2006). Similarly, a consultative green paper (DH, 2005) outlines the need for a health care service designed around the needs of the patients rather than the patients needs being forced to fit the services already provided. The focus is on improved choice and improving long term health with greater emphasis on health promotion, prevention of ill health and health support. Furthermore there are clear messages for improving public health in the interim report by Lord Darzi, **Our NHS, Our Future** (DH, 2007) where the six key goals for health improvement are linked to both social and behavioural factors. These social factors are known as the social determinants of health and are seen to be the factors that influence people's health (CSDH, 2005). The final report of Lord Darzi: **High quality: care for all** (DH, 2008) underpins these goals for improving health with plans for investment in well-being and prevention services.

The use of HNA for education

Learners in health and or social care are often asked to look at a group relating to their placement area. Practitioners employed in primary care may be required to investigate the area and the health of the population where they are based. This is intended to support them in both in becoming familiar with the area but also in developing the skills necessary to research and collate information which they can then draw on to plan services to address or meet identified need.

Determinants of health

The notion of health needs incorporates the wider social and environmental influences on health of individuals and populations, often known as the determinants of health. The well known model by Dahlgren and Whitehead (1991) (See Fig. 14.1) captures the Influences on health, describing them as socio-economic, cultural and environmental living and working conditions, social and community influences and influences brought about through individuals behavioural, genetic and lifestyle factors. The availability of good quality healthcare and access to services is also recognized in determining long-term health and influencing health outcomes.

Other models such as the one by Najman (2001) illustrate how the causal pathways originate from the social, cultural and economic characteristics of society, travelling through differing lifestyle/ behavioural options be they health enhancing or damaging, influenced by various genetic and constitutional factors to finally ending up as a particular vision of health whether for the individual or the population group.

These models illustrate how determinants of health influence individual health along the lifespan. The social position of the individual impacts or enhances their life chances, their development, their behaviour and their access to health education and available services for health.

Health needs

In relation to health need there are two main forms of interpreting health needs: objective and subjective.

Objective interpretation

This is when need is framed within the notion of universal concept and this can be through the perspective of another i.e. the health professional, the organization, the recognized expert.

Subjective interpretation

This is when need is judged by the individual and everyone has a right to have their health protected.

Approaches to defining and assessing need

Health needs are also defined as from a sociological, epidemiological, health economist or consumerist approach and all four of these accounts influence how need is assessed and then how services are targeted to meet the identified need.

Sociological account

Health needs can be described drawing on the typology presented in the seminal work of Bradshaw (1972) :

Felt need

This is defined by clients, patients, service users or communities in terms of what they feel they need or what they want. The difficulty may be that the notion of need could be inflated by unrealistically high expectations or Bradshaw (1994) suggests that individuals may not know what they need or may not wish to express their need.

Expressed need

This is often a felt need that is acted upon and turned into a demand. Patients may feel they need service provision and ask or demand that this is provided. Bradshaw (1994) suggests that not all felt needs are turned into expressed needs as some individuals do not have access to professionals who can influence services and others do not raise issues of concern, but accept whatever is offered to them.

Normative need

This is defined by the professional or expert. The need is measured against a standard set by the expert or associated professional body. The difficulty with this is the standard set rarely takes influencing factors on individual health into account and suggests that despite individuals being well paced to manage their own health, there are experts, more able and qualified to advise individuals how to manage their lifestyles. Experts by definition will have their own areas of expertise and subsequently their own ideas of prioritizing need, hence expert measurement of need can be subjective.

Comparative need

This is need that arises in comparison to other similar members of the community. It may be used to assess individuals for provision of services but comparative assessment is about comparing similar characteristics to ensure equitable provision and needs are not always easily measured against each other.

Epidemiological account

This account uses quantitative data on morbidity and mortality which allows measurement of ill health both in terms of lives lost and quality life years lost. It may also use population census data and data providing statistics on deprivation and determinants of health. The data may incorporate variables such as employment status, gender, ethnicity and single parent numbers and this information combined to give an overall score.

An epidemiological account interprets need not on the data outlining the size of the problem, but on the ability of the identified problem to be improved by intervention. The subsequent anticipated health gain can be represented in adding years to life (reducing premature mortality) and/or adding life to years (enhancing the quality of life and improving health).

The difficulties this presents are in that the data may be not fully accurate nor may it be complete, it may be out of date in relation to the problem and it may be subjected to bias because whoever commissioned the primary data collection and the purpose for which it was collected may not be the same as the purpose for which it is to be used secondarily.

Health economist account

This is need defined in the context of cost effectiveness, supply and demand. Often articulated as 'wants', 'demands' and 'preferences' and the focus is on gaining the greatest benefit for every pound spent and value for money. Resource allocation is the key issue and this is targeted at groups identified as 'at risk' and as a consequence is deemed to be cost effective health care intervention.

There are methodological and ethical difficulties in measuring life improvement and individual benefit identified (Bowling, 2004) in both examining methodology that can accurately measure survival and quality of life but also ethically determining the notion of quality of life.

Consumerist account

This more recent addition is a category that takes the view of the individuals and communities that use the services. It originally referred to an approach where individuals would be asked for their opinion on a particular service, with data collected through the form of survey or focus groups. However it may now be seen to include other groups form the local population such as interest groups which may in some way be seen as representative of public opinion. Recent government documentation, **Creating a Patient-Led NHS** (DH, 2005) highlighted the need for services to fit around the need of the patient rather than the patient being obliged to fit around the service provided for all. This was seen as instrumental in improving health and preventing ill health. The views and experiences of individual service users, carers, service user organizations, statutory and voluntary sector service providers are deemed valuable and essential in informing and shaping strategic development and planning of services.

Public health guidance for strengthening community engagement has been issued (NICE, 2008) to support those working with communities. The guidance outlines the ways in which differing levels of community engagement affect health both in the short and long term and how directly or indirectly this will shape the commissioning and delivering of services.

Undertaking health needs assessment

Who might undertake a HNA?

Health needs assessment can be undertaken by a wide variety of individuals, on behalf of a broad range of organizations. These extend from those employed at regional levels and local levels including nurses at all levels including chief nurses to health professionals, working in local trusts, including those employed within the local community and the voluntary sector. Health needs assessment therefore can potentially involve a wide team of participants and involvement of the public. It is essential that an easy to understand language is used, avoiding technical jargon and acronyms, in discussion and to describe the requests for information as the process moves through the varying stages.

Tools for undertaking HNA

There are a wide variety of tools that have been developed to enable health needs assessment to take place. Health needs assessment is not a single, one off, activity (Mitcheson, 2008) nor is it simple, but it is a purposeful activity which takes skill and understanding to gather and analyse the information that will shape service delivery. The skill in gathering the information is in understanding the complexity and care must be taken to avoid employing a mechanistic approach to HNA with too structured an instrument as this has been found to limit the successful identification of clients needs and prohibits clients participating fully in the process (Mitcheson and Cowley, 2003).

Client and service users input into HNA

There is strong emphasis placed on client participation by Cowley and Billings (1999) stating that the uniqueness of an individuals health dictates that it cannot be seen as a separate entity, it is unique to the individual. Building individual health capacity for health enhancement is identified as equally as important as ensuring resources are available. Links into personal empowerment and culturally shaped behaviours are also identified as enhancing health creating resources and improving public health (Cowley and Billings, 2001). This illustrates the necessity to assess health needs from a population based approach rather than adopting a top down directive of intervention, if potentially detrimental culturally shaped behaviour is to be addressed by interventions.

There are five steps that have been set out by (HDA, 2005:21):

Step 1: Getting started,

Step 2: Identifying health priorities,

Step 3: Assessing health priority for action,

Step 4: Planning for change,

Step 5: Moving on/ review.

Step 1: Getting started

- What population and why?
- Which population are you intending to assess?

The term population can refer to a group within a defined geographical area or a particular community, for example a group of patients attached to a GP surgery. It may be individuals who have been diagnosed with a certain condition or it may be users of a particular service.

What are you trying to achieve?

The rationale for choosing your population is crucial in assisting you to decide what you are trying to achieve and setting the boundaries for what you can hope to achieve. This can be supported by having clear aims and objectives from the beginning of what you hope to achieve through the health needs assessment. Your aims and objectives should also be examined in relation to their ability to be achieved through the health needs assessment of your chosen population. It may also be possible that another organization has already performed a level of assessment on this population and the results can be available to inform or influence your decisions.

Who needs to be involved?

For learners in health and social care and for staff employed in primary care, the purpose of performing a health needs assessment may be for the intention of enhancing their practice or for the purpose of educational assessment. Both of which can then be used to highlight identified need in an attempt to improve services.

For others it will be achieved through collective effort for a common purpose and will have a project leader to coordinate and manage the process. There may be a stakeholder group which will include representation from all groups involved and service users. If the health needs assessment is commissioned for organizational or policy purpose then the managers and policy makers will need to be involved in decision making.

Overall, those who need to be involved are the individuals that can assist you in investigating the health of the population and generate the required information.

What resources do I need?

Resources are varied and if you are performing the health needs assessment for your own work or the purpose of your educational programme, remember that time, even if it is your own, costs money and effort. Also you may have to travel to access the services or population you wish to investigate. Once there, will you see people in their own homes? (if applicable) or arrange for them to come to you and if so, who is funding this aspect of the project?

If it is a collective effort, then you need time, a place to meet, data recording and storage facilities and specialist skills in data analysis, interpretation and writing up findings. Backfill time at work for staff involved may also be a requirement to allow them to be released to work on the health needs assessment project. Finally the project needs to be cost analysed and the timescale planned accordingly to ensure successful completion of the project.

Step 2: Identifying health priorities

To identify the health priorities of your chosen population refer back to why you have chosen your population. This rationale, based on who you chose, why you chose them and what you hope to achieve, will influence your identification of health priorities. For example if you are looking at individuals who have been diagnosed with a certain condition or users of a particular service then you have a clear idea of what you are attempting to investigate in relation to that particular population.

Alternatively, if you are performing a health needs assessment for your own practice or educational assessment, then you may be looking at the bigger picture, from which the health priorities will evolve through the process of health needs assessment.

To enable you to build a picture of the population you may choose to perform a profile often known as community or population profiling. A community profile has been described as:

A comprehensive description of the needs of a population that is defined, or defines itself, as a community, and the resources that exist within that community, carried out with the active involvement of the community itself, for the purpose of developing and action plan or other means of improving the quality of life of the community.
Hawtin, *et al.,* 2007:11

This definition indicates that community profiling can be performed by the community rather than on the community by individuals and outside agencies. It can also be performed to build community capacity through the input of resources designed to develop, confidence, leadership and skills through collective effort. The community can work together to develop their individual and collective potential.

Profiling assists with the identification of health needs, through the identification and comparison of a wide range of health data and is a method through which needs are assessed (Billings in Cowley, 2002: 113 and 115).

There are a variety of methods suitable to support you in achieving your community profile and these depend again on your original rationale for your choice of population and what you are hoping to achieve. You may use primary data or secondary data. Primary data refers to data you collect for your specific purpose, such as holding focus groups or interviews with your chosen population to provide you with information to assist in health profiling. Whereas secondary data refers to data that is already available, gathered by someone else for a different purpose such as quantitative data found in census, health, housing, education and crime records or qualitative data such as reports or community responses to other initiatives.

Main features you will wish to consider are:

1. How many members make up your chosen population?
2. How you are going to define their actual location, be it geographical or attached to a fixed location/ organization.
3. Where you will be able to access available data about them, through the internet or by visiting local government offices or other agencies.
4. How similar are the group and do they have any differences?

You may wish to draw information to build the picture up further relating to housing, education, health services provision and access and other determinants of health.

Another method to assist you in building a picture of your population would be through the process of participatory rapid appraisal. This approach is rapid as the method suggests and takes place over a short period of time often two to three weeks. In this time the method attempts to engage with the chosen population through a variety of methods such as interview, focus groups, observation, often supported by secondary data. This data is then assembled, analysed and evaluated.

When gathering data relating to your population, whether through community profiling, rapid participatory appraisal or another method, it is important to take into account those members of your population you may have inadvertently excluded. These may be members who are difficult to identify and consequently engage with but they are critical to the bigger picture of your community profile. These individuals may be excluded through social or health inequality or there may be language or communication barriers, but without their contribution to the final picture, the impact of your findings may be diminished.

Step 3: Assess a health priority for action

This involves evaluating the findings from your study of the population and using that information to decide what you health priority or priorities are going to be. This may have been decided at the start of your study and again relates directly to your original rationale of why you chose that population. You may have a specific remit relating to one aspect of the populations health and well-being that you are exploring, within the context of their wider environment from the start of your HNA.

Through analysis and evaluation of your findings, the health need identifiable as the main health priority, should start to become clear. This will be accompanied by an agreed understanding of all the members of the team as to what the main health priority is. Consideration needs to be given next to the larger picture and the question: what are the associated health conditions with that priority? For example, is the chosen health priority linked to a predisposing behaviour or environmental influence such as smoking and CHD.

The next step should be exploring possible interventions that could be beneficial in addressing the agreed main health priority. What are your agreed and defined target population and subsequently, what changes can be implemented to improve the health and well-being of that population. The choice of intervention will undoubtedly have resource implications and the level of successful impact leading to health improvement will be measured on cost effectiveness and positive impact. The rationale for this is that not all interventions will be suitable, for a variety of reasons and the chosen activity must have the ability to bring about significant improvement to health at a reasonable level of cost. There may be changes that could be made to existing services that would bring about improvement in health at little or no cost and these should be considered alongside other interventions.

Step 4: Action planning for change

This involves thinking about what you set out to do and how you can bring it about, utilising the information you have gathered. To do this effectively, it may be useful to work through some steps.

1. What are you wanting to achieve?
   You may want to consider the a range of issues e.g. what was your reason for performing the HNA? Did you have a specific aim in identifying health problems or inequalities? Or did you wish to research your chosen population to look for health needs?

2. What did you find out about health needs and priorities and what can be done to bring improvement to health?
   The health needs you identified will have now been prioritized into what you consider are the categories relevant for your study. These needs will be the ones that can bring about improvement in health with significant impact on the population health. They will need to be acceptable to the population, in as much as they must be locally available, tailored to meet their needs, for example there is little point delivering health promotion for parents with small children at midday, if the parents wish their children to take

a midday nap. It would be wise for planning for this and any group activity, to ask the group or a sample of suitable individuals with similar characteristics, what would be the best time, day of the week, location and any other impinging factors. Similarly there is little point in providing a service for older members of the population, who you may have assessed as non car owners, and then expecting them to travel to the next town. Basically, all these feasibility issues need to be thought through. Availability and accessibility of public transport is a very relevant issue in planning services for change and health improvement for members of the population that may need transport to get themselves to the venue.

3. What have others done in similar circumstances?
   It would be a good idea to expand your knowledge base about what you think are your priorities through conducting a review of available literature. Looking specifically at what others in similar areas have provided, how they evaluated their interventions and their outcomes. You can do this through using journals, websites and library resources that are electronically available. You may be able to contact some other project leaders and discuss your plans for health improvement in light of their experiences. You may also be able to link with local organizations that could have possible input into your project.
   It may be possible to plan a meeting inviting members who can represent your chosen population, individuals from other organizations and stakeholders in the results of your study to enable you to plan joint action.

4. Plan your actions
   Plan the steps you need to take, in light of the information your have gathered through your HNA and enlisting the views of others. Decide who will take responsibility for differing aspects, who will do what? Set the time plan for implementing the action. Decide who is going to gather evaluation data and how they are to do this. This will be done in direct proportion to your available resources. You may have a team, or there may be just you involved.

5. Deliver the intervention
   Deliver the planned intervention to your target audience whether it is a live intervention or a written study for the purpose of interest to your employer or educational assessment.

Step 5: Moving on/project review

This involves looking back and evaluating the project, reviewing whether your aims and objectives were achieved, in total or in part. What were you successful with? Were there any challenges? Look at the evaluation you received, were the comments favourable? Did you omit anything? What was the general feedback like? Would there be anything you would now do differently?

Evaluate the success of the HNA through requesting feedback either from the target population, the assessor or the relevant organization.

Finally, identify further action to be taken through writing up your recommendations.

The benefits of the HNA step-by-step process

The process of HNA enables information to be gathered about a defined target population, usually a community group, or population area but can commence at individual level. Working through the HNA process step-by-step, provides the data and information that when analysed, identifies and highlights the areas of health need and the determining factors, influencing these health issues. This then informs the planning and provision of services that will improve health.

The collective action of the process, influences life span and quality of life for individuals and communities, it is reassuring for the public who can envisage improvement in their own health and that of the community and it provides confidence to the public in their health and social care services, reassuring them that public money is both well targeted and its value for money, measurable.

Summary of Section Two: health needs assessment of populations

In the opening section of this chapter, the authors discussed the importance of an accurate, holistic assessment in the care of an individual patient, and described this process in some depth. The skills required in maintaining increasing numbers of people with long-term conditions in the community, preventing unnecessary hospital admission by identifying and responding to early signs of deterioration, have never been more in demand. This chapter explicitly recognized that there are therefore, exciting opportunities for clinical leadership in this area, as the role of the nurse develops to encompass aspects of care increasingly required in contemporary healthcare settings e.g. advanced physical assessment.

The chapter then moved on to explore the concept of 'health need assessment', drawing on sociological, epidemiological, consumerist and economic perspectives. There was a focused analysis of the process, from the initial identification of the target population and morbidity under consideration, through each stage to implementation and review. The practical means of utilizing this information and involving the community in developing equitable, accessible, patient-led health care provision was considered. This population-based

approach to health needs assessment was therefore proposed as a means of reducing inequality, enhancing patient choice, promoting the effective use of resources, thereby moving the emphasis away for health from care provision towards prevention.

 Online Resource Centre

For more information on health needs assessment visit the Online Resource Centre —
http://www.oxfordtextbooks.co.uk/orc/linsley/

References

Audit Commission (1999). *First assessment: a review of District Nursing Services in England and Wales*. London: Audit Commission.

Bach, S. & Grant, A. (2009). *Communication and Interpersonal Skills for Nurses*. London: Learning Matters.

Baid, H. (2006). The process of conducting a physical assessment: a nursing perspective. *British Journal of Nursing* 15(13): 710–714.

Baid, H., Bartlett, C., Gilhooly, S., Illingworth, A., & Winder, S. (2009). 'Advanced physical assessment: the role of the district nurse.' *Nursing Standard*. 23(35):42–46.

Benner, P. (2001). *From Novice to Expert. Excellence and Power in Clinical Nursing Practice.* London: Prentice Hall.

Bickley, L. S. (2007). *Bates' Guide to Physical Examination and History Taking*, (9th ed.). Philadelphia: Lippincott.

Billings, J. (2002). Profiling health needs. In: S. Cowley (ed.) *Public Health in Policy and Practice*. London: Balliere Tindall.

Bowers, K. & Barrett, S. (2009). Wound-related pain: features, assessment and treatment. *Nursing Standard*. 24(10): 47–56.

Bowling, A. (2004). *A Review of Quality of Life Measurement*. (3rd edn.). Maidenhead, Berks: Open University Press.

Bradshaw, J. (1994). The conceptualization and measurement of need: a social policy perspective. In: J. Popay, & G. Edwards (eds.) *Research the People's Health*. London: Routledge.

Bradshaw, J. (1972). A taxonomy of Social need. In: G. Maclachlan (ed.) *Problems and progress in Medical Care*. (6th edn.) Oxford: Oxford University Press.

Brogan, M. (1996). 'The sexual needs of elderly people: addressing the issue'. *Nursing Standard*. 10(24):42–45.

Bryans, A. & McIntosh, J. (1996). 'Decision-making in community nursing: an analysis of the stages of decision-making as they relate to community nursing assessment'. *Journal of Advanced Nursing*. 24:.24–30.

Bryans, A. & McIntosh, J. (2000). 'The use of simulation and post-simulation interview to examine the knowledge involved in community nursing assessment practice'. *Journal of Advanced Nursing*. 31 (5):1244–1251.

Burrows, D. & Baillie, L. (2009). 'Managing Pain and Promoting Comfort'. In: L. Baillie. (ed.) *Developing Practical Adult Nursing Skills*. (3rd edn.). London: Hodder Arnold.

Button, D., Roe, B., Webb, C., Frith, T., Colin-Thone, D. & Gardner, L. (1999). *Continence Promotion and Management by the*

Primary Health Care Team. Consensus Guidelines. London: Whurr.

Commission on Social Determinants of Health (2005). *Action on social determinants of health: learning from previous experiences.* Background paper prepared for the CSHD Geneva: WHO. Dahlgren, G. &Whitehead, M. (1991) *Policies and Strategies to Promote Social Equity in Health.* Stockholm: Insitute for Further Studies.

Cowley, S. Billings, J. R. (2001). Resources revisited: salutogenesis from a lay perspective. *Journal of Advanced Nursing* 29(4):994–1004.

Cox, C. (2004). *Physical Assessment for Nurses.* Oxford: Blackwell Publishing.

Department of Health (2000). *The NHS Plan. A Plan for Investment: A Plan for Reform.* London: Her Majesty's Stationery Office.

Department of Health (2001). *Involving Patients and the Public in Health Care.* London: The Stationery Office.

Department of Health (2004). *Choosing Health: Making Healthy Choices Easier.* London: Her Majesty's Stationery Office.

Department of Health (2005). *Creating a Patient-Led NHS.* London: Her Majesty's Stationery Office.

Department of Health (2006). Our Health, Our Care, Our Say. London: Her Majesty's Stationery Office.

Department of Health (2007). *Our NHS, Our Future. The Interim Report* by Lord Darzi. http://dh.gov.uk

Department of Health (2008). *High Quality Care for All. Next Stage Review, Final Report.* by Lord Darzi. London: The Stationery Office.

Department of Health (2001a). *Seeking consent: working with people with learning disabilities.* London: DH.

Department of Health (2003). *Winning Ways: Working together to reduce Healthcare Associated Infection in England.* London: DH.

Department of Health (2006). *The Expert Patient: A New Approach to Chronic Disease Management for the 21ˢᵗ Century.* London: DH.

Department of Health. (2000). *Good Practice in Continence Services.* London: DH.

Department of Health. (2001b). *Medicines and Older People. Implementing medicines related aspects of the NSF for Older People.* London: DH.

Department of Health. (2009). *Reference guide to consent for examination or treatment.* (2nd edn.). London: DH.

Docherty, B. (2002). Cardiorespiratory physical assessment for the acutely ill. *British Journal of Nursing.* 11(11):750–758.

Doherty, W. (2006). 'Intermittent self-catheterization: a change in practice or just a series of developments?' *Journal of Community Nursing.* 20(9):38–44.

Hawtin, M. Hughes, G. &Percy Smith, J. (2007). *Community Profiling: A revised edition.* Maidenhead: Open University Press.

HDA (2005). Health needs assessment: a practical guide. NICE. www.nice.org.uk October 1 2008 taken on after the HDA transferred functions to NICE referring to the quote taken by them from J. Hooper, P. Longworth (1998). Health Needs Assessment in Primary Care Workbook. Version 2, HDA.

Herbert, R., A. & Rowswell, M. (1992). 'Maintaining body temperature'. In: S. Redfern(ed.). *Nursing Elderly People* (2ⁿᵈ ed.) London: Churchill Livingstone.

Holland, K. (2004). 'An introduction to the Roper-Logan-Tierney model for nursing, based on Activities of Living'. In: K. Holland, J. Jenkins, J. Soloman, & S. Whittam, (eds.) *Applying the Roper,*

Logan, Tierney Model in Practice. London: Churchill Livingstone.

Hoskins, R.A.J. & Smith, L.,N. (2002). 'Nurse-led welfare benefits screening in a General Practice located in a deprived area'. *Public Health.* 116:214–220.

Hutson, M. & Millar, E. (2009). 'Record Keeping'. In: H. Iggulden, C. MacDonald, & K. Staniland (eds.) *Clinical Skills. The Essence of Caring.* London: Open University Press.

IMD (2004). *The English Indices of Deprivtion.* London: Neighbourhood Renewal Unit, Office of the Deputy Prime Minister.

Indices of Deprivation (2000). *Measuring Multiple Deprivation at the Small Area Level.* London: DETR.

Jenkins, J. (2004). 'Sleeping'. In: K. Holland, J. Jenkins, J. Soloman,& S. Whittam (eds.) *Applying the Roper, Logan, Tierney Model in Practice.* London: Churchill Livingstone.

Johnson, C. (2005). 'Manual Handling risk assessment—theory and practice'. In: J. Smith. (ed.) *The Guide to The Handling of People.* (5ᵗʰ edn). London: BackCare.

Keleher, H., Parker, R., Abdulwadud, O. & Francis, K. (2009). 'Systematic review of the effectiveness of primary care nursing'. *International Journal of Nursing Practice.* 15:16–24.

Marsh, L. (2009). 'Assessing and Meeting Nutritional Needs'. In: L. Baillie. (ed.) *Developing Practical Adult Nursing Skills.* (3ʳᵈ edn). London: Hodder Arnold.

McCormack, P. (1997). 'Undernutrition in the elderly population living at home in the community: a review of the literature'. *Journal of Advanced Nursing.* 26:856–863.

Mitcheson, J. (2008). *Public Health Approaches to Practice.* Cheltenham: Nelson Thornes.

Mitcheson, J. Cowley, S. (2003). Empowerment or control? An analysis of the extent to which client participation is enabled during the health visitor/ client interactions using a structured health needs assessment tool. *International Journal of Nursing Studies.* 49: 413–426.

Morris, K. (1999). 'Tackling the taboo of urinary incontinence'. *The Lancet* 353 (9147): 128.

Najman, J, M. (2001). A general model of the social origins of health and well being In: R. Eckersley, J. Dixon &B. Douglas (eds.) The Social Origins of Health and Well Being. Cambridge: Cambridge University Press.

National Gold Standards Framework Centre (2006). *'The Gold Standards NHS Framework'.* [Online] Walsall/NHS End of Life Programme. Available from: http://goldstandardsframework. nhs.uk/AdvanceCarePlanning/ACPandGSF [Accessed 18.04.10]

NHS (2009). *'Liverpool Care Pathway for the dying Patient' (LCP)* [Online] National End of Life Care Programme. Available from: http://endoflifecare.nhs.uk/eolc/lcp.htm [Accessed 02.05.10]

Nazarko, L. (2002). *Nursing in Care Homes.* (2ⁿᵈ edn.). London: Blackwell.

National Institute for Health and Clinical Excellence (2003). *The use of pressure-relieving devices (beds, mattresses and overlays) for the prevention of pressure ulcers in primary and secondary care. Clinical Practice Guidelines No 7.* [Online] London. NICE Available from: http://guidance.nice.org.uk/nicemedia/ live/10928/29181/29181.pdf [Accessed 13.04.10]

National Institute for Health and Clinical Excellence (2008). Community Engagement. NICE Public Health Guidance 9. NICE. www.nice.org.uk. Accessed 25 August 2008.

Norton, C. (1996). (ed.), *Nursing for Continence.* (2ⁿᵈ edn.). Beaconsfield: Beaconfield Publishers.

Nursing and Midwifery Council (2008a). *The Code. Standards for conduct, performance and ethics for nurses and midwives.* London: NMC.

Nursing and Midwifery Council (2008b). *Standards for medicines management.* London: NMC.

Nursing and Midwifery Council (2009). *Record Keeping: Guidance for nurses and midwives.* London: NMC.

Orem, D. (1995). Nursing: Concepts of Practice. (5th edn.). Philadelphia: Mosby

Peate, I. (2007). *Becoming a Nurse in the 21st Century.* London: Wiley.

Pierce, E, Cowan, P. & Stokes, M. (2001). 'Managing Faecal retention and incontinence in neurodisability'. *British Journal of Nursing* 10(9): 592–601.

Price, C. I.M. Han, S.W. Rutherford, I.A. (2000). Advanced nursing practice: an introduction to physical assessment, British Journal of Nursing 9(22): 2292–2296.

Pritchard, E. (1999). 'Dementia. Part 2: person-centred assessment'. *Professional Nurse* 14(9):657.

Rasmor, M. & Brown, C. (2003). Physical Examination for the Occupational Health Nurse, *American Association of Occupational Health Nursing Journal* 51(9): 390 401.

Roberts, D. (2004). 'Dying'. In: K. Holland, J. Jenkins, J. Soloman, & S. Whittam, (eds.). *Applying the Roper, Logan, Tierney Model in Practice.* London: Churchill Livingstone.

Roe, B. & Mae, C. (1999). 'Incontinence and sexuality: findings from a qualitative perspective'. *Journal of Advanced Nursing*30(3):573–579.

Rollnick, S., Mason, P. & Butler, C. (2000). *Health Behaviour Change. A Guide for Practitioners.* London: Churchill Livingstone.

Roper, N., Logan, W. & Tierney, A. (1996). *The Elements of Nursing: Based on a Model of Living.* (4th edn.). London: Churchill Livingstone.

Rose, K. (1994). Structured and semi-structured interviewing. *Nurse Researcher*1(3):23–32.

Royal College of Nursing & National Institute for Health and Clinical Excellence (2005). *Pressure ulcers: The management of pressure ulcers in primary and secondary care. Clinical Guideline 29.* [Online] London: NICE. Available from: http://www.nice.org.uk/nicemedia/live10972/29885.pdf

Sackett, D.L., Rosenberg, W.M., Muir Grey, J.A., Haynes, R.B. & Richardson, W.S. (1996). 'Evidence based medicine: what it is and what it is not'. *British Medical Journal* 312: 71.

Staniland, K. & Gascoigne, F. (2009). 'Food and nutrition' In: H. Iggulden, C. MacDonald, & K. Staniland(eds.). *Clinical Skills. The Essence of Caring.* London: Open University Press.

Stevens, A. (1998). Health Needs Assessment Needs Assessment; from theory to practice. *British Medical Journal* 316: 1448–1452 accessed via http://www.bmj.com/cgi/content/full/316/7142/1448 on 31/07/08

Talley, N. & O'Connor, S. (1998). *Clinical Examination* (3rd edn.) Australia: MacLennan and Petty Pty Limited.

Todorovic, V., Russell, C., Stratton, R., Ward, J. & Elia, M. (2003) (eds.). *The MUST explanatory booklet.* [Online] Redditch BAPEN Available from: http://www.bapen.co.org.uk/pdfs/must/must_explan.pdf [Accessed 13th April 2010].

Walker, S. (2004). 'Controlling body temperature'. In: K. Holland, J. Jenkins, J. Soloman, & S. Whittam, (eds.). *Applying the Roper, Logan, Tierney Model in Practice.* London: Churchill Livingstone.

Walker, S.H. (2009). 'Continence, bowel and bladder care'. In: H. Iggulden, C. MacDonald, & K. Staniland, (eds.) *Clinical Skills. The Essence of Caring.* London: Open University Press.

Walsh, M. & Ford, P. (1992). *Nursing Rituals. Research and Rational Actions.* Manchester: Butterworth Heinemann.

Wanless, D. *et al.* (2004). *Securing good health for the whole population.* London: HM Treasury & Norwich: The Stationery Office.

Waterlow, J. (1985). *The Waterlow Score.* [Online] Waterlow, J. Available from: http://www.judy-waterlow.co.uk/downloads/Waterlow%20Score%20Card-front.pdf [Accessed 13th April 2010]

Webb, C. (1992). 'Expressing sexuality'. In: S. Redfern (ed.). *Nursing Elderly People.* (2nd ed.). London: Churchill Livingstone.

West. S. L. (2006). Physical assessment: whose role is it anyway. Nursing in Critical Care 11(4):161–167.

Whittam, S. (2004). Working and playing. In: K.Holland, J. Jenkins, J. Soloman, & S. Whittam (eds.). *Applying the Roper, Logan, Tierney Model in Practice.* London: Churchill Livingstone.

Wilde, M.H. (2003). 'Meanings and Practical Knowledge of People with Long-term Urinary Catheters.' *Journal of Wound, Ostomy and Continence Nursing.* 30(1):33–39.

Wilkins, R.L, Krider, S. J. & Sheldon, R. L. (2000), *Clinical Assessment in Respiratory Care.* Philadelphia:Mosby.

Chapter 10

Planning interventions: meeting the needs of individuals and communities

Grace Spencer

Introduction

This chapter outlines some of the key principles of planning interventions commonly used in public health. Both strategic population level interventions and individual nurse-patient approaches to planning are discussed. Illustrating population and individual approaches will point to the multi-levelled nature of public health planning and will help the reader to identify the different ways in which health may be promoted to meet the health needs of the individuals and communities with whom you work.

Common terms used in public health planning are defined in the chapter and key components of successful planning interventions identified. This includes defining and identifying aims, objectives, and methods. In addition, various approaches to public health planning and some frequently used models are outlined. These approaches further illustrate notions of community participation and collaboration, multi-agency and partnership working. These terms are defined and identified for their significance to planning interventions and draw further attention to some of the ways in which political, economic and organizational issues may impact upon health and well being. An understanding of such issues, including critical atten-

tion to the wider determinants of health (see Chapter 2) and processes of needs assessment (see Chapter 9), is considered central to the successful planning and related effectiveness of any intervention at meeting the health related needs of individuals and communities.

By the end of this chapter the reader will understand the key principles of planning interventions and begin to consider how best to evaluate these interventions. This will enable you to develop the necessary skills to plan and implement a health promotion intervention whether you are working with individuals, groups or communities; and in a variety of different settings and contexts, whether that might be whilst studying at university, working on placement, or perhaps the reader's own local community.

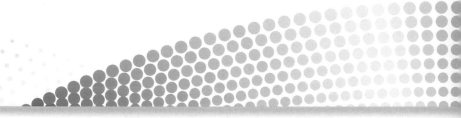

Case Study *Planning a health promotion intervention*

As part of the Government's public health **policy**, Kate has been asked to **plan** a health promotion **intervention** that promotes young people's health.

Her **aim** is to increase young people's awareness of the factors influencing their own health and well-being. In **collaboration** with the school nursing team, the **Healthy School's** coordinator, and youth services Kate identifies the following **objectives**:

(i)   To increase young people's awareness of sexual health services,

(ii) To reduce the number of young people smoking,

(iii) To reduce the amount of alcohol consumed by young people,

(iv) To encourage young people to eat more fruit and vegetables as part of their diet,

(v)   To increase young people's participation in physical activity and sport.

Her **strategy** will be to work in schools using different **methods** including group work, poster displays, campaigns, and social skills training to promote young people's health.

Discussion points

Before reading this chapter, write down what factors Kate might need to consider when planning this health promotion intervention. You may wish to discuss this with your peers or colleagues and generate a **thinking shower** in order to identify your initial thoughts and ideas.

Ask yourself:

• What does Kate need to do?

• What resources might she need and how will she get them?

• Who will she work with?

• What does Kate need to know about her target population?

• How will Kate know if the intervention has been successful at achieving its aim of promoting young people's health?

• How will Kate promote the health of young people marginalized from school?

Hints:

Have a look at the Government's recent policy outlining its overall aim and strategy for promoting young people's health to help you identify what Kate might consider when planning her health promotion intervention. You might want to think about how to access or work with different groups of young people. For example, how would you promote the health of looked after children, or those excluded from school? Working with local youth services might help you consider how best to promote the health of hard to reach groups.

Kate's aim and objectives are ambitious. However, by carefully and systematically working through this activity you will begin to understand the different components and complexities of public health planning. Remember that health promotion planning is challenging and you may wish to come back to

this activity at different stages in your nursing programme and career to help you identify the various components and challenges involved in promoting health.

Promoting health amongst other population groups

This activity can also be used to plan a health promotion intervention with many different population groups depending on your area of clinical practice. Other groups might include men, older people, pregnant women, or individuals with long-term conditions such as coronary heart disease, asthma or diabetes. The readings and activities in this chapter will help you to think through what specific factors you will need to consider when working with any population group. As you work through the activities in this chapter, it is important to remember that public health planning is a multifaceted and complex task and requires critical attention to the wider determinants of health (see Chapter 2) and methods of needs assessment (see Chapter 9.).

Relevant further reading on recent Government policy can be found at the end of this chapter.

What is health promotion planning?

'Effective planning requires anticipation of what will be needed along the way towards achieving the goal. This statement implies that the goal is defined, as are the necessary steps involved in reaching the goal. Perhaps most importantly, it requires an understanding of the steps and how they interrelate'.
Dignan and Carr, 1992: 4

Before considering how you might plan a health promotion **activity** or intervention, it is necessary to understand what is meant by **planning**. Planning simply refers to a process that identifies a course of action which leads to the achievement of a particular outcome (Tones and Green, 2006). Systematic planning is a key ingredient for successful health promotion programming. Hubley (1993: 207) identifies four questions underpinning health promotion planning:

1. Where are we now?

2. Where do we want to go?

3. How will we get there?

4. How will we know when we get there?

The first stage of planning involves reviewing existing practice and identifying health related needs. Assessing health needs helps determine what might be the main focus or aim of the planning intervention. An aim is a broad statement of what is to be achieved. For example, in the next Activity, Kate's aim is to increase young people's awareness of the factors influencing their own health and well-being. After identifying the aim, it is then necessary to set more specific objectives. In contrast to the broad statement of what is to be achieved, objectives are precise measurable statements of what is to be achieved by an activity. For example, Kate identifies five specific objectives or targets to achieve her overall aim of promoting young people's health.

After setting aims and objectives, and following Hubley's (1993) questions, the next stage of health promotion planning is deciding which methods will be used to achieve the stated aim and objectives. A method simply refers to the techniques, approaches or activities used to achieve the aim and objectives. For example, in the Case Study Kate might use a variety of different methods such as poster displays, workshops, and skills training. When identifying what methods will be used it is important to consider not just what resources are available, but also how effective the chosen methods are at achieving the stated aims and objectives.

The final stages of the planning process include plans for an evaluation of the effectiveness of the intervention. Chapter 12 discusses approaches to evaluation but it is important to identify from the outset how the relative success of the intervention might be assessed and evaluated. This will ensure a comprehensive and stage-wise plan is devised and implemented.

Activity box

Review the points you made previously on Kate's health promotion intervention for young people's health. From your thinking shower, do you think you have answered Hubley's four questions underpinning health promotion planning?

In order to do this you will need to consider which type of context or **setting** you are planning your intervention. For example; the setting could be a school, a hospital, or the local community.

1. Where are we now?

- What health promotion activities and interventions are currently in place to promote young people's health?
- How does the school environment and school nursing team currently meet the aim and objectives set out in the case study?

2. Where do we want to go?

- You will need to review Kate's aim and objectives here. These objectives are part of the Government's public health agenda to promote young people's health. Have a look at the Government's visions of 'where do we want to go' to help you.

- Relevant further reading on recent Government policy can be found at the end of this chapter.

3. How will we get there?

- What methods could Kate use to achieve the given aim and objectives?
- You may find some ideas for promoting young people's health at www.healthyschools.gov.uk and www.nhs.uk/change4life

4. How will we know when we get there?

- This is your evaluation of the intervention. How will you know Kate's aim and objectives have been achieved? How will you evaluate increases in knowledge or any changes in health related behaviour by young people?
- See Chapter 12 on evaluating health promotion interventions to help you identify how you might best evaluate the success of the intervention.

Try to organize your initial thoughts and ideas from Case Study 10.1 under each of the questions. This will enable you to logically structure the planning process. Remember that evaluation of your intervention is a key component of the planning process and should not be left to after the event.

Individual and population health promotion planning

Planning can take different forms and may also be approached from different levels. For example, individual planning may involve the nurse and patient identifying together particular lifestyle factors that present health risks to the individual. These may include factors such as smoking, lack of regular exercise, or a diet high in sugar or saturated fat. Through the identification of health **risk factors**, the nurse can work with the patient to plan a healthy lifestyle based on current evidence and health advice. Community level planning may involve collaboration with local groups and service providers to identify and remove barriers to healthy lifestyles such as increasing access to sporting and leisure facilities.

Activity box

Individual health promotion planning

Write down, or discuss with your peers, a time when you have been involved in **targeting** health promotion messages at the individual level during your placements.

Nursing practice in all areas involves health promotion planning. On medical wards you are likely to nurse patients with acute and chronic health conditions such as asthma, diabetes

Table 10.1 Levels of health promotion planning and interventions

Level	Example of planning interventions at that level
Individual	Individual advice on physical activity to support lifestyle change and increase in physical activity.
Community	Working with local businesses and voluntary services to promote access to sport and leisure facilities and activities in the local community.
Regional	A regional media campaign highlighting the benefits of an active lifestyle and physical exercise.
National	Lobbying Government to increase funding and sponsorship for sports equipment and facilities.
International	International bodies such as the World Health Organization's (WHO) global strategy on diet, physical activity and health. See www.who.int/dietphysicalactivity

Adapted from Hubley and Copeman (2008)

and cardiovascular disease. Working in surgical areas will involve planning post-operative care which may include wound care, nutritional support and chest and ambulatory physiotherapy. In the community, planning care may involve an assessment of the home environment and available support. As part of the planning process you may also work with a number of allied health professionals as part of the multidisciplinary team.

- Drawing upon your experiences from practice, how has nursing care been planned, implemented and evaluated in these areas to promote the patient's health and well being?

- What were some of the challenges of planning health promotion for the individuals you have worked with whilst on placement?

- What professionals were involved in the planning of health promotion?

You may have identified working with other health professionals such as the physiotherapist, dietician, occupational therapist or clinical specialists such as a stoma nurse or diabetes specialist nurse. From your community placements you may have identified a number of health professionals working within primary care such as community nurses, school nurses or a specialist community public health nurse.

Collaborative working, a key component of much recent Government policy (Scottish Executive, 2003; DH, 2004), is a central element of planning successful public health interventions at the individual, community and population level. For example, in the case study activity and when planning her health promotion intervention for young people's health, Kate may wish to work in partnership with school nurses, sexual health advisors, the SEAL (Social and Emotional Aspects of Learning) coordinator, youth workers, counsellors, and various school staff involved in delivering the **Personal Social and Health Education (PSHE)** curriculum.

In contrast to individual level planning, population level planning aims to improve the overall health of the population often through addressing wider social and economic factors that militate against health and well-being. Planning a population level public health intervention often takes a strategic approach and is typically large scale involving a number of individuals and groups. For example, vaccination policies and campaigns such as the MMR and the Human Papillomavirus (HPV) programmes are examples of large scale population interventions to prevent disease and promote health through targeting particular groups within the population (see www.nhs.uk.mmr and www.nhs.uk/hpv for information and examples of these population measures to prevent disease and promote health).

Further examples of population planning interventions may include changes to health related policy such as the introduction of a smoking ban or lobbying the alcohol industry to increase costs of alcohol to promote safe and responsible drinking patterns amongst the population as a whole (see www.smokefreeengland.co.uk and www.drinkaware.co.uk for examples of policy related planning interventions).

Planning may also be approached using a 'top-down' or 'bottom-up' strategy. Top-down planning refers to interventions that address issues that are defined and guided by professionals and are often based on government priority areas. For example, a smoking cessation intervention might be based on professional and political concern for the adverse effects of smoking on individual and population health.

In contrast, bottom-up planning takes individual and community perspectives as the starting point. Bottom-up strategies involve the development of partnerships with communities who identify and respond to their own needs (see Laverack and Labonte, 2000). Through careful assessment of individual and community needs, priorities and recommended action are identified and implemented by individuals and communities themselves. This is sometimes referred to as an **empowerment** approach to planning (Laverack, 2005). The notion of **advocacy** is often highlighted as a means through which nurses and health professionals can represent the views of individuals, groups and communities with whom they work using a bottom-up approach to planning.

These different approaches and levels of planning point to the importance of appropriate targeting of health promotion messages. As you might expect, the role of the health care professional can be quite different when working from a top down perspective to that of a bottom up approach. Should nurses and health professionals target health promotion interventions at the individual or population level?

Much health care is based on understanding why an individual is sick and responding appropriately. Some critiques of this approach would argue this has resulted in a sustained focus on identifying individual risk factors in order to prevent disease and promote health and thus, does little to address the fundamental causes of ill health which may include economic, political, social and organizational factors (see Chapter 2 for a detailed discussion of the wider determinants of health). Consequently, individual approaches are often considered symptomatic, rather than radical, interventions. Many advocates of a population approach seeking to address the wider determinants of health draw upon the well known Geoffrey Rose (1992) hypothesis to support their arguments for targeting public health interventions at the population level.

arguments and approach to planning interventions (see Townsend *et al.*, 1992; and Acheson, 1998).

'The essential determinants of the health of society are thus to be found in its mass characteristics: the deviant minority can only be understood when seen in its societal context, and effective prevention requires changes which involve the population as a whole'
Rose, 1992: vii

Thus, the population approach recognizes the need to take action at the societal level.

Review questions:

- What implications does the Geoffrey Rose hypothesis have for public health and nursing?
- Would it change your approach to public health planning?
- Review Kate's health promotion aim and objectives according to Rose's ideas. How would you plan a population level intervention to promote young people's health?

Box 10.1 Geoffrey Rose hypothesis

'The primary determinants of disease are mainly economic and social, and therefore its remedies must also be economic and social...'
Rose, 1992: 129

Geoffrey Rose was a Professor of **Epidemiology** whose work most notably demonstrated the need and benefits of addressing population health rather than targeting particular 'high risk' individuals or groups. According to Rose, public health planning often identifies high risk groups, such as smokers, heavy drinkers or drug users, on which to base appropriate interventions. However, Rose argued that high risk groups represent the extremes of the population and thus, constitute a relatively small proportion of people. As a result, targeting responses, for example the screening and treatment of high risk individuals, does little to affect the overall health of the population.

Largely drawing upon epidemiological data on cardiovascular disease, Rose argued that population level characteristics such as factors influencing and shaping the socio-economic and political environment in which people live need to inform public health interventions. For Rose, the most effective way of promoting public health is to examine, and change, the population as a whole through focusing attention on factors adversely affecting the population's health. This is termed a **mass population strategy**. Factors addressed from this approach may include an assessment of the political, economic and social determinants of health. Sustained evidence of inequalities in health arising from socio-economic factors support Rose's

Health promotion planning models

As demonstrated, effective public health planning is based on a systematic and comprehensive approach using a variety of methods to select the most appropriate course of action to promote individual and population health. In order to plan effective health promotion interventions at the individual or population level, a number of planning models have been developed.

For example, Dignan and Carr's (1992) planning model commences with a community analysis and assessment of needs. This bottom-up approach to planning enables the identification of key issues to be addressed in order to identify target areas to be assessed. Other approaches to health promotion planning include the **PABCAR model** proposed by Maycock *et al.* (2001); and the implementation of logical frameworks, or **LogFrame matrix**, often used by aid programmes (see Nancholas, 1998; and Bell, 2001 for a summary of these approaches).

Following a model provides a systematic approach to planning and can help identify and provide a comprehensive review of required action to bring about changes to health. Furthermore, by working through the planning process using a model or framework you will begin to recognize and identify some of the key skills required for effective health promotion planning. These key skills include advocacy, communication, collaboration, teaching, team-work, leadership, organization and time management strategies. As you may recognize, these key skills underpin many areas of professional nursing practice.

By way of example of how to plan interventions to meet the needs of individuals and communities, two commonly used models in health promotion are detailed here: Ewles and Simnett's (2003) seven stage planning model, and the precede-proceed model developed by Green and Kreuter (1991). By following the various phases and stages of these models you will begin to develop the necessary skills for effective planning.

Ewles and Simnett (2003) Planning Model

Ewles and Simnett's (2003: 84) seven-stage flowchart for effective health promotion planning and evaluation is a commonly used planning model in public health. The model outlined by Ewles and Simnett may be used for a number of different health promotion interventions and involves a cyclical process with feedback loops (see Fig.10.1). By way of example of how to use this model, Kate's health promotion aim to promote young people's health is drawn upon to illustrate how you might plan a health promotion intervention. You may wish to adapt the example based on the ideas and suggestions you have already identified in the previous activities.

Stage 1 Identify needs and priorities

As indicted previously, the first stage of the planning process involves the identification of health needs in order to respond to health priorities. The process of assessing needs is complex

and is addressed in detail in Chapter 9. However, when planning any health promotion activity or intervention, it is important to consider who is identifying health needs. Identifying health needs may be influenced by whether your health promotion activity is based on top-down priorities such as areas identified in Government policy; or bottom-up as identified by the patients or groups you are working with. Once you have identified clear needs and priorities you can then begin to set your aims and objectives.

Activity box

Identifying needs and priorities

Firstly you will need to consider what aspect of health you will focus on. You may approach this in different ways. For example, you may draw upon key health related issues identified in current Government policy such as obesity, smoking or 'binge drinking'. You may wish to conduct or draw upon a health needs assessment that systematically identifies the health needs of the local population you are working with. This may highlight particular groups with identified health needs such as young people, women, men or various ethnic groups.

An alternative, and bottom-up approach, would be to ask individuals and communities themselves what they consider to be most important to promote their health and well-being. This approach can be very illuminating and may identify different aspects and understandings of health and priorities for health promotion planning and intervention (see Spencer, 2008 for an example of this approach with young people).

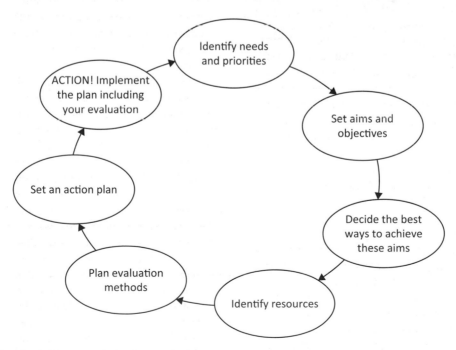

Fig. 10.1 Ewles and Simnett's (2003) planning model.

Activity

Write down the areas you consider important for health promotion. Then ask your peers, tutors, mentors, friends and family what they consider to be a health need and a health promotion priority.

Compare your responses:

- Are the responses similar?
- How do professional perspectives differ from lay perspectives, i.e. the views and opinions of your friends and family?
- What might be some of the implications for planning your intervention of any similarities or differences in these responses?

Stage 2 Set aims and objectives

Recall that the aim is your overall statement about what you want to achieve. Your objectives are more specific and point to desired outcomes or results. The acronym **SMART** is often used as a way to set objectives:

S Specific
M Measurable
A Achievable
R Realistic
T Time limited

At this stage you need to ask yourself what am I trying to achieve? And, importantly, why? It is always important to make sure that these aims and objectives will address the health needs and priorities you have identified, but also that they are realistic and achievable. This helps you to consider **why** you are doing something, and not just **what** you are doing. Factors such as time and resources need to be considered as they present limits to what your aim and objectives might be.

Your objectives maybe health related, for example reducing the number of young people who smoke; educational related, for example increases in knowledge of the risks of alcohol consumption or a change in attitudes or developing young people's personal skills; or policy related, for example the introduction of a school travel plan encouraging young people to walk and cycle to school (Ewles and Simnett, 2003).

Activity box

Set aims and objectives

Once you have decided on your focus you will then need to consider your aim and purpose.

- What do you hope to achieve?
- Do you want to raise awareness of a particular health issue?

- Are you seeking to change young people's health related behaviour?
- Perhaps you might want to raise money for a local charity that supports community health in your locality?
- Do you want to work with or collaborate with other agencies?

You may consider one or more of these aims, but remember that health promotion planning takes time.

Activity

Using the SMART acronym, identify your aims and objectives for a health promotion activity or intervention aimed at promoting young people's health.

Remember your aims and objectives should be Specific, Measurable, Achievable, Realistic, and Time limited.

Stage 3 Decide the best way of achieving the aims

Kate's aim to promote young people's health may be achieved in a number of different ways. For example, she may wish to give out leaflets, organize some health education workshops in schools, or perhaps work in collaboration with local businesses to promote alcohol safety and exercise plans. Ewles and Simnett (2003: 90) highlight six questions to consider when deciding the best way of achieving aims:

- Which methods are most appropriate and effective for your aims and objectives?
- Which methods will be acceptable to the clients?
- Which methods will be easiest?
- Which methods are cheapest?
- Which methods are most acceptable to the people involved?
- Which methods do you find comfortable to use?

Deciding which methods are most appropriate and effective for achieving your aims and objectives should be based on current available evidence. **Evidence-based practice** is a **term** commonly used in health and nursing care and remains an important concept in public health planning interventions (see Tones and Tilford (2001) for an evaluation of the effectives of health promotion and the National Institute for Health and Clinical Excellence [NICE] for national guidance on promoting good health according to best evidence www.nice.org.uk).

You may decide that a number of methods are needed to achieve your aim, and again these might be planned and targeted at the level of the individual, group, community or population as a whole. The next activity box illustrates a number of different methods that may be used to promote

young people's physical activity at the various levels of health promotion planning. Can you identify which level of intervention the methods are addressing? In other words, do they seek to promote the health of the individual, community or population as a whole? Are the methods aiming to change behaviour, increase awareness or knowledge, or prompt social change?

Activity box

Methods for promoting physical activity

- Teaching sessions in PSHE and science on the role of physical activity in health,
- Leaflets and posters promoting physical activity,
- After school sports clubs such as football, netball, rugby and tennis,
- Development and implementation of a school travel plan,
- Secure bicycle storage at schools,
- Working with local sports groups to engage young people in sports out of school,
- Lobbying local leisure facilities to provide appropriate and affordable sporting activities for young people,
- Ensuring the school curriculum offers opportunity for all young people to engage in at least two hours of physical activity a week according to national guidance,
- Providing open safe spaces and equipment for young people to engage in sports and exercise.

Activity

Now consider what methods you will use to achieve the aims and objectives you have set in Stage 2 of the planning process.

Stage 4 Identify resources

Availability and access to resources are central to successful health promotion planning. If resources are scarce or limited this may present limits to what is achievable. Resources available may include materials such as posters, leaflets, teaching equipment; but also yourself and your peers, the individuals, groups and communities you work with, other professionals, existing services and policies.

You may find a number of resources from your university, health clinics and practice areas, the health authority and local health promotion service. Funding is an important issue for planning and you may need to consider the costs of your planned activity. Costs may arise from travel, any necessary training, provision of material resources and equipment. Remember costing is an important element of ensuring your objectives are achievable and realistic.

Activity box

Identify resources

Activity

Identify what resources might be needed for your intervention and where you might find them. Remember resources can be costly and you will need to consider the cost of your intervention and where and how you will obtain any necessary funding for the intervention.

Stage 5 Plan evaluation methods

How will you know if your programme has been effective at achieving its aim? It is important to consider how you will evaluate your programme before it is implemented. Evaluation may be conducted in a number of ways and approaches are detailed in Chapter 12. However, you may wish to consider whether, and how, you will measure knowledge, attitude or behaviour change? You might want to ask people their views on the programme by designing a questionnaire or running a focus group discussion. An effective evaluation will help you plan for your next intervention by conducting a systematic assessment of what worked well and identifying what you might do differently in the future.

Stage 6 Set an action plan

An action plan identifies what must be done and by whom in order to implement and evaluate the programme. By writing down what action needs to be taken and when, you can monitor the progress made and what else needs to be done. An example of an action plan is given in the next activity box.

Activity box

Setting an action plan

1. Arrange a planning meeting with key individuals to identify aims, objectives and methods to be used.
2. Liaise with individuals and community groups via telephone, email, letter and face-to-face meetings.
3. Make arrangements for venue and obtain any necessary permission.
4. Obtain resources and any available funding.
5. Organize planning meeting before the event to confirm final arrangements.
6. Put intervention into action. This might include setting up a stand or facilitating a group workshop in a local community centre.
7. Evaluate success of intervention.

When developing your action plan, it is important to set relevant timescales. Each part of the planning process takes time and involves a number of individuals and **stakeholders**. Stakeholders can include health practitioners, employers, funding bodies, policy makers and the public or population group you are working with. Public health interventions are usually required to be accountable and report back to these stakeholders. Time to arrange and hold meetings and report progress to stakeholders must be carefully worked into the action plan.

Stage 7 Action!

This is when all the hard work involved in planning your health promotion intervention is put into action! It is important to note down any key points arising from the implementation as part of your evaluation and also to inform future events.

As Fig. 10.1 illustrates, this model involves a cyclical process with continuous feedback loops at each stage of the planning process. As you plan your health promotion intervention, remember to constantly review each stage as you gather more information to help you plan your intervention. This constant review and feedback will help you to continuously reflect on the progress made and incorporate new ideas as they are generated throughout the planning process.

Precede-proceed (Green and Kreuter, 1991)

The precede-proceed model developed by Green and Kreuter (1991) and has been extensively used in health promotion. **PRECEDE** is an acronym for:

P **P**redisposing,
R **R**einforcing,
E **E**nabling,
C **C**auses in,
E **E**ducational,
D **D**iagnosis, and
E **E**valuation.

PROCEED is an acronym for:

P **P**olicy,
R **R**egulatory,
O **O**rganizational,
C **C**onstructs in
E **E**ducational and
E **E**nvironmental
D **D**evelopment.

The components of the **PRECEDE** enable the identification

of community health needs in collaboration with individuals and communities. This component of the model builds on theories of community development and participation such as those advocated within bottom-up or empowerment based interventions (for examples of this approach see Laverack and Labonte, 2000; and Laverack, 2005).

The **PROCEED** element enables the practitioner to move beyond health education to assess and affect organizational and environmental determinants of health. This includes policy development to develop healthy systems more conducive to healthy lifestyles. It therefore adopts a multi-levelled approach to health promotion planning.

The model identifies nine phases to planning and involves the assessment of the multiple determinants of health such as those highlighted by the Geoffrey Rose hypothesis. It makes suggestions for possible solutions and involves a collaboration of professionals to ensure a comprehensive approach to planning. This comprehensive approach enables the application of the model in a variety of settings such as schools, communities, and patient care settings such as hospitals. A key element of the model is the active participation of clients themselves.

Phase 1 Social diagnosis

Phase 1 identifies population health concerns and draws upon methods of needs assessment to assess subjective health concerns of individuals and communities. The aim is to gain an understanding of social problems as perceived by individuals and communities themselves and to draw the links between these concerns and specific health problems which become the focus of health promotion work. Methods used for social diagnosis may include questionnaires, focus groups, interviews, and community forums.

Phase 2 Epidemiological diagnosis

Phase 2 considers some of the wider factors and determinants of health which impact upon the subjective perceptions identified in phase one. The focus of this phase is on identifying factors that are associated with health problems and quality of life. Identifying such factors helps to establish priorities for health promotion and draw together different professionals involved in the promotion of health. Epidemiological diagnosis may include an examination of morbidity and mortality statistics.

Following Phases 1 and 2, programme objectives are determined.

Phase 3 Behavioural and environmental diagnosis

This phase involves the identification of factors linked to health problems identified in phase three. This may include age,

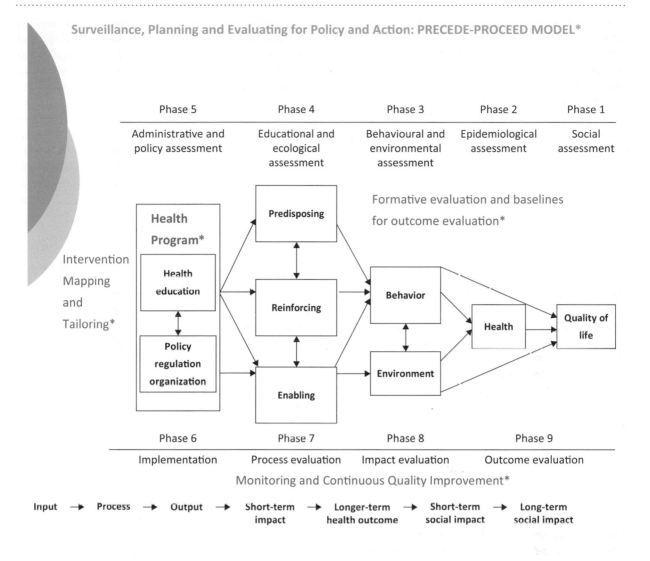

Fig. 10.2 Green and Kreuter's precede-proceed model. Green, L.W. and Kreuter, M.W. (4th edn. in press).

gender, existing morbidity, access to health facilities and individual behaviours linked to the health problems. Behavioural diagnosis involves identifying health practices linked to the social and epidemiological diagnoses. Environmental diagnosis is an analysis of social and environmental factors that link to behaviour.

Phase 4 Educational diagnosis

This phase involves an assessment of the cause of behaviours identified in phase three. Three causes are identified: predisposing factors, enabling factors, and reinforcing factors. Predisposing factors include any characteristics motivating the behaviour such as knowledge, beliefs, attitudes and values. Enablers refer to environmental characteristics that facilitate action and include accessibility, skills, availability. Reinforces include sanctions (positive or negative) that follow the behaviour and thus serve to strengthen the motivation

for the behaviour. These include peers, family, colleagues, and teachers.

Identifying causal factors that may be targeted for behavioural change is the main goal in this phase. This identifies the factors that will initiate behaviour change.

Phase 5 Administrative and policy diagnosis

This phase involves an analysis of existing policies, administrative and organizational concerns that may hinder or facilitate the implementation of a programme. This may involve an assessment of resources and budgets available and the coordination of departments and organizations involved in the programme.

Phase 6 Implementation of the programme

Phase 6 is the putting into action, or implementation, of the health promotion programme.

131

Phases 7–9 Evaluation — process, impact and outcome

Phases 7–9 involves an evaluation of the programme and involves an assessment of the **process, impact** and **outcome** of the programme.

Process evaluation is an assessment of the effectiveness of the way in which the programme was implemented. Impact evaluation measures the effectiveness and success of the programme in terms of achieving its objectives and changes to predisposing, enabling and reinforcing factors. Outcome evaluation measures the overall achievement of the aims and objectives. This can take a long time as changes to health and the social environment may not be evident until many months or years after the implementation of the programme.

As you can see, the precede-proceed model is a systematic and detailed approach to public health planning. It seeks to address all factors influencing health and well-being at a number of different levels. The model illustrates the complexity of the planning process and the various elements and components involved in health promotion.

Discussion points

How might you use Green and Kreuter's precede-proceed model in your area of practice?

Review your case study based on promoting young people's health. Can you organize your ideas using the model? This is a complex model and involves a multi-levelled assessment of the various components of health promotion planning.

- What areas do you now need to review as part of your planning to ensure you have a comprehensive plan?

- Have you considered all seven phases in your planning?

Try to assess the points you have made previously and organize these according to the precede-proceed model. What else do you need to consider in your planning? This is challenging and takes time, but will also show you how much work is involved in successful planning.

Finally, write up a reflection on your planning experiences and public health intervention. Ask yourself what worked well? What worked less well? What would you do differently next time? It is always important to review each step of the planning process to help you assess the success of the intervention and consider how you might do things differently in the future. This will help improve your planning skills for future interventions.

Summary

This chapter has outlined the key principles and complexities of successful health promotion planning. Key terms used in planning have been defined and further illustrated through the use of practice examples and activities. Individual and population level interventions have been discussed and the distinction between top-down and bottom-up strategies exemplified. A number of approaches to planning have been identified and two common planning models used in health promotion practice, Ewles and Simnett's (2003) seven-stage planning model and Green and Kreuter's (1991) precede-proceed model, have been outlined. The chapter has argued that effective public health planning is based on a systematic approach using a variety of methods to select the most appropriate course of action to promote individual and population health.

 # Online Resource Centre

For more information on Planning interventions visit the Online Resource Centre —
http://www.oxfordtextbooks.co.uk/orc/linsley/

Further reading

Department of Health (2004) *Choosing Health: Making Healthy Choices Easier.* London: The Stationery Office, Ch 3.

Department of Health/Department of Children, Schools and Families (2009) *Healthy Lives Brighter Futures — The Strategy for Children and Young People's Health and Well Being.* London: The Stationery Office. Available at www.dh.gov.uk

Scottish Executive (2003) *Improving Health in Scotland: The Challenge.* Edinburgh, The Stationery Office.

Scottish Executive (2007) *Delivering a Healthy Future: An Action Framework for Children and Young People's Health in Scotland.* London: Scottish Executive. Available at www.scotland.gov.uk

Summaries and full documents of Government policies are available at Department of Health www.dh.gov.uk

Scotland's Health on the Web www.show.nhs.uk

National Public Health Service for Wales www.nphs.wales.nhs.uk

References

Acheson, D. (1998). *Independent Inquiry into Inequalities in Health: A Report.* London: The Stationery Office.

Bell, S. (2001). *LogFrames: Improved NRSP Research Project Planning and Monitoring* Hemel Hempstead: Department for International development/ NRSP.

Department of Health (2004). *Choosing Health: Making Healthy Choices Easier.* London: The Stationery Office..

Department of Health/Department for Children, Schools and Families (2009). *Healthy Lives, Brighter Futures — The Strategy for Children and Young People's Health.* London: The Stationery Office.

Dignan, M. B. & Carr, P. A. (1992). *Program Planning for Health.* (2nd ed.). Malvern, PA: Lee & Febiger.

Ewles, L., Simnett, I. (2003). *Promoting health: A Practical Guide.* (5th edn.). London: Balliere Tindall.

Green, L. W. & Kreuter, M. W. (1991). *Health Promotion Planning: An Educational and Environmental Approach.* Mountain View, CA: Mayfield.

Green, L. W. & Kreuter, M. W. (4th edn. in press). *Health Promotion Planning: An Educational and Environmental Approach.* Mountain View, CA: Mayfield.

Hubley, J. (1993). *Communicating Health: An Action Guide to Health Education and Health Promotion.* London: Macmillan.

Hubley, J. & Copeman, J. (2008). *Practical Health Promotion.* Cambridge: Polity Press.

Laverack, G. & Labonte, R. (2000). A planning framework for community empowerment goals within health promotion. *Health Policy and Planning.* 15 (3): 255-62.

Laverack, G. (2005) *Public Health: Power, Empowerment and Professional Practice.* Basingstoke: Palgrave Macmillan.

Maycock, B., Howat, P. & Slevin, T. (2001). A decision-making model for health promotion advocacy: the case for advocacy of drink driving control measures. *Promotion and Education.* 8(2): 59-64.

Nancholas, S. (1998). 'How to do (or not to do)…a logical framework', *Health Policy and Planning.* 13 (2): 189-193.

Rose, G. (1992). *Rose's Strategy of Preventative Medicine.* Oxford: Oxford University Press.

Scottish Executive (2003). *Improving Health in Scotland: The Challenge.* Edinburgh: Scottish Executive.

Scottish Executive (2007). *Delivering a Healthy Future: An Action Framework for Children and Young People in Scotland.* Edinburgh: Scottish Executive.

Spencer, G. (2008). Young people's perspectives on health related risks. *Educate* 8 (1): 15-28.

Tones, K. & Green, J. (2006). *Health Promotion: Planning and Strategies.* London: Sage.

Tones, K. & Tilford, S. (2001). *Health Promotion: Effectiveness, Efficiency and Equity.* (3rd ed.). Cheltenham: Nelson Thornes.

Townsend, P., Davidson, N. & Whitehead, M. (1992). *Inequalities in Health: The Black Report and the Health Divide.* (2nd ed.). London: Penguin Books.

Chapter 11

Implementing interventions: delivering care to individuals and communities

Ian Loveday and Paul Linsley

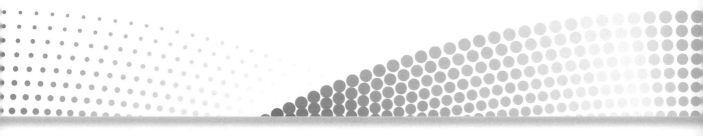

Introduction

The pursuit of public health is an important aspect of every nurse's practice and as such warrants close consideration. The following chapter looks at the spectrum of services through which the nurse may contribute to this agenda and what it is deliver care to individuals and communities. It recognizes the move from hospitals providing increasingly specialized care to home and community treatment options and the importance of prevention rather than cure. The chapter explores the diversity and challenges for nurses providing public health interventions and the many ways in which nurses can promote and help protect good health and well-being.

A shift in focus

Nursing practice in the UK has changed dramatically over the last 20 years, and this pace of change shows no sign of slowing down (DH, 2010; RCN, 2007). Nurses in acute settings manage an increasingly complex range of health care interventions that incorporate advances in technology (see Chapter 7) and disease management, while nurses in primary care settings

manage an increasing burden of chronic diseases and facilitate patient self management of their health. The focus of health care has moved from hospital to community settings and has a far greater emphasis on health promotion for maintaining good health and well-being than has been seen previously (DH, 2010). The current changes in health care delivery which focus on cost containment, managed care and home-based services have caused nurses to once again focus on their unique contributions to the care of individuals and the communities in which they work.

A key turning point was seen with the publication of the Wanless reports in 2002 and 2004 which identified an over-reliance on acute hospital care and recommended more primary and community-based care with public involvement in health improvement. This change in focus was echoed in the NHS Improvement Plan (DH, 2004), which further signaled the need for major cultural change to address this move from sickness to health. The reports also recognized that the role of the nurse was changing and that they were undertaking work traditionally carried out by doctors.

There has for some time been a formal commitment to increasing the contribution nurses make to public health but it is only now that it is starting to gain momentum. Since the publication of the Acheson report into health inequalities in 1988, the need for a radical approach to improving the health of the population has been recognized. In 1998 an official statement of intent to examine the role of nurses within the public health arena was published by the European and UK Chief Nursing Officers. This was later further enforced in the **Munich Declaration** (WHO, 2000) when ministers pledged to 'enhance the roles of nurses and midwives in public health, health promotion and community development'.

It was recognized however, that this would not be possible without an accompanying shift in the focus of the workforce. Choosing Health (DH, 2004) made direct reference to the need to 'develop training and support for all NHS staff to develop their understanding and skills in promoting health and to foster and expand a comprehensive range of community health improvement services'. This focus on prevention was further reiterated in a number of key policy documents including, The Future Nurse: the RCN vision (RCN, 2004), The Future Nurse: the future for nurse education (DH, 2007) and Modernizing Nursing Careers: setting the direction (DH, 2006). Developments in health care delivery including an ailing health care system and large-scale public dissatisfaction, higher activity levels, expanding roles for clinicians with increased accountability, technological developments and international recommendations to reorientate health care systems have all expedited these changes.

Box 11.1 The UK's key public health policy drivers

- Department of Health (1999). Saving Lives: our healthier nation.
- Department of Health (1999). Making a Difference: strengthening the nursing, midwifery and health visiting contribution to health and health care.
- Department of Health (2004). Choosing health.
- Department of Health (2006). Our health, our care, our say.
- Scottish Executive (2003). Improving health in Scotland.
- Welsh Assembly Government (2002). Well being in Wales.
- Department of Health, Social Services and Public Safety (2005). A healthier future: a 20-year vision for health and well being in Northern Ireland 2005–2025.

Increasingly, specialist nurses are working outside hospital providing care to patients with long-term conditions in their homes and providing specialist advice to other community staff. For many, nurses provide the first point of contact with the health care services through NHS Direct, NHS walk-in centres and practice nurses based within GP surgeries.

District and school nurses, health visitors and others who have a long history of working in the community are adapting their roles to meet the changing needs of patients and clients.

The role of the nurse in delivering care to individuals

Central to the role of the nurse is the planning and delivery of care (NHS Confederation, 2009). Responsibilities include assessment and treatment within the scope of professional nursing practice, communication with third parties, referral to physicians and other health care professionals, and provision or supervision of prescribed nursing care. Nursing includes the promotion of health, the prevention of illness, and the care of people who are ill. Additionally advocacy, promotion of a safe environment, research, participation in shaping health policy and in-patient and health systems management, and education are also key nursing roles (Schober and Affara, 2007).

The goal of any nursing care is to maximize the patient's positive interactions with the environment, promote a level of wellness, and enhance the patient's independence (Ferrell and Coyle, 2008). As a health care practitioner, the nurse assesses the overall system of care and develops a plan for ensuring that health needs are met. This is called the nursing process (White, 2002). The phases of the nursing process are assessment, diagnosis, planning, implementation and evaluation. Validation, the checking out of information with the patient, is part of each step, and all phases may overlap or occur simultaneously. It is an interactive, problem-solving process that respects the individual's autonomy and freedom to make decisions and be involved in nursing care.

In the assessment phase, information is obtained from the patient in a direct and structured manner through observations, interviews, and examinations. Nurses play a pivotal role in helping patients adapt to the community setting whether it be their own home, the home of a relative or friend, a voluntary care facility or private nursing home (Adams and Thomas, 2001). An assessment tool or nursing history form can provide a systematic format that becomes part of the patient's written record. This format enables the nurse to assess the patient's level of functioning and serves as a basis for diagnosis, outcome identification, planning, implementation, and evaluation of nursing care. Using specific data collection format helps ensure that the information is obtained. It also reduces repetition of the patient's medical history and provides a source of information available to all health care team members (White, 2002). The assessment tool the nurse uses to collect data should be derived from a conceptual model of nursing (see Chapter 9).

Many nursing interventions in the community setting are the same as in the acute or outpatients setting. However, in this case the nurse is a guest in the patient's home and must be mindful of this at all time. By receiving nursing care in the home the patient experiences a sense of comfort and control often lacking in the acute or outpatient environment, and the nurse has a unique opportunity to assess factors in the home that may impinge on the patient's ability to cope. The nurse can assess the influence of family, friends, the physical environment, and the patient's financial resources and ways of coping.

The challenge is to develop a rapport with the patient and so create an atmosphere which allows an effective consultation to take place. Neighbour (2005) describes this as connecting and it forms the first step of a five stage consultation model. There are many published models to guide the process of the clinical encounter. Neighbour's (2005) work has been widely cited as being influential (Moulton, 2007). The five stages of Neighbour's (2005) models can be applied in different settings the stages are:

1. Connecting,
2. Summarize,
3. Handover,
4. Safety net,
5. Housekeeping.

It is during the connecting stage that rapport is built with the patient, their concerns explored and a large proportion of the history is gained. This takes place through listening and asking open questions, enabling the patient to describe their experience of their illness. The best results can often be achieved when the nurse overcomes the desire to interrupt the patient and allows them to describe their experiences in their own terms. It can often be tempting to interrupt the patient's narrative and focus on a particular element, the risk in doing this however, is that the consultation then focuses on the point of interest which may not be the patients principle problem. Open questions may then be followed by more directed closed questions. (Douglas, *et al.,* 2006). As Purcell (2003) notes successful history taking requires the skills of the conversationalist in creating an atmosphere of empathy and the ear to detect the subtleties of communication.

The second stage of Neighbour's (2005) model involves summarizing the information gained back to the patient; this serves to ensure that information is correct. It is possible that the clinician may not be clear about details; this particularly applies to the time and order in which events occurred. Through summarizing the details of the patients concerns the clinician can confirm the information they have received (Moulton, 2007). It is also the case that when information is summarized or echoed back to the patient in this manner patients will often add useful further detail.

The third stage, handing over, involves the creation of a management plan. After writing a tentative management plan, nurses must validate this plan with the patient. Patient involvement in the development of a management plan is of the up most importance. A joint planning gives patient control over their care and increases the chances they will achieve the plan's goals. This saves time and effort for both as they continue to work together. It also communicates to the patient a sense of self-responsibility in getting well. The patient can tell the nurse that a proposed management plan is unrealistic regarding financial status, lifestyle, value system, or perhaps, personal preference. Usually there are several possible approaches to a patient's problem. Choosing the one most acceptable to the patient improves the chances of success.

The management plan focuses on improving the patient's ability to manage the activities of daily living (Castledine and Close, 2009). If the patient is too frail to work with the nurse in developing the management plan the nurse should involve the caregivers wherever possible. Taking time to listen and involve caregivers validates their concerns and opens the door to further discussion of how to cope with these feelings so they will be able to continue providing patient care. This is particularly true of those looking after people with dementia for example.

Once goals are agreed on, the nurse must state them explicitly. The more specifically the goals of treatment are stated, the more attainable these goals are. These goals also guide later nursing actions and enhance the evaluation of care. Goals should be written in behavioural terms. Goals should realistically describe what the nurse wishes to accomplish within a specific time span. Before defining expected outcomes, the nurse must realize that patients often seek treatment with goals of their own. These goals may be expressed as relieving symptoms or improving functional ability. Sometimes a patient cannot identify specific goals or may describe them in general terms. Translating non-specific goals into specific goal statements is not easy. The nurse must understand that the patient's coping resources and the factors that influence them.

One of the most important tasks facing the nurse and patient is to assign priorities to goals (Wardrope, Laird and Driscoll, 2004). Often, several goals can be pursued simultaneously. Those related to protecting the patient and preventing deterioration in health are given priority. When identifying expected outcomes and goals, the nurse must keep the proposed time sequence firmly in mind.

Once the goals are chosen the next task is to outline the plan for achieving them.

If a goal answers the question of what, the management plan answers the question of how and why. The plan chosen will depend on the nursing assessment and diagnosis, the nurse's theoretical orientation and the nature of the goals pursued.

The nursing management plan applies theory from nursing and treated biological behavioural and social sciences to the unique responses of the individual patient. This assumes that as the nurse identifies patient needs, appropriate resources will be consulted. Good planning increases the chances of successful implementation. Such factors as available people, equipment, resources, time, and money must be considered as nursing actions are planned. In most situations there is more than one way to accomplish the sated goals. It is helpful when planning care to identify alternative nursing actions that are also appropriate to the goal. If this is done, the nurse is not left floundering if the first approach fails. Considering several alternatives makes the implementation phase of the nursing process highly flexible.

Implementation is the actual delivery of nursing care to the patient and the response to that care. Interventions should be evidence-based and to aid the practitioner there are a range of organizations that publish guidelines based on best evidence. Skilled nursing requires a commitment to the ongoing pursuit of knowledge that will enhance professional growth. The National Institute for Health and Clinical Excellence (NICE) has produced guidance on a wide range of subjects. While publications relating to controversial and expensive drugs and treatments receive much media attention, other guidance exists on issues as diverse as managing fever in children, asthma care in adults and the management and treatment of depression. Evidence based interventions become more problematic when the evidence available is inconclusive or in some cases contradictory. This is often the case in even minor conditions such as tonsillitis; Collins and Pinch (2005) discuss the fact that despite tonsillectomy has been recorded as surgical procedure since the time of the Roman Empire there is still little agreement on when it should be performed.

Safety-netting is a vital part of any clinical consultation and any management plan should deal with this in a precise manner. Safety-netting refers to the instructions on what to do if a patient's condition worsens. Neighbour (2005) argues that safety netting should be a wider process that not only involves patient education but also the clinicians diagnostic process. Neighbour (2005) states that the practitioner should ask themselves three questions with respect to the patient newly formed diagnosis;

'If I'm right what do I expect to happen?'
'How will I know if I'm wrong?'
'What would I do then?'
Neighbour (2005: 204)

In considering these questions the safety net becomes more than just a statement to the patient at the end of the consultation. Rather it influences the management plan as a whole; if the diagnosis is uncertain then it may be appropriate to plan a repeat consultation as part of the management plan. It is not enough to give vague advice **'to return if necessary'**. Advice should be specific and take into account alterative diagnosis, places the patient could attend and whom they should contact for advice. In some cases written advice is available in the form

of leaflets or cards. Written advice is particularly useful where the patients condition may change, written advise will allow the patient and family to make a more informed decision on returning. A common example of written advice is the **'head injury card'** which is used in a range of settings. The final stage of the model is housekeeping, this refers to issues around the health and the well-being of the clinician. Issues that arise in one consultation can spill over into the next if steps are not taken to deal with them before moving on.

When evaluating care the nurse should review all previous phases of the nursing process and determine whether the expected outcomes for the patient have been met. Key words for the evaluation phase of the nursing process are mutual, competent, accessible, effective, appropriate efficient and flexible. The nurse must make many decisions throughout the process, including the following:

• What was the evidence base appropriate to this patient situation?
• Was my data collection adequate?
• Were my nursing diagnosis accurate and based on the analysis and synthesis of relevant data, the application of theory, and the appropriateness of nursing treatment?
• Were the expected outcomes and plan of care relevant and mutual showing appropriate priorities and the consideration of all relative alternatives?
• Were my nursing interventions effective and efficient?
• Were the expected outcomes achieved and, if not, did I make changes?
• Was the patient satisfied with the nursing care received?

Finally, evaluation is a continuous, active process that begins early in the relationship and continues throughout.

The role of the public health nurse in delivering care

Public health has been defined as 'organized social and political effort for the benefit of populations, families and individuals' (Mason and Clarke, 2001). Nurses have much to contribute

> ### Box 11.2 Primary care
> Primary care is an approach to care that includes a range of services designed to keep people well, from promotion of health and screening for disease to assessment, diagnosis, treatment and rehabilitation as well as personal social services. The services provide first-level contact that is fully accessible by self-referral and have a strong emphasis on working with communities and individuals to improve their health and social well being (DH, 2001).

to the promotion and delivery of public health whatever branch of nursing they may be, whether working in a community or hospital setting (WHO, 2000).

Public health and primary care services are primarily delivered by community health and social care staff of which nurses make up the largest proportion. Public health nurses fulfill the public health's essential services by implementing interventions to address public health problems and opportunities identified through a community and individual assessment (American Public Health Association, 2006). Those nurses working within public health integrate community involvement and knowledge of the entire population with the personal clinical understandings of health and illness gleaned from the experiences of individuals and families within the population. The public health nurse can apply her knowledge of strategies to choose the intervention(s) that meets the needs of a particular community, family or individual (Department of Health Social Services and Public Safety, 2003). The nurse is the agent who translates and applies the knowledge of health and social sciences to individuals and population groups through specific interventions, programs and advocacy. He or she also articulates and translates health and illness experiences of diverse, often vulnerable, individuals and families to the health planners and policy makers (WHO, 2000).

Public health nurses provide a range of health care services in the community. They are usually based in your local health centre and are assigned to cover specific geographical areas. They provide services in schools, in health centres, in day care and other community centres and in people's homes. Some nurses work in local government health departments as general practice nurses in neighborhoods. In some health departments, the community intervention role of public health nurses is not well established and their work is confined to home visits and clinic work. Their primary role is that of **case manager** and they have a varied caseload of individuals and families whom they assist with illness-oriented concerns, such as communicable diseases and health problems of mothers and children.

Public health nursing is the practice of promoting and protecting the health of populations using knowledge of nursing, social and public health sciences. In order to do this public health nurses (Health Resources and Services Administration, 2005):

- Assess the health and health care needs of a population in order to identify sub-populations, families and individuals who would benefit from health promotion or who are at risk of illness, injury, disability or premature death.
- Develop a plan with the community to meet the identified needs taking into account available resources.
- Implement the plan at the community, family or individual level.
- Evaluate the impact of the intervention.
- Use the results of the evaluation to influence and direct current delivery of care, deployment of health resources and the development of local, state and national health policy and resources to promote health and prevent disease.

Public health nurses recognize that the community and environment in which people live can affect their ability to make healthy lifestyle choices and can affect whether or not such choices exist at all (Stanhope and Lancaster, 2000). Thus, public health nurses may spend a significant portion of their time on ensuring healthy living conditions in the neighborhoods where they work and on improving the health status of the entire community, not just that of individuals. Examples of community issues on which the public health nurse may work are reducing tobacco sales to minors, fluoridation of drinking water, identifying and reducing workplace hazards, immunization of all children against communicable diseases, and reducing the risk of drowning through community education, pool

Box 11.3 The aims of delivering public health through nursing services

- Increase life expectancy by influencing healthy behaviours,
- Reduce health inequalities — for example, targeting vulnerable populations to improve health outcomes and access services,
- Improve population health — for example, reducing obesity, alcohol abuse, improving sexual health behaviour.
- Increase awareness of positive healthy behaviours in communities,
- Promote and develop social capital,
- Engage with individuals, families and communities to influence the design and development of services,

RCN (2007)

Box 11.4 Community

Communities are comprised of individuals who share a common goal and are bonded by location, interdependent social groups, interpersonal relationships and culture. The culture of the community gives rise to values, norms, beliefs and a sense of attachment for its members. Clark (1996) describes community as a group of men and women who share some kind of bond, who interact with each other, and who operate collectively in respect of common concerns.

safety, and construction regulation. In doing so the public health nurse systemically enhances the quality and effectiveness of nursing practice and attains knowledge and competency that reflects current nursing and public health practice (Helvie, 1998).

Any interaction or intervention should be planned carefully. The overall goal should be to assist people with health gain and live successfully within the community. It should clearly state what is expected of the person and specific actions that will be taken to meet them. This plan is reflective of the nursing process. According to Moxley (1989) the major components of such a plan include the following:

- Specification of problem areas to be addressed,
- Identification of goals,
- Identification of the service and supports needed to achieve goals,
- Identification of the people or agencies who will undertake specific activities to achieve the objectives of the plan,
- Specification of a timeline for the completion of each objective,
- Identification of changes expected to result form the completion of each objective.

Improving the health of families and communities requires more than responding to the manifestations of illness or the outcomes of risk. Rather, it requires that public health nurses focus on the underlying causes of illness, injury, premature death, and disability — the social determinants of health (see Chapter 3). This model suggests a powerful co-mingling and interplay of risk and supportive factors. The physical environment, genetics, individual biologic and behavioral response, access to health care, level of prosperity, stress, early life and experience, social support, social exclusion, work environments, unemployment, addiction, availability of food and transportation have all been linked to health outcomes (WHO, 2003).

Public health nurses are able to assist individuals and families to take action to improve their health status. Often this takes the form of teaching about healthy lifestyle choices in the home, in the workplace, and in community settings. Public health nurses assist people in applying improved health behavior choices to their everyday lives. Examples of personal behaviors that can contribute to health problems are tobacco use, improper diet, lack of physical exercise, unsafe sexual practices, and driving while intoxicated. By proving community care nurses need to mobilize and coordinate resources around the needs of the patient to maximize the patient's potential to stabilize, cope and gain as much independence as possible.

Many (if not all) of these are provided by the statutory health care services although there needs to be recognition given to the growing contribution that the voluntary health care section makes to maintaining people in the community.

Box 11.5 Through a wide spectrum of services, nurses can:

- Identify individual and population health need, using assessment.
- Target their services at vulnerable individuals and communities.
- Contribute to and develop services that protect the public's health — for example, immunization, emergency planning and communicable disease prevention.
- Share health information to encourage individuals, families and communities to become more active in developing healthy lifestyles.
- Prevent ill health and promote health enhancing activities by working with families and individuals.
- Promote and develop action to tackle the underlying causes of ill health.
- Lead partnership working for health and other key organizations.
- Advocate for health gain in relation to all public activities — for example, housing, leisure, transport, shopping and the environment.
- Be catalysts for health, creating new resources and collaboration to sustain good health in local groups and communities, such as schools or prisons.
- Challenge vested interests that threaten public health.
- Access hard-to-reach groups, engaging them around their health hopes and fears.

RCN (2007)

Activity box

Make a list of as many services within your local community providing public health support. You may be surprised at the number which you arrive at. Try to make time to visit some of these and learn more about what they have to offer, both the individual and community.

Levels of interventions

Interventions may be directed at the entire population within a community, the systems that affect the health of those populations, and/or the individuals and families within those populations known to be at risk (Minnesota Department of Health, 2001).

Population-based community-focused practice

This intervention changes community norms, community attitudes, community awareness, community practices, and community behaviors. They are directed toward entire populations within the community or occasionally toward target groups within those populations.

Community-focused practice is measured in terms of what proportion of the population actually changes.

Population-based systems-focused practice

This intervention changes organizations, policies, laws, and power structures. The focus is not directly on individuals and communities but on the systems that impact health. Changing systems is often a more effective and long-lasting way to impact population health than requiring change from every single individual in a community.

Population-based individual-focused practice

This intervention changes knowledge, attitudes, beliefs, practices, and behaviors of individuals. This practice level is directed at individuals, alone or as part of a family, class, or group. Individuals receive services because they are identified as belonging to a population-at-risk.

Interventions at each of these levels of practice contribute to the overall goal of improving population health status. Public health professionals determine the most appropriate level(s) of practice based on community need and the availability of effective strategies and resources. No one level of practice is more important than another; in fact, most public health problems are addressed at all three levels, often simultaneously. Consider, for example, smoking rates, which continue to rise among the adolescent population. At the community level of practice, public health nurses coordinate youth led, adult supported, social marketing campaigns intending to change the community norms regarding adolescents' tobacco use. At the systems level of practice, public health nurses facilitate community coalitions that advocate city councils to create stronger ordinances restricting over-the-counter youth access to tobacco. At the individual/ family practice level, public health nurses teach middle school chemical health classes that increase knowledge about the risks of smoking, change attitudes toward tobacco use, and improve 'refusal skills' among youth 12–14 years of age.

Prevention rather than cure

Whenever possible, public health programs emphasize prevention. The work of public health nurses is defined as 'primary prevention', which means preventing disease, injury, disability and premature death. According to Turnock (1997), there are three levels of prevention and these are as follows:

Primary prevention

This level both promotes health and protects against threats to health. It keeps problems from occurring in the first place. It promotes resiliency and protective factors or reduces susceptibility and exposure to risk factors. Primary prevention is implemented before a problem develops. It targets essentially well populations. Primary prevention promotes health, such as building assets in youth, or keeps problems from occurring, for example, immunizing for vaccine-preventable diseases.

Secondary prevention

This level detects and treats problems in their early stages. It keeps problems from causing serious or long-term effects or from affecting others. It identifies risks or hazards and modifies, removes, or treats them before a problem becomes more serious. Secondary prevention is implemented after a problem has begun, but before signs and symptoms appear. It targets populations that have risk factors in common. Secondary prevention detects and treats problems early, such as screening for home safety and correcting hazards before an injury occurs.

Tertiary prevention

This level limits further negative effects from a problem. It keeps existing problems from getting worse. It alleviates the effects of disease and injury and restores individuals to their optimal level of functioning. Tertiary prevention is implemented after a disease or injury has occurred. It targets populations who have experienced disease or injury. Tertiary prevention keeps existing problems from getting worse, for instance, collaborating with health care providers to assure periodic examinations to prevent complications of diabetes such as blindness, renal disease failure, and limb amputation.

Health care screening and surveillance

Disease and other health event investigation systematically gathers and analyzes data regarding threats to the health of populations, ascertains the source of the threat, identifies cases and others at risk, and determines control measures. The threats may be actual or potential. While investigation traditionally focuses on contagious diseases, it also may be used with chronic diseases, injury, and other health events. The investigative process consists of identifying and verifying the source of the threat; identifying cases, their contacts, and others at risk, determining control measures, and communicating with the public, as needed (WHO, 2008).

Nurses play an important part in this through health care screening and surveillance. Screening identifies individuals with unrecognized health risk factors or asymptomatic disease conditions in populations.

Three types of screening are described in the literature:

- **Mass:** a process to screen the general population for a single risk—such as cholesterol screening in a shopping centre,or for multiple health risks —such as health risks within an industry or place of work **(community level)**.

- **Targeted:** a process to promote screening to a discrete subgroup within the population—such as those at risk for HIV infection **(individual/family level)**.

- **Periodic:** a process to screen a discrete, but well, sub-group of the population on a regular basis, over time, for predictable risks or problems; examples include breast and cervical cancer screening among age-appropriate women, well-child screening, and the follow along associated with early childhood development programs **(individual/family level)**.

> ## Nursing Practice box
>
> The practice nurse provides screening and referral for health conditions. Health screenings can decrease the negative effects of health problems by identifying individuals with potential underlying medical problems early and referring them for treatment as appropriate. Early identification, referral to other health care professionals, and use of appropriate community resources promote optimal outcomes. Screening includes but is not limited to vision, hearing, and BMI assessments (as determined by local policy).

Activity box

Apart from breast cancer screening for women, write a list of any other diseases, conditions or developmental abnormalities that you know are the focus of screening tests. In each case, state which group is screened and whether the example is a population screening programme or high risk screening. Then read our comments below.

Surveillance, as opposed to screening, focuses on significant health threats such as contagious diseases but is also used with other health events such as chronic diseases, injury, and violence. Like investigation of disease and other health events, surveillance collects and analyzes health data. Unlike

investigation, however, surveillance is an ongoing process which detects trends and seeks to identify changes in the **incidence** (that is, the occurrence of new cases over a set period of time) and **prevalence** (that is, the combined number of old and new cases at any one point in time).

Health promotion

Of importance to primary prevention is the concept and practice of health promotion (see Chapter 3). Nurses have a key role in not only delivering but devising health promotion interventions and strategies. Health promotion is not only concerned with fostering the motivation, skills and confidence (self-efficacy) necessary to take action to improve health. It also includes the communication of information concerning the underlying social, economic and environmental conditions impacting on health, as well as individual risk factors and risk behaviours, and use of the health care system. In this way, health promotion may involve the communication of information, and development of skills which demonstrates the political feasibility and organizational possibilities of various forms of action to address social, economic and environmental and determinants of health (again see Chapter 3).

> ## Nursing Practice box
>
> The school nurse provides health promotion by providing health information to individual students and groups of students through health education, science, and other classes. The school nurse assists on health education curriculum development teams and may also provide programmes for staff, families, and the community. Health education topics may include nutrition, exercise, smoking prevention and cessation, oral health, prevention of sexually transmitted infections and other infectious diseases, substance use and abuse, immunizations, adolescent pregnancy prevention, parenting, and others.

Partnership working

Improving the public's health is a key role for all nurses, yet it is acknowledged that this is not an activity that lies solely within the health domain. It is important to remember that nurses work within multidisciplinary teams who also have the interest and aim of promoting health within those that they care for. A core competency of public health nursing is the ability to establish partnerships. For example, public health nurses and community registered general nurses liaise with family doctors (GPs), practice nurses, hospitals, hospices and other health service providers to ensure that the needs of the patient are met by the overall health service. They also work as a team with other public health professionals such as environmental health specialists, health educators, epidemiologists, public health physicians, and nutritionists. As members of this team, they work with local communities to assess and prioritize the major health problems and work on a plan to alleviate or eliminate these problems and the conditions that contribute to their development.

Effective care and treatment requires innovative approaches, coordination and cooperation amongst services. Nurses make important contributions to the availability, quality, and accessibility of health services by advancing collaborative working. From liaisons with primary care providers to educational programmes, nurses may better serve their patients by encouraging collaborative working relationships among health and social care providers, the informal care giving network (including community organizations and self help groups), and the statutory health care providers. By integrating and sharing available resources from each these domains, nurse may improve the overall delivery of care.

The nurse as public health advocate

As part of partnership working, the nurse has a responsibility to act as a public health advocate.

Advocacy has been defined as:

'A combination of individual and social actions designed to gain political commitment, policy support, social acceptance and systems support for a particular health goal or programme'
WHO, (1995)

Such action may be taken by and/or on behalf of individuals and groups to create living conditions which are conducive to health and the achievement of healthy lifestyles. Advocacy is one of the three major strategies for health promotion and can take many forms including the use of the mass media and multi-media, direct political lobbying, and community mobilization through, for example, coalitions of interest around defined issues. Health professionals have a major responsibility to act as advocates for health at all levels in society. Helping people receive all available services and influencing providers to improve existing services and develop new ones is a fundamental role of the nurse.

Public health nurses are granted a societal privilege to practice, therefore have a responsibility to understand, learn, and take individual and collective action on health disparities. Public health nurses are, therefore, advocates for health equality and social justice. Public health nursing leaders advocate for structures within state and local health departments that foster participation by public health nurses in systems and community interventions, not just with individuals and families. Information about communities, and the importance of ethnicity, language, and culture, needs to be translated and interpreted to policy makers in a way that encourages doing 'the right thing' (Christoffel, 2000).

The role of the nurse in developing public health guidance

Public health guidance makes recommendations for populations and individuals on activities, policies and strategies that can help prevent disease or improve health. The guidance may focus on a particular topic (such as smoking), a particular population (such as schoolchildren) or a particular setting (such as the workplace).

Each public health nurse must see his or her role as more than custodial of current policies and programs. Rather, public health nurses must constantly be aware of opportunities to improve programs and services to better serve communities and population groups at increased risk of illness, injury, premature death, and disability.

The public health nurse is constantly evaluating his/her own nursing practice in relation to professional practice standards and guidelines, ethics, relevant statutes, rules and regulations and against the unmet and evolving needs of the populations served. The goals for health improvement and health equity can be supported through thorough, objective evaluation of what works and what does not work, and through subsequent alterations in policy and practice. The public health nurses' role as stewards of public investment demands it, as does the public trust (Hofrichter, 2006).

Summary

The nurse has a pivotal role in delivering care to individuals and communities. Public health nurses recognize that the community and environment in which people live can affect their ability to make healthy lifestyle choices and can affect whether or not such choices exist at all. Thus, public health nurses may spend a significant portion of their time on ensuring healthy living conditions in the neighborhoods where they work and on improving the health status of the entire community, not just that of individuals. Community-based partnerships and coalition activities have become an accepted part of the overall strategy for maintaining people within their own home and community. Choosing interventions that work in general and that are well matched to local culture, needs, and capabilities and then implementing those interventions well are vital steps for improving people's health and well being. In setting priorities for interventions to meet local objectives, nurses should considered such local information as resource availability, administrative structures, and the cultural, economic, social, and regulatory environments of organizations and health agencies. In meeting the public health agenda the nurse must be able to apply their knowledge of strategies to choose the intervention(s) that meets the needs of a particular community, family or individual.

 # Online Resource Centre

For more information on implementing interventions visit the Online Resource Centre — http://www.oxfordtextbooks.co.uk/orc/linsley/

References

Adams C. & Thomas E. (2001). The benefit of integrated nursing teams in primary care. *British Journal of Community Nursing,* 6 (6): 271–274.

American Public Health Association (2006). *The Public Health Workforce Strategy. Left Unchecked Will We Be Protected?* Issue Brief. Washington: APHA

Castledine G. & Close A. (2009). (eds.). *Oxford Handbook of Adult Nursing.* Oxford: Oxford University Press.

Christoffel K. K. (2000). Public Health Advocacy: Process and Product. *American Journal of Public Health,* 90 (8): 722–726.

Clark M. J. (1996). *Nursing in the Community,* revised edition. Stanford, CT: Appleton and Lange.

Collins H, Pinch T. (2005). *Dr Golem: how to think about medicine.* Chicago: University of Chicago Press.

Department of Health (2001). *Primary care, general practice and the NHS Plan.* London: DH.

Department of Health (2004). *The NHS Improvement Plan: putting people at the heart of public services.* London: DH

Department of Health (2006). *Modernizing Nursing Careers: setting the direction.* London: DH.

Department of Health (2010). *Front line care. Report by the Prime Minister's Commission on the Future of Nursing and Midwifery in England 2010.* London: DH.

Department of Health, Social Services and Public Safety (2003). *Community Health nursing. Current Practice and Possible Futures.* Belfast: Castle Buildings.

Douglas G., Nicol F. & Robertson C. (2006). *Macleod's Clinical Examination.* : London: Elsevier Churchill Livingstone.

Ferrell B. R. & Coyle N. (2008). *The Nature of Suffering and the Goals of Nursing.* Oxford: Oxford University Press.

Heath Resources and Services Administration (2005). *Public health workforce study. Bureau of Health Professions.* Rockville, Maryland.

Helvie, C. O. (1998). *Advanced Practice Nursing in the Community.* Thousand Oaks, CA: Sage Publications.

Hofrichter R. (2006). (ed.). *Tackling Health Inequalities Through Public Health Practice. A Handbook.* London: W. K. Kellogg Foundation.

Mason C. & Clarke J. (2001). *A Nursing Vision of Public Health. All Ireland Statement on Public Health and Nursing.* Belfast: DHSSPSt and Dublin: DoHC.

Minnesota Department of Health. Division of Community Health Sevices: Public Health Nursing Section (2001) *Public health nursing interventions.* Application to public health practice. Minneapolis: MDH.

Moulton L. (2007) *The Naked Consultation: A Practical Guide to Primary Care Consultation Skills.* Oxford: Radcliffe Publishing.

Moxley, R. (1989). *Case Management.* Beverly Hills, CA: Sage Publications.

Neighbour R. (2005). *The Inner Consultation.* Oxford: Radcliffe

NHS Confederation (Employers) (2009). *Discussion paper 3: The role of the nurse.* London: NHS Employers.

Purcell J. (2003). *Minor injuries a clinical guide for nurses.* London: Churchill Livingstone.

Royal College of Nursing (2007). *The Future Nurse: the future for nurse education. A discussion paper.* London: Royal College of Nursing.

Schober M. & Affara F. (2007). (eds.) *International Council of Nursing: advanced nursing practice.* London: Blackwell Publishing.

Simon C., Everitt H., & Kendrick T. (2005). *Oxford handbook of general practice.* Oxford: Oxford University Press.

Stanhope M. & Lancaster J. (2000). *Community and Public Health Nursing,* revised edition. St. Louis, MO: Mosby.

Turnock, B. (1997). *Public Health: What it is and how it works.* Gaithersburg, MD: Aspen Publishers, Inc.

Wanless D. (2002). *Securing our Future Health: taking a long term view.* London: Her Majesty's Stationery Office.

Wanless D. (2004). *Securing Good Health for the Whole Population.* London: Her Majesty's Stationery Office.

White L. (2002). *Documentation and the Nursing Process: A Review.* London: Delmar Cengage Learning.

World Health Organization (1995). *Advocacy Strategies for Health and Development: Development Communication in Action.* Geneva: WHO.

World Health Organization (2000). *Munich Declaration: Nurses and midwives: a force for health 2000.* Geneva: WHO.

World Health Organization (2003). The *Social Determinants of Health: The Solid Facts.* Geneva: WHO.

World Health Organization (2008). *Communicable disease alert and response for mass gathering.* Geneva: WHO.

Chapter 12

Evaluating interventions: focusing on measuring impact at both the individual and community level

A. Niroshan Siriwardena

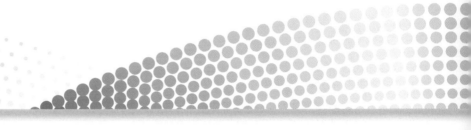

Introduction

This chapter seeks to outline the basic concepts and skills needed when evaluating clinically-led (including nurse led) health care and health promotion (or prevention) interventions. It starts by seeking to explore why we might undertake an evaluation and, after defining the term *evaluation*, describes different types of evaluation. Next, it seeks to clarify the differences and overlaps between clinical audit, evaluation, improvement or research. The main body of the chapter describes the ten key steps which need to be considered for a successful evaluation, explains how these steps can be used to construct a logic model evaluation and elaborates on how a variety of different methods can be used to answer different questions within the evaluation framework. The methods for evaluation and quality improvement are compared to see how the latter can be used as part of the process of evaluation. Finally there is a section on health systems, complexity and complex interventions because it is important to see health promotion as a multifactorial intervention in the context of the wider health system.

Deciding to undertake an evaluation

There are a number of reasons why you might wish to conduct an evaluation of your work. It may be for personal reasons such as continuing professional development, recertification or simply out of individual interest and for individual growth borne out of curiosity. You may have been asked to evaluate a service or health promotion (prevention) activity to demonstrate its usefulness, for marketing to service users or for commissioners, deciding whether to continue with the current approaches, or when considering whether to design or purchase new models of provision.

Evaluation of policy or health promotion interventions has not been traditionally considered to be within the scope of routine nursing or other clinical practice. When it does happen it is still often arrived at as an afterthought rather than being considered integral to the assessment of existing services or development of new modes of delivery. However, as health promotion, preventive health and care delivery continue to evolve, as new roles emerge and develop in the workforce, and as organizations and teams reorganize and reconfigure to improve care, evaluation becomes an increasingly important part of practice. There is a need to determine whether services and health promotion interventions are of the highest quality, that is to say they are safe, effective and efficient, and geared to enhancing the patient experience by being timely, accessible and patient centred (Institute of Medicine, 2001; Darzi of Denham, 2008). However, as commissioners of health services focus on purchasing health promotion, prevention and clinical care that is not only of high quality but also builds in continuing improvement, then evaluation that is focused on quality improvement will increasingly become an essential component rather than an afterthought of service specification.

Evaluation may therefore be defined as the 'systematic assessment of a health project or initiative, programme, policy, personnel, technology, or organization in order to establish or improve its effectiveness, efficiency, safety and acceptability'. It is about examining whether we and the health services we are providing are doing the right thing and doing things right (NHS Institute for Innovation and Improvement, 2005).

An evaluation can be focused on health service users at various levels including that of an individual patient or carer, group or population; or it can look at services from the perspective of the health practitioner, their team and practice or the wider organization. The introduction focuses on why is it important to measure the impact of new interventions and approaches, when and where we should focus our evaluation efforts, what should be measured and how it should be assessed and, importantly, how evaluation should relate to improvement and implementation of change.

Evaluation is sometimes categorized according to whether it informs the design of an intervention (formative evaluation), assesses process and structure (process evaluation) or outcome or impact of services or activities (outcome evaluation). Formative evaluation informs the nature or design of a service or intervention, often through the collection of data from the target audience. Conducting focus groups to test the language, tone and style of health promotion posters is an example of this. Process evaluations describe the structure and processes employed such as techniques (or equipment) used, how they are implemented, who they involve and the pathway of care that is involved. Outcome evaluations look at the direct effects on service users or the recipients of health promotion, such as satisfaction with services, uptake of activities (e.g. exercise promotion, dietary advice) or concordance with advice or treatment. Impact evaluations look at longer term consequences for patients, staff or other services including positive, negative and unintended effects as well as costs.

Clinical audit, evaluation, improvement or research

There is sometimes confusion between the different activities of clinical audit, evaluation, quality improvement and research.

Part of the confusion lies in the simple fact that there is overlap between these activities. The most important difference from a practical point of view is that research generates new knowledge and, through the internal and external validity of the findings, is generalizable to settings other than where it was conducted. Audit, evaluation and improvement activities do not necessarily have these features of newness and generalizability. As a consequence of this, and because research has the potential for harm, it is deemed to require ethical approval and should follow the standards of the International Conference on Harmonization of Good Clinical Practice (ICH-GCP) Guideline. However, it is important to remember that the other activities also have important ethical considerations.

Clinical audit involves assessment of practice against criteria derived from evidence and standards based on published performance, previous achievement or consensus with the aim of implementing change to bring about improvement. It is usually specific to the site and time at which it was carried out although larger regional, national or multinational audits can sometimes generate new knowledge or, in the case of large scale audits, be generalizable. Clinical audit is just one quality improvement method.

Quality improvement involves (usually) 'small scale cycles of interventions that are linked to assessment and that have the goal of improving the process, outcome, and efficiency of complex systems of health care' (Casarett et al., 2000). Quality improvement can generate knowledge about novel methods or combinations of improvement methods and be generalizable for issues such as organizational performance, gaps in performance and the effectiveness of improvement methods depending on the scale of the improvement project.

Evaluation aims to inform the nature of and to measure the quality of health promotion interventions or current provision of care or a newly introduced service. Interventions can be introduced as part of an evaluation but these are interventions based on established guidance or good practice rather than experimental techniques without established evidence, and usually involve analysis of existing data or data from questionnaires or assessment against practice. Evaluation can form part of a quality improvement process and it can employ clinical audit as an improvement method. When conducted properly evaluation aspires to be systematic and rigorous, just as research and audit do, and it may use similar methods of quantitative or qualitative data collection and analysis. It is sometimes said to differ in its practical nature and its focus on judgment or improvement although evaluations using so-called quasi-experimental designs or action research methods also fall within the scope of research. Quasi-experimental designs include time series designs which analyse quantitative changes over time (using statistical methods such as process control or regression) and non-randomized control designs where changes in the service being evaluated are compared with a 'control' service. Action research is a method whereby researchers collaborate with service providers (practitioners) to implement and evaluate change.

It can be seen that evaluation, improvement (including clinical audit) and research, have characteristics which are particular each to themselves, but also contain some features which are common to all. Although there will be examples which fall clearly into one category or another there are others which include elements of all and it becomes a matter of judgment as to how it should be classified. If there is any doubt, it should be possible to get advice from a research ethics committee or a research management and governance department. If an evaluation is deemed to require research ethics approval then it should adhere to current standards of research governance and have independent ethics approval. Even if it does not, there are still ethical issues that need to be considered and addressed and which will often need organizational approval, so it is important that advice is sought from the appropriate research office and that any proposed evaluation is discussed with senior staff in the organization.

> **Box 12.1** The ten steps to a successful evaluation
>
> **Step 1** Decide whether you need to conduct an evaluation,
>
> **Step 2** Define your evaluation question,
>
> **Step 3** Involve stakeholders,
>
> **Step 4** Gather realistic resources,
>
> **Step 5** Choose evaluation methods,
>
> **Step 6** Develop foundations for action,
>
> **Step 7** Formulate reporting and communication framework,
>
> **Step 8** Assess and develop expertise,
>
> **Step 9** Follow governance and ethics processes,
>
> **Step 10** Put together an evaluation plan.
>
> Marsh and Glendenning, 2005

Key steps in evaluating health systems

When planning an evaluation there are a number of steps that need to be considered whatever the scale or focus of the evaluation (Box 12.1). A number of schemes have been developed but the following framework, developed by Marsh and Glendenning for primary care (Marsh and Glendenning, 2005) is particularly helpful.

The first step in any evaluation is to be clear about the rationale for undertaking it. The possible reasons are to determine the quality of care being provided by an individual, team or service where quality can include the effectiveness, efficiency, safety or patient focus of that care; to ensure that the aims of care are being met in terms of the service being delivered or the care being experienced; to provide information for service users, commissioners, health care providers or other stakeholders about the quality of services being provided; and finally to establish the basis for future improvements.

Evaluation of individual or team care is often conducted primarily for personal development, to provide evidence for clinical supervision or reaccreditation and as part of a personal portfolio. Even if this is the case, an evaluation can provide powerful information about the quality of care being provided and help to shape and improve future services or interventions. Arguably the most important purpose of evaluation is to help make decisions on whether the right care is being provided or whether this can be improved.

The evaluation question will depend on whether you are interested in the structure, process, outcome or impact. Structure refers to the way care is organized and this includes personnel, facilities and equipment, operating protocols and guidelines and the training programmes which underpin these to enable health care staff to operate effectively. The processes are the patterns and schedules of individual work, how they link and integrate between team members and how these integrate across organizations to enable the pathways of care that service users need to follow. Outcomes refer to immediate or short-term effect on services users in terms of their choices, satisfaction, health benefits, adverse effects or quality of life. Impact assessment looks at longer term benefits and adverse consequences beyond the direct effects of the care or services or interventions delivered.

If evaluation is ultimately about making decisions on the quality of care and how to better this, then involving other stakeholders is a key consideration unless, possibly, one is just evaluating personal care. However, all evaluations can create worry and anxiety and therefore should make careful consideration of other stakeholders. This will often include team members and managers but in wider evaluations could include users and commissioners of the service. 'Ownership' of the evaluation among relevant stakeholders is the key to gaining support for a robust design, valid conclusions, involvement in improvement and potential resources for its conduct. The resources required for an evaluation can range from personal or work time for small scale individual or team evaluations, to considerable time, funds and expertise for large scale evaluations involving one or more organizations, regions or countries.

For such larger-scale evaluations it can also be helpful to be clear about the underpinning theoretical framework for the evaluation (Grol *et al.*, 2007). Examples of theoretical frameworks include psychological theories such as the theory of planned behaviour where behavioural decisions are based on

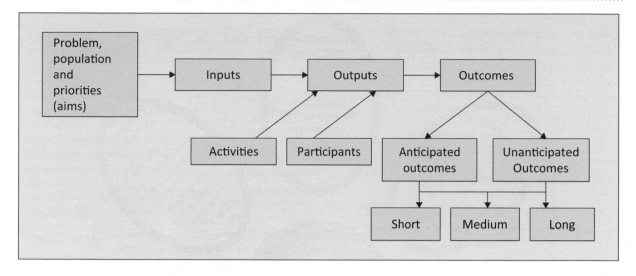

Fig. 12.1 Outline logic model for an evaluation.

analysis of available information to make rational choices (Ajzen, 1991); social worlds theory emphasizes the tension and conflict between the different players involved (Rhydderch *et al.*, 2004); organizational behavioural and organizational developmental models attempt to understand human factors involved in organizational change (Garside, 1998); systems theory emphasizes the interconnectedness of different components of a system (Nolan, 1998); and complexity theory which includes ideas of interaction, unpredictability, adaptation, co-evolution, and self-organization (Plsek and Greenhalgh, 2001).

More than one theoretical framework can also be called upon for explanation in terms of the problem being addressed, the population being studied and the aims of the programme or intervention, as well as the anticipated inputs, outputs and outcomes being considered. These can be represented as a logic model (Thurston *et al.*, 2003) which can help you to formulate a more detailed evaluation timeline and plan as well as the communication strategy for the evaluation (Fig. 12.1).

Let's consider the following scenario. A new sexual health service has been running for a year. Your local primary care organization is planning to commission an evaluation of the service. The service is run in primary care by two nurses, and a lead general practitioner supported by a specialist in genitourinary medicine for a local community comprising several general practices. Fig. 12.2 shows the proposed logic model for such an evaluation.

Evaluation methods

The method chosen for an evaluation depends on the evaluation question being asked. In particular, are we interested in measuring impact at the level of the services user, the patient or their carer or are we trying to look at the effect on wider

groups or communities? Also, are we interested in looking at the structure, processes or outcomes of care or interventions? A variety of methods can be used and examples of these are described below.

> **Box 12.2** Examples of conventional clinical evaluation methods
>
> **Process/structure**
> 1. Equipment, staff, guidelines, protocols,
> 2. Process and pathway mapping,
> 3. Process performance measurement against indicators.
>
> **Outcome/impact**
> 1. Cost analysis,
> 2. Intermediate (proxy) or true health outcome measures,
> 3. Adverse event analysis.
>
> **Both**
> 1. Patient or staff questionnaires.
> 2. Interviews (single or group), observation, textual analysis.

We may seek to answer different evaluation questions using a variety of techniques including questionnaires, interviews (individual or group; structured, semi-structured or unstructured), observational methods to collect quantitative or qualitative data, review of written documents (minutes of meetings, policy), or analysis of quantitative data (on processes or costs).

147

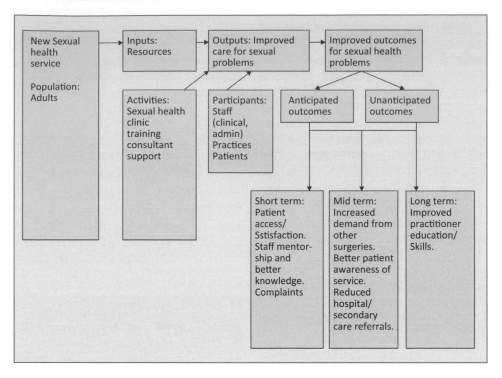

Fig. 12.2 Outline logic Model for evaluation of a new sexual health service.

Patient satisfaction questionnaires have been validated and used for gaining information on patient satisfaction as a basis for improving care (Harris *et al.*, 1999; Mead *et al.*, 2008). Although there is limited evidence on the effectiveness of individual feedback to clinicians (Cheraghi-Sohi and Bower, 2008), questionnaires can provide a useful basis for quality improvement initiatives by identifying potential barriers to uptake of health interventions (Siriwardena, 1999). However, they are limited by the constraints inherent on instruments which are only able to access information on the questions that are asked.

Interviews are another well tried and tested method which help to understand gaps in services, identify opportunities for enhancing care and help to determine how this can be done with a patient focus (Siriwardena *et al.*, 2008). A particular type of interview, the 'discovery interview', has been developed to access patient and carer narratives with the aim of evaluating health systems from a user perspective in order to improve services.

In one study which sought to evaluate breaches in confidentiality in general practice waiting rooms and the reason for these an ethnographic method was used. A researcher gained consent to sit in the waiting area of family doctor surgeries and observe the content of confidentiality breaches and the features of the environment which led to or prevented breaches occurring This enabled feedback to the practices involved and general practices more widely about the potential for breaches of confidentiality and how to overcome these (Scott *et al.*, 2007).

Multi-method approaches to evaluation which include anthropological techniques such as participant or non-participant observation, together with interviews and quantitative analysis are increasingly being used for evaluating complex communitywide services or interventions (Aronson *et al.*, 2007).

Quality improvement methods

There are a number of improvement methods and techniques which could also be used for evaluation at an individual or team level (Siriwardena, 2009). Each has advantages and disadvantages. There is an overlap with evaluation techniques and in some respects the differences between these are artificial. All of these techniques, if carried out well, can lead to better understanding of the process of care, and the potential through introducing change for improved outcomes for patients, increased professional satisfaction and enhanced inter-professional communication and team working.

The quality improvement methods, although they have been well used and described in industry and despite their introduction and application to health services (Plsek, 1999b) have not diffused widely into clinical thinking.

Clinical audit

Clinical audit consists of the 'systematic, critical analysis of the quality of medical care, including the procedures used for diagnosis and treatment, the use of resources and the

Box 12.3 Clinical improvement methods

Audit and improvement cycles
- Clinical audit,
- Significant event analysis,
- Plan-do-study-act cycles.

Analysis of barriers and facilitators to improvement
- Discovery interviews, focus groups,
- Participant and non-participant observation (ethnography),
- Critical to quality (CTQ) trees.

Change management
- WIFM ('What's in it for me') charts,
- SWOT or SCOT analysis,
- Force field analysis.

Transformation methods
- Process redesign.

Measurement for change
- Benchmarking,
- Confidence charts or funnel plots,
- Run/control charts.

resulting outcome for the patient' (Secretaries of State for Health, 1989). Audit requires the measurement of care ('how are we doing?') against established criteria and standards ('what should we be doing?') against which performance can be measured but the audit cycle critically requires change to be implemented for improvements ('how can we improve') in performance to occur ('have the changes we have made led to improvement?'). Feedback and improvement are integral to the audit process and those whose performance is being measured should be involved in the process of change.

Clinical audit is a technique that has been promoted for nearly twenty years, but unfortunately is often conducted badly (McKay *et al.,* 2006) or applied inappropriately (Foy *et al.,* 2005). This may be because of lack of expertise in design or analysis, inadequate communication or teamwork and deficient resources or support (Johnston *et al.,* 2000). In particular there is often an emphasis on data collection without an appropriate weight attached to bringing about change through the cycle or spiral of improvement which lies at the heart of clinical audit. Although the effects of clinical audit in improving quality of care have been intensely debated systematic reviews have found moderate positive effects for published, and therefore well conducted, audits (Holden, 2004; Thomson O'Brien *et al.,* 2000).

Significant event audit

Significant event audit is another technique that is frequently used to evaluate care and bring about improvements in health care processes (Pringle, 2000). A significant event is a method of case-based auditing where events are cases identified as those which might provide lessons for health care staff to improve the organization or delivery of care. Cases can be identified where care has been excellent as well as that in which negative outcomes have occurred which is why the term 'significant event' is preferred to 'critical incident'. The types of cases are many and varied and can be clinical or administrative.

Cases can include new or missed diagnoses, deaths whether unexpected or following palliative care, complaints or patients leaving the list to register elsewhere. Cases are brought to a significant event meeting where all the members of team including those who have been directly or indirectly involved in it are brought together to discuss it. The case is presented by the member of staff who is closest to it and they are given an opportunity to describe the good points of care as well as offer recommendations for improvement. Other members of the team are then offered the chance to comment on good practice as well as suggestions for change. Finally, the agreed action points from the meeting are summarized and minuted so that they can be actioned in order to improve care. One of the advantages of significant even audit is that lessons and solutions can be discussed and shared with the whole team. The technique also has an immediacy and emotional content which conventional audit lacks. If conducted properly, significant event audit is a powerful tool for improving communication, team building and quality improvement (Westcott *et al.,* 2000).

Plan-do-study-act cycles

Plan, do, study, act (PDSA) cycles are another means of rapidly implementing and testing evidence-based or commonsense changes to processes of care on a small scale which because they have been trialled, enable changes to be spread more easily and effectively (Langley, 1996). There are four stages of the PDSA cycle.

- The first step involves planning the change to make sure that the change is appropriate, evidence-based and can be implemented easily. The key question is what are we trying to accomplish and how will we do this?

- The next step is to do, or make the change that has been planned.

- This is followed by studying the effect of the change using numerical or qualitative data. Even with small scale changes, the effect over time on processes of care can be measured and analysed using statistical process control techniques which are relatively easy to learn and understand.

149

- The final stage is to act, which consists of agreeing and implementing the previous change(s) or repeating the cycle with further changes depending on what was learnt as a result of study.

It can be seen from this that PDSA cycles are a useful means of evaluating while introducing rapid changes to health care processes in order to bring about improvement (Plsek 1999a).

Discovery interviews

Focus groups and individual interviews are an important technique for gathering data about the experiences of patients and staff and how services and the experience of both can be improved. One development from the traditional semi-structured interview is the 'discovery interview' (NHS Modernization Agency, 2003). This is a technique for listening to the stories of patient and carer experiences of the care that they have received in order to understand this from a user perspective specifically directed at improving care. This enables healthcare staff to gather data to inform patient-focused improvements (Wilcock *et al.,* 2003).

Root cause analysis

Root cause analysis is a specific type of significant event analysis which aims to find solutions to improve care through a systematic review of written and oral evidence which establishes underlying causes and therefore potential solutions to problems identified as adverse or untoward events (Burroughs *et al.,* 2000). The theory being applied is that for improvement methods to be effective we need to address root causes. There are a number of ways of analysing root causes but most involve defining the problem, gathering evidence systematically using tried and tested categories for identifying possible root causes and the underlying reasons for these and deciding which causes are amenable to change to produce improvement. This leads to recommendations, the effect of which can be further evaluated (Woloshynowych *et al.,* 2005).

Causes can be categorized adopting industrial language, for example:

- 6Ms (machine, method, materials, maintenance, man and mother nature (environment),
- 8Ps (price, promotion, people, processes, place/plant, procedures, product),
- 4Ss (surroundings, suppliers, systems and skills), reasons can be further explored by repeatedly asking why ('the 5 whys').

Ohno and Ohno, (1988).

These can be linked and shown pictorially using pathway representations, such as cause and effect diagrams, to establish the root of a particular problem.

Cause and effect diagrams

A basic model for a cause and effect is sometimes called a fishbone or Ishikawa diagram (Fig. 12.3). The central line is the patient pathway, which is affected by patients themselves, but also by the other inputs into the health system which they are travelling through (Volden and Monnig, 1993).

Pareto analysis

The Pareto (or 80/20) principle, in simple terms, explains that a relatively small number of key causes, will lead to most of the important outcomes, e.g. 80% of problems are due to 20% of potential causes.

The first step of a Pareto analysis is to list the causes in decreasing order of frequency (as a percentage) and to arrange these on the x-axis of a chart (Fig. 12.4). The next step is to plot the cumulative percentages on the y-axis of the chart. Then a line is drawn from the 80% mark on the y-axis parallel to x-axis in order to find the point of intersection with the curve on x-axis and this is used to distinguish key factors from less important causes (Ziegenfuss, Jr. and McKenna, 1995).

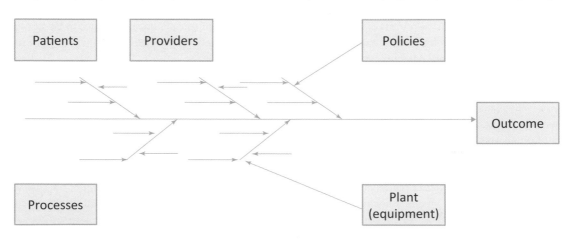

Fig. 12.3 Cause and effect ('fishbone') diagram.

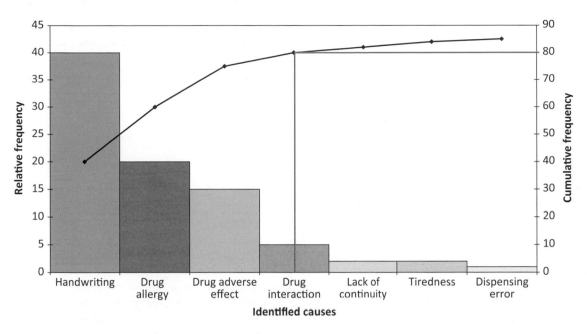

Fig. 12.4 Pareto diagram showing causes of prescribing adverse events. Siriwardena, A.N. (2009).

Process mapping and redesign

Process mapping is a way of describing the patient journey. The technique involves identifying each step of the journey from the patient's perspective. One way to do this is to write the steps down on stick-it notes and then to combine these to represent each component of the pathway that the patients needs to take in travelling through the system of care. Many pathways are complex, often far more complex for the patient than is anticipated or needed, and these can be visualized using the notes on a large board or table. One way to show this is by using a spaghetti diagram to show complex pathways. Another type of diagram shows the pathway with different job roles, team activities or processes separated into 'swim lanes' (Fig. 12.5). The components of a process which are critical to quality (CTQ) can be represented as a CTQ tree (Fig. 12.6). Once a process map is defined and drawn is often possible to redesign the process through simplification by taking out unnecessary steps or by introducing additional steps in order to make a process safer or better. The goal is to ensure that the right treatment is given by the right person at the right time and place. (Great Britain.NHS Modernization Agency, 2005b).

Change management

One aspect of evaluation which is critically important to successful quality improvement is the human dimension of change (Great Britain.NHS Modernization Agency, 2005a),

Ownership of change is particularly important for professionalized groups in health care such as doctors and nurses. They are at the front line of care and able to promote or subvert change, an ability which as been described as the inverted pyramid of care. An understanding of strengths, challenges (weaknesses), opportunities and threats as well as individual and group drivers and barriers to change is critical to successful improvement efforts. This approach has a theoretical basis in the ideas of 'forcefield theory' which states that reducing forces resisting change is more effective than strengthening driving forces (Lewin, 1947).

Benchmarking

Comparing individual and organizational performance is important for evaluating and identifying gaps in performance. The traditional way of ranking teams or organizations in order of performance, as a league table (Fig.12.7), is often unhelpful for a number of reasons. If performance is measured as a rate (percentage) these can vary widely and be considerably influenced greatly by small numbers of patients. Because fifty percent of participant teams or organizations are above and below the average, and those at either end may also be close to this, it is often difficult to determine whether performance is unusual compared to the mean and to draw a cut off between those that are performing at or around the average and those that are truly different. This sometimes leads teams to maintain mediocrity rather than pursue perfection.

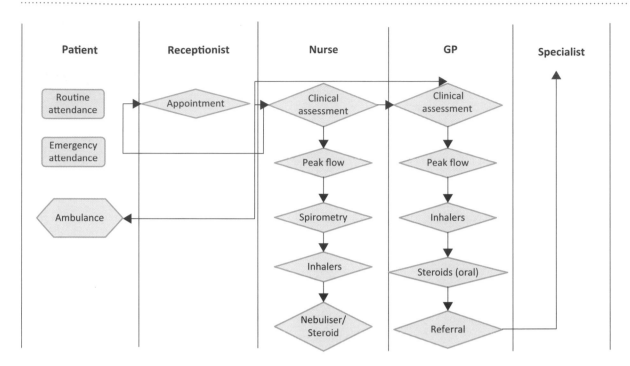

Fig. 12.5 Swim lane diagram for asthma care. Siriwardena, A.N. (2009).

Over the past few years health services have begun to use measurement methods originally developed in industry, such as statistical process control, for comparing and benchmarking institutional performance (Mohammed *et al.,* 2008). An example of a funnel plot is shown displaying the same data as represented in the league table above (Fig. 12.8).

The centre (blue) line on the chart shows the average of the underlying data and the outer curved (red) lines three standard deviations above and below the mean delineate the control limits (the bell of the 'trombone'). The upper and lower control limits (indicated in red on the chart) take into account the natural, random or expected variation as well as differences due to variation in sample size. They account for

over 99.9% of the data (this is known as 'common cause variation') and therefore performance should fall within those limits. Points which fall above or below the control limits are categorized by convention as outliers and indicate 'special cause variation' for which an explanation should be looked for.

Outliers in data do not necessarily mean that there is good or bad practice but do identify a need to look further for special causes. There are usually identifiable causes for special cause variation, for example differences in organizational systems or data quality. Interpretation depends on the indicator being measured. In cases where NHS trusts are outliers showing higher performance, this could identify areas of good

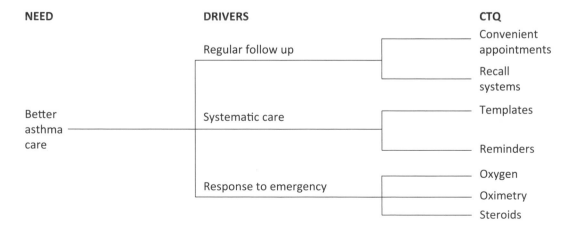

Fig. 12.6 Critical to quality (CTQ) tree for asthma.

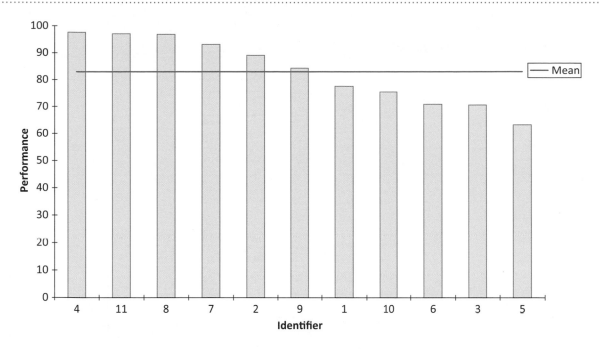

Fig. 12.7 Graph showing institutional performance for aspirin administration to patients with ST-elevation myocardial infarction.

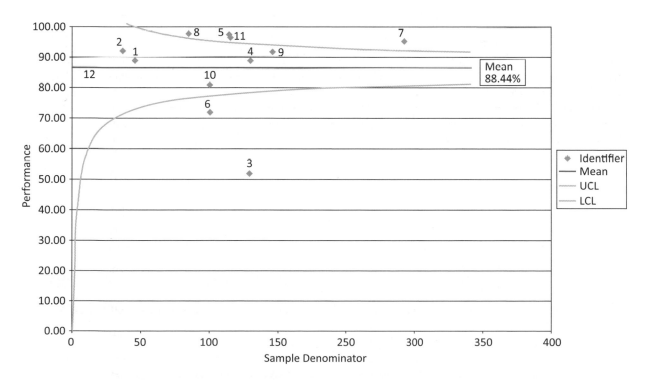

Fig. 12.8 Funnel plot showing institutional performance for aspirin administration to patients with ST-elevation myocardial infarction. Siriwardena, A.N., Shaw, D., Donohoe, R., Black, S. Stephenson, J. (2010).

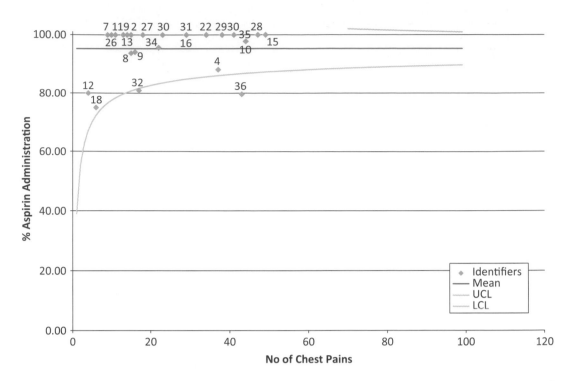

Fig. 12.9 Funnel plot showing clinical team performance for aspirin administration to patients with chest pain. Siriwardena, A.N. (2006).

practice which could be shared with other trusts. By identifying these differences and looking for explanations we can begin to understand what might be possible in terms of improvement and to look at further ways of changing practice to improve performance.

The same method can be used to compare team performance, even when numbers of cases seen are small, and thereby to identify, investigate and support teams where performance is outside the normal variation expected (Fig. 12.9).

Control charts

Statistical process control plots plotted against time in one team or organization can also show where improvements have occurred in response to planned interventions (Fig. 12.10). The graph shows monthly changes in prescribing data for one practice. The mean line is shown in green. Upper and lower control limits are shown in (dashed) red lines. 'Common cause' (natural) variation is demonstrated between October 2006 and December 2007 and following a collaborative to reduce hypnotic prescribing one can see a large fall in prescribing to below the lower control limit, signifying a 'special cause' (or unusual) variation.

For both types of statistical process control chart we are trying to improve performance and reduce the variation or unpredictability of the process (Berwick, 1991). Feedback is often an important component and driver of improvement (Thomson O'Brien *et al.,* 2000) and enhancing feedback by using statistical process control techniques can have a powerful effect.

Large scale evaluations

Larger scale evaluation will require more complex techniques and resources. These may include quasi-experimental designs such as time series or non randomized control group designs and may also include a cost analysis (Ukoumunne *et al.,* 1999). These techniques require statistical and health economic advice and expertise and are outside the scope of this chapter.

Health systems, complexity and complex interventions

Whichever health services sector one happens to be working in or evaluating, it is increasingly apparent that we are not operating in isolation but that we form part of a wider healthcare system (Nolan, 1998). The health care system is 'the sum

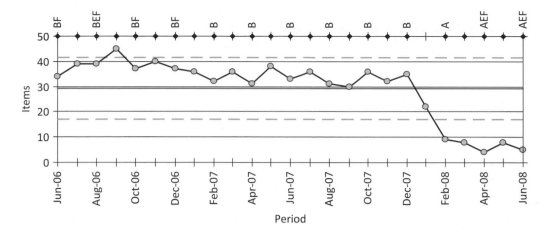

Fig. 12.10 Prescribing of hypnotic benzodiazepines over time. Siriwardena, A.N., Apekey, T., Tilling, M., Ørner R.J., Quershi, M.Z., Dyas, J., Middleton, H. (2008).

total of all the organizations, institutions and resources whose primary purpose is to improve health' (World Health Organization, 2008). Because individual components of health systems whether at the level of the health care worker, team, or organization are closely and often inextricably interrelated, they often exhibit features of **complex systems**, and these are important in understanding health care systems.

Complex systems involve many interacting elements. The interactions are often unpredictable, sometimes working through feedback loops, which lead to non-linear and uncertain effects. Individual components of complex systems are able to adapt to changes and because they are related to each other can co-evolve and self-organize (Kernick, 2006). These notions are important in the development of evaluations as well as in critical understanding of their conclusions.

Many interventions, whether these are delivered to individual patients or to populations involve more than one health technology. For example if you are encouraging a mother to have her child vaccinated with the measles, mumps rubella vaccine or an older patient to be immunized against influenza you might use a combination of methods to encourage vaccine uptake such as a reminder to clinicians or patients, a patient group direction, a recall system, a protocol or communication method (Siriwardena et al., 2002). Therefore in many clinical settings we are more often dealing with multiple or complex interventions, which involve a number of components, often interacting with each other, rather than a single simple intervention (Hulscher et al., 2001).

An ever more important element of complex systems is the health care team. Health care is more often than not delivered by teams, whether this is a community nursing team, a primary care team, rapid response team or other group of staff who work closely together to care for particular groups of patients. Moreover, teams increasingly tend to be multidisciplinary rather than uni-professional and this provides the opportunities for a greater range of skills to be brought to bear on a problem as well as introducing the potential problems of professional barriers, difficulties at the interface between teams and failure to take responsibility for an individual patient (Ferlie et al., 2000).

Summary

This chapter has explored the nature of evaluation and proposed a number of evaluation tools for developing an integrated approach to evaluation (and quality improvement) which focuses on measuring impact at both the individual and community level in a systematic way. Many of these techniques can be used by nurses or other professionals (many of whom will nowadays be working in multidisciplinary teams) to understand and improve the care that they are delivering to patients.

The approach to evaluation will need to understand whether an intervention is directed at individual service users (patients or carers), practitioners, teams, or organizations. It will also need to take a planned and structured approach using a logic model and an evaluation framework.

Fundamentally important to evaluation will be what is meant by health improvement in the context of planned changes to services and an understanding of potential benefits as well as unintended consequences at an individual or organizational level when introducing change in a complex health system.

Online Resource Centre

For more information on the influences on evaluating interventions visit the Online Resource Centre — http://www.oxfordtextbooks.co.uk/orc/linsley/

References

Ajzen I. (1991). The theory of planned behavior. *Organizational Behavior and Human Decision Processes* 50, 179–211.

Aronson R.E., Wallis A.B., O'Campo P.J., Whitehead T.L., & Schafer P. (2007). Ethnographically informed community evaluation: a framework and approach for evaluating community-based initiatives. *Matern.Child Health J* 11, 97–109.

Berwick D.M. (1991). Controlling variation in health care: a consultation from Walter Shewhart. *Med.Care* 29, 1212–1225.

Burroughs T.E., Cira J.C., Chartock P., Davies A.R., & Dunagan W.C. (2000). Using root cause analysis to address patient satisfaction and other improvement opportunities. *Jt.Comm J Qual.Improv.* 26, 439–449.

Casarett D., Karlawish J.H., Sugarman J. (2000). Determining when quality improvement initiatives should be considered research: proposed criteria and potential implications. *JAMA* 283, 2275–2280.

Cheraghi-Sohi S., & Bower P. (2008). Can the feedback of patient assessments, brief training, or their combination, improve the interpersonal skills of primary care physicians? A systematic review. *BMC.Health Serv.Res.* 8, 179.

Darzi of Denham A.D. (2008). 'High quality care for all: NHS Next Stage Review final report.' London: Stationery Office

Ferlie E., Fitzgerald L., Wood M. (2000). Getting evidence into clinical practice: an organizational behaviour perspective. *J Health Serv.Res.Policy* 5, 96–102.

Foy R., Eccles M.P., Jamtvedt G., Young J., Grimshaw J.M., & Baker R. (2005). What do we know about how to do audit and feedback? Pitfalls in applying evidence from a systematic review. *BMC.Health Serv.Res.* 5, 50.

Garside P. (1998). Organizational context for quality: lessons from the fields of organizational development and change management. *Qual.Health Care* 7 Suppl, S8–15.

Great Britain.NHS Modernization Agency. (2005a). 'Improvement leaders' guide : managing the human dimensions of change.' London: DH.

Great Britain.NHS Modernization Agency. (2005b). 'Improvement leaders' guide : process mapping, analysis and redesign.' London: DH.

Grol R.P., Bosch M.C., Hulscher M.E., Eccles M.P., & Wensing M. (2007). Planning and studying improvement in patient care: the use of theoretical perspectives. *Milbank Q.* 85, 93–138.

Harris L.E., Swindle R.W., Mungai S.M., Weinberger M., & Tierney W.M. (1999). Measuring patient satisfaction for quality improvement. *Med.Care* 37, 1207–1213.

Holden J. D. (2004). Systematic review of published multi-practice audits from British general practice. *J.Eval.Clin.Pract.* 10, 247–272.

Hulscher M.E., Wensing M., van der W.T., & Grol R. (2001). Interventions to implement prevention in primary care

(Cochrane Review). *Cochrane Database.Syst.Rev.* 1, CD000362.

Institute of Medicine (2001). 'Crossing the quality chasm: a new health system for the 21st century.' National Academy Press: Washington, D.C.

Johnston G., Crombie I.K., Davies H.T., Alder E.M., & Millard A. (2000). Reviewing audit: barriers and facilitating factors for effective clinical audit. *Qual Health Care* 9, 23–36.

Kernick D. (2006). Wanted —-new methodologies for health service research. Is complexity theory the answer? *Fam.Pract.* 23, 385–390.

Langley G.J. (1996). 'The Improvement guide: a practical approach to enhancing organizational performance.' San Francisco: Jossey-Bass.

Lewin K. (1947). Frontiers in group dynamics. *Human Relations* 1, 4–41.

Marsh P., & Glendenning R. (2005). 'The primary care service evaluation toolkit.' Leeds: National Co-ordinating Centre for Research Capacity Development.

McKay J., Bowie P., & Lough M. (2006). Variations in the ability of general medical practitioners to apply two methods of clinical audit: A five-year study of assessment by peer review. *J Eval. Clin.Pract* 12, 622–629.

Mead N., Bower P., Roland M. (2008). The General Practice Assessment Questionnaire (GPAQ) — development and psychometric characteristics. *BMC.Fam.Pract* 9, 13.

Mohammed M.A., Worthington P., Woodall W.H. (2008). Plotting basic control charts: tutorial notes for healthcare practitioners. *Qual.Saf Health Care* 17, 137–145.

NHS Institute for Innovation and Improvement (2005). Improvement leaders' guide. Evaluating improvement. Coventry: NHS.

NHS Modernization Agency (2003). 'A guide to using discovery interviews to improve care.' Leicester: Department of Health.

Nolan T.W. (1998). Understanding medical systems. *Ann.Intern. Med.* 128, 293–298.

Ohno T., & Ohno T. (1988) 'Toyota production system: beyond large-scale production.' Portland, OR: Productivity Press. Plsek P. (1999a). Innovative thinking for the improvement of medical systems. *Ann.Intern.Med.* 131, 438–444.

Plsek P.E. (1999b). Quality improvement methods in clinical medicine. *Pediatrics* 103, 203–214.

Plsek P.E., & Greenhalgh T. (2001) Complexity science: The challenge of complexity in health care. *BMJ* 323, 625–628.

Pringle M. (2000). Significant event auditing. *Scand.J Prim.Health Care* 18, 200–202.

Rhydderch M., Elwyn G., Marshall M., & Grol R. (2004). Organizational change theory and the use of indicators in general practice. *Qual Saf Health Care* 13, 213–217.

Scott K., Dyas J.V., Middlemass J.B., & Siriwardena A.N. (2007). Confidentiality in the waiting room: an observational study in general practice. *Br.J Gen.Pract.* 57, 490–493.

Secretaries of State for Health WNIaS (1989). 'Working for patients. The health service: working for the 1990s. Cm 555.' London: Her Majesty's Stationery Office.

Siriwardena A.N. (1999). Targeting pneumococcal vaccination to high-risk groups: a feasibility study in one general practice. *Postgrad.Med.J* 75, 208–212.

Siriwardena A.N. (2009). Using quality improvement methods for evaluating health care. *Qual.Prim.Care* 17, 155–159.

Siriwardena A.N., Apekey T., Tilling M., Ørner R.J., Qureshi M.Z., Dyas J., & Middleton H. (2008). Developing a psychosocial intervention for sleep problems presenting to primary care (REST: Resources for Effective Sleep Treatment). In 'The future of primary care. Southampton University 15–17 September 2008'.

Siriwardena A.N., Rashid A., Johnson M.R., & Dewey M.E. (2002). Cluster randomized controlled trial of an educational outreach visit to improve influenza and pneumococcal immunization rates in primary care. *Br J Gen Pract* 52, 735–740.

Thomson O'Brien M.A., Oxman A.D., Davis D.A., Haynes R.B., Freemantle N., & Harvey E.L. (2000). Audit and feedback: effects on professional practice and health care outcomes. *Cochrane.Database.Syst.Rev.* CD000259.

Thurston W.E., Graham J., & Hatfield J. (2003). Evaluability assessment. A catalyst for program change and improvement. *Eval. Health Prof.* 26, 206–221.

Ukoumunne O.C., Gulliford M.C., Chinn S., Sterne J.A.C., & Burney P.G.J. (1999). Methods for evaluating area-wide and organization-based interventions in health and healthcare: a systematic review. *Health Technol.Assess.* 3.

Volden C.M., & Monnig R. (1993). Collaborative problem solving with a total quality model. *Am.J Med Qual.* 8, 181–186.

Westcott R., Sweeney G., & Stead J. (2000). Significant event audit in practice: a preliminary study. *Fam.Pract* 17, 173–179.

Wilcock P.M., Brown G.C., Bateson J., Carver J., & Machin S. (2003). Using patient stories to inspire quality improvement within the NHS Modernization Agency collaborative programmes. *J Clin. Nurs.* 12, 422–430.

Woloshynowych M., Rogers S., Taylor-Adams S., & Vincent C. (2005). The investigation and analysis of critical incidents and adverse events in healthcare. *Health Technol.Assess.* 9, 1–143, iii.

World Health Organization. (2008). *Health systems*. Geneva: WHO.

Ziegenfuss J.T., Jr., & McKenna C.K. (1995). Ten tools of continuous quality improvement: a review and case example of hospital discharge. *Am.J Med Qual.* 10, 213–220.

Part 4

Key areas of health need

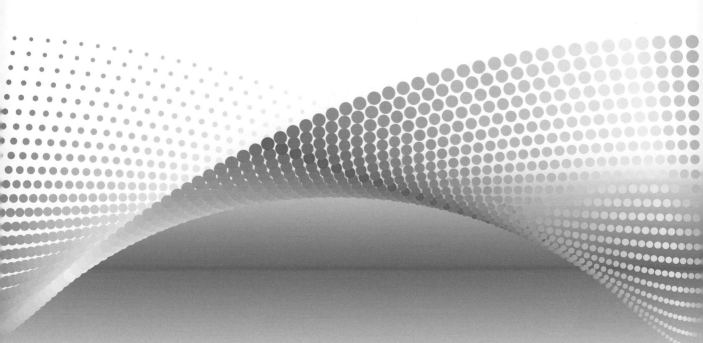

Chapter 13
Smoking and smoking cessation

Vicki Linsley

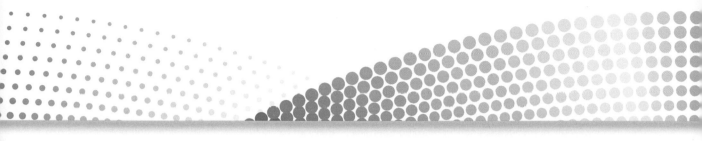

Introduction

Smoking has become a global health issue and this is reflected in a number of government documents, health campaigns and international initiatives such as 'Smoking Kills: a white paper on Tobacco' (Department of Health, 1988) 'Beyond Smoking Kills' (Action on Smoking and Health, 2008) and 'Report on the global tobacco epidemic' (WHO, 2009). The risks associated with smoking were notably published by Fletcher and Peto in 1977 and this remains a landmark study often cited in current research. They identified risks which mainly involved premature death and respiratory disease. We now know that smoking can cause other health and social problems not only an increased risk of lung cancer but increased risk of other cancers, chronic obstructive pulmonary disease (COPD), vascular disease and also social inequality (due to cost of tobacco and dependency upon it)(Edwards, 2004). Some of these issues will be discussed in more depth later in the chapter.

This chapter provides a profile of smoking, its prevalence, the effects upon the individual and those close to them and the steps that are currently being employed to help those that want to stop. It looks at the role of the nurse in supporting those that have taken the decision to stop and the possible consequences of either choosing not to stop or being unable to stop.

Case Study 13.1: Michael

Michael is a 57 year old man who has been a smoker since the age of 14. Like many smokers he is not happy with his habit and would like to stop. He has booked an appointment with the practice nurse in order to get some help and advice. He has had a morning cough for about ten years and has lately noticed that although he can walk for long distances on the flat he struggles to walk up slight inclines at anything but a slow pace. He has been trying to pass this off as an ageing process but he is now unable to keep up with his wife and other friends of a similar age. He fears that his breathing problems may be smoking related having recently seen a series of television advertisements.

He is worried that his practice nurse or doctor might consider his illness to be 'self inflicted' but he defends this by explaining that he started smoking at a young age as it was common and accepted as the norm amongst his friends and family; also its harmful effects were not known at that time.

Discussion points

What information should the nurse gather during this initial consultation?

What should s/he do with this information? i.e. How would it be recorded? How would it be used?

Why do people smoke?

Smoking is one of the most difficult addictions to break (Royal College of Physicians 2000). Scientists estimate that cigarettes are more addictive than cocaine, heroin, or alcohol (Royal

College of Physicians, 2000). Globally **COPD** is the fourth most common cause of death (Shahab *et al.*, 2006). In the UK approximately 114,000 premature deaths per year are attributed to smoking with one quarter of them being due to lung cancer and one fifth due to **COPD** (Peto *et al.*, 2000). With all this information available and with current health promotion initiatives, why do people choose to start smoking and to continue to smoke?

There are many different reasons why people start to smoke and also many reasons why they choose to either continue smoking or to try and stop smoking.

A persons social circumstance should be considered when supporting them to stop smoking as the reasons for starting to smoke are, to some degree, influenced by age, social class and occupation (Office for National Statistics, 2007). For example many years ago the majority of now elderly male smokers would have started to smoke during National service when cigarettes were part of their issued rations and smoking was seen as not only the norm but also good for relaxation, settling nerves and helping to clear the chest! Women of a similar age started to smoke when they began to join traditionally male employment in such areas as ammunition factories and manufacturing industries rather than staying at home to look after their husbands and families.

Smoking in the 1930s and 1940s onwards was also glamorized in films and media; it was promoted as having health benefits as well as being sociable, attractive and acceptable. Many Hollywood stars of the period were paid to endorse certain brands of cigarettes as being stylish, and in the case of female actors, as a means to stay thin. The advertising of tobacco in the form of cigarettes and cigars continued in printed media, point of sale displays, shop front logos and sporting events after the advertising of cigarettes was banned from television in 1965. This form of television advertising has also now been banned in most of the developed world and was influenced in the UK by the **Tobacco Advertising and Promotion Act** (2003) and within Europe by a EU directive which is weaker than the UK Act. A UK Act is enforceable by law whereas a EU directive is advisory. Tobacco advertising had a big influence the uptake of smoking. For years, the industry has focused on making smoking glamorous through advertising in films, television, and billboards. The link with sport and event sponsorship has also been very prominent with formula one car racing team sponsorship, tennis, horse racing, football and rugby all having sponsored events in the past.

Most people who continue to smoke do so because either they can't stop (due to physical addiction or emotional/psychological dependence) or because they have no desire to stop (Lader and Goddard, 2004). Smoking can be an enjoyable experience for many smokers who despite the evidence of smoking related disease and pressure from friends, family, health professionals and media campaigns choose to continue smoking.

Nicotine is a highly addictive substance that makes people feel energised and alert, it gives smokers a 'rush' after smoking and can lead to withdrawal symptoms when people try to quit

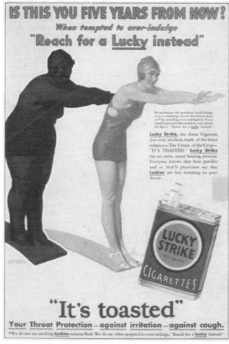
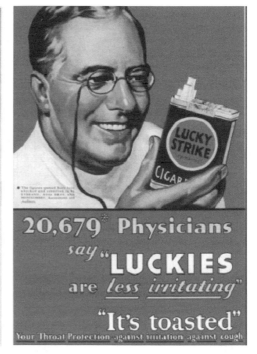

Lane Library, Stanford School of Medicine

Fig. 13.1 Old advertisements made no mention of any ill effects (other than throat irritation) which we now attribute to the smoking of tobacco and may be perceived as promoting the health benefits of smoking!

(Royal College of Physicians, 2000). The following list includes the most commonly experienced withdrawal symptoms; although not all people who are trying to stop smoking will experience all, or even many, of them (Roy Castle Foundation, accessed 15/04/09) :-

- The craving to smoke,
- Irritability/mood swings/feelings of emptiness/heightened anxiety,
- Dizziness/light headiness,
- Headaches,
- Inability to concentrate,
- Sleeplessness,
- Tiredness/feeling of exhaustion,
- Upset stomach,
- Mouth Ulcers/taste disturbance,
- Sore tongue,
- Worsened cough/offensive sputum,
- Tingling sensations,
- Constipation.

Nicotine replacement therapy in the form of patches, gum or lozenges can help to reduce some cravings but can also have some side effects such as gastrointestinal disturbances, headache, dizziness, flu like symptoms and dry mouth (BNF, 2009). The best success rate for smoking cessation involves support either as part of a group or on an individual basis either with or without nicotine replacement therapy (National Institute for Health and Clinical Excellence, 2006). Only 3% of smokers succeed in quitting using will power alone and only 20% of those who embark upon a course of treatment will succeed in abstaining for one year (Thorax, 1998). Most smokers with a serious desire to quit will need to make more than one attempt to stop (Thorax, 1998. National Institute for Health and Clinical Excellence, 2006).

Case Study 13.2: Michael (cont. from pp. 161)

Make a list of the places including web pages, where Michael could access smoking cessation support and advice.

What therapies or medication could be offered to him? Look in the BNF or MIMMs to find out about side effects of these treatments.

Packaging and media is becoming more sophisticated and is being aimed at specific target audiences such as Silk Cut super slim cigarettes which are aimed at young girls who would like to be 'super slim'. As recently as 2008 these super slim cigarettes have been re-packaged in 'perfume type boxes' and promoted as being elegant and sophisticated like the expensive perfumes they mimic (Action on Smoking and Health, 2006). Although advertising may be strictly controlled, media reporting about the big tobacco companies gives them indirect media coverage and therefore a type of free advertising (Action on Smoking and Health, 2006) (although it may be an article about the negative effects of smoking not everyone who sees the pictures will read the article). This type of advertising has been going on for many years and is sometimes referred to as brand sharing or brand stretching. For example the Marlboro clothing range is advertised in very similar backgrounds and style to their cigarette advertisements and is therefore advertising their brand of Marlboro country cigarettes.

Since direct advertising of tobacco was banned from television in 1965 (under powers granted by the television act 1964) sports sponsorship and brand stretching has been a major way of tobacco companies influencing the public via television. This kind of sponsorship and brand stretching was banned in 2003 within the United Kingdom following the implementation of the 'tobacco advertising act, 2003'. Motor sport sponsorship (Formula 1) was allowed to continue until July 2005. Such legislation is common within the developed world but is minimal within developing countries and the World Health Organization reports that 'Progress on implementing bans on tobacco advertising, promotion and sponsorship has stalled, leaving more than 90% of the world without protection from tobacco industry advertising' (WHO, 2009). This has in effect diverted the tobacco companies towards trying to sell more tobacco in the developing world. This is partially to compensate for the reduction in smoking within the developed world. Targets for smoking reduction within the whole of the UK were set out in a Department of Health white paper: 'Smoking Kills' (1998) have been met, and in some cases exceeded so that new, more ambitious targets have been set in 'Beyond Smoking Kills' (Action on Smoking and Health, 2008).

Many teenagers start smoking due to peer pressure and previous social exposure to smoking. They may also smoke to feel more mature, because their parents smoke or as a form of rebellion against parental authority (Royal College of Physicians, 1992). It has been shown that children are more likely to smoke if their parents or older siblings do (Royal College of Physicians, 1992).

The smoking habit can sometimes develop into a source of emotional support i.e. a means of coping with stress, anxiety or boredom; as such it is often cited by people who return to smoking after a period of abstinence (Lantz, 2003. Gilbert and Spielberger, 1986). Smoking is a social activity as well as physically addictive (due to the nicotine content). Many people who smoke do so as a way to start conversations and interact at parties or in crowded places. This is known as 'social smoking', and it usually involves alcohol as a complement (Goddard, 2006).

Often the hardest obstacle to overcome when trying to stop smoking is being surrounded by people (either friends, family or workmates) who still smoke and/or having a routine which previously fitted around existing smoking habits such as smoking upon waking, after every cup of tea or whilst out socializing (Steele, 1993). The physical addiction of smoking and nicotine dependency is hard to break but so are the habits and rituals of years (Steele, 1993). Many people claim that smoking keeps them thin, but the truth is that smoking reduces the sense of taste, so many people who smoke simply eat less because they don't enjoy food as much (Perkins, 1993).

The gaseous phase also contains:

- Benzene (used as a solvent in chemical manufacture
- Hydrogen cyanide
- Formaldehyde (used to preserve dead bodies. Know to cause cancer)
- Acetone (used as a solvent in nail polish)
- Ammonia (used in dry cleaning fluids)
- Cadmium (used in batteries)

British American Tobacco, updated 2009

Box 13.1 Facts about smoking

Tobacco smoke

More than 4000 chemical substances, which may be present as gas or particulate state, have been identified in tobacco smoke. Some are toxic, some **mutagenic** and at least 43 are known **carcinogens**. The burning of tobacco from a cigarette releases mainstream and sidestream smoke: mainstream smoke is generated from the burning cone when the smoker draws on the cigarette and it travels down through the column of tobacco to the mouthpiece. Side stream smoke is emitted from the smouldering cigarette between puffs and can account for 85% of the smoke in a room. The constituents of sidestream smoke are different and are more toxic than mainstream smoke. (United States Environmental Protection Agency, 1992)

Chemicals which are particulate in nature include:

- Tar which is drawn into the lungs when the smoker inhales. Cigarette smoke condenses once inhaled and 70% of the tar in smoke is deposited in the lungs.
- Nicotine which is an addictive substance. When the smoker inhales, nicotine is absorbed into the bloodstream and affects the body within about eight seconds. The effects include:
  - an increased in blood pressure,
  - an increase in heart rate,
  - vasoconstriction.

The gaseous chemicals include carbon monoxide is the same gas that is emitted from car exhausts and is the main gas formed when a cigarette is lit. It is found as a concentration of 1–5% at the filter of the cigarette and this concentration is well within the toxic range for that chemical. Carbon monoxide binds to haemoglobin more readily than oxygen and this means that the blood can carry less oxygen. For some smokers, with end-stage respiratory disease, long-term oxygen therapy may be prescribed, although care must be taken to fully assess the benefits and risk of giving current smokers oxygen.

Epidemiology
Smoking rates

As shown in Table 13.1 below, the prevalence of cigarette smoking in adults in the UK has gradually fallen from 1974 onward. Although men are still more likely than women to smoke cigarettes, the gap has narrowed. In 1974, 51% of men and 41% of women smoked (almost half the adult population). The latest figures show that the prevalence of smoking has fallen significantly to 22% of men and 20% of women (about one fifth of the adult population) in 2007 (Office for National Statistics, 2007).

Smoking prevalence fell steadily from 1974 to 1992, and remained broadly flat between 1992 and 1998. Since 1998 smoking prevalence among all adults has fallen, including a slight fall in prevalence among manual groups.

Looking at the percentage of adults who have never or only occasionally ever smoked, there has been gradual increase of non-smoking amongst both men and women since 2000. The most recent data available shows the rate (of never smoking) to be 47% for men and 52% for women (Office for National Statistics, 2007).

Box 13.2 Recent findings from the General Household Survey

The Department of Health has produced a summary bulletin of the most recent findings from the General Household Survey (GHS). The General Household Survey is a multi-purpose continuous survey carried out by the Social Survey Division of the Office for National Statistics (ONS) which collects information on a range of topics from people living in private households in Great Britain.

Table 13.1 Percentage of population who smoke (Office for National Statistics, 2007)

%	1974	1980	1986	1992	1998	2004	2005	2006	2007
Men	51	42	35	29	30	26	25	23	22
Women	41	37	31	28	26	23	23	21	20
All	45	39	33	28	28	25	24	22	21

Summary bulletin:

• Cigarette smoking is still most prevalent among adults aged 20 to 34. In 2005/6, 31% of adults aged 20 to 24 and 26% of adults aged 25 to 34 were smokers compared with 12% of those aged 60 and over.

• The number of cigarettes smoked per day by men has steadily fallen from its highest of 21.6 in 1975 to 14 per day in 2007. The number of cigarettes per day for women has steadily risen from 6.8 in 1949 to 13 per day in 2007. Men and women are apparently almost equal now in terms of number of cigarettes per day smoked.

• In 2007 two thirds (66 per cent) of cigarette smokers in Great Britain said that they wanted to give up. 17% of smokers have their first cigarette within five minutes of waking (35% who smoke 20 or more per day smoke within five minutes of waking compared to 3% of those who smoke less than ten per day). Smoking within five minutes of waking is accepted as a rough guide to the degree of dependency on smoking/nicotine.

Adapted from: General Household Survey, 2007

Table 13.2 Prevalence of smoking by socio-economic classification based on current or last job of the household reference person, Great Britain 2007

	Men %	Women %
Large employers and higher managerial	13	15
Higher professional	12	10
Lower managerial and professional	19	16
Intermediate	20	17
Small employers / own account	22	20
Lower supervisory and technical	25	22
Semi-routine	31	27
Routine	31	27

Adapted from: DH Status Report (2005)

Smoking prevalence by social class

Smoking prevalence among manual groups is consistently higher than in non-manual groups and in the adult population as a whole.

Since 1998 the gap in smoking prevalence between manual groups and the average for all adults has not changed significantly in absolute or relative terms. This also applies to the gap between manual and non-manual groups.

A recent survey by National Centre for Social Research and the National Foundation for Educational Research was conducted to monitor smoking, drinking and drug use among secondary school children aged 11–15. Information was obtained from 9,715 pupils in 313 schools throughout England during the autumn term of 2004 (Fuller *et al.* 2005). The percentage of young people who are regular smokers (defined as those who smoke at least one cigarette a week) has fluctuated since 1982, but has remained stable since 1999 at between 9% and 10% with a fall to about 6% in 2007. There are differences by age however. In the early 1980s, equal proportions of girls and boys smoked regularly. Since the mid 1980s, girls have been consistently more likely to smoke than boys. In 2004, 10% of girls were regular smokers compared with 7% of boys (Fuller *et al.* 2005).

Scottish figures (SALSUS, 2007) show similar trends in that girls are now slightly more likely to smoke than boys but smoking in general amongst school age young people has declined.

International comparisons

When we look at the actual number of cigarettes consumed annually, the most recent data available from the European Health for All database (HFA-DB) pertains to 2000 and is shown in Fig. 13.2. The UK has lower rates than many other European countries. In Spain, The Netherlands and Switzerland annual consumption per person exceeds 2000 where in the UK the rate is just over 1100.

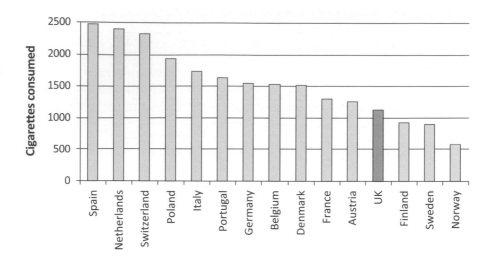

Fig. 13.2 Number of cigarettes consumed per person per year, selected European countries. Adapted from European Health for All database, WHO (2010) http://data.euro.who.int/hfadb/.

Effects of smoking on health

Lung function

Lung function declines gradually with age, but some smokers demonstrate a more rapid deterioration of lung function than non-smokers (Fletcher and Peto, 1977). This can have an impact on pre-existing lung conditions such as Asthma and Chronic Obstructive Pulmonary Disease (COPD). Research by Fletcher and Peto in 1977 illustrated the natural progression of lung decline over time. They compared non-smokers (and those not susceptible to the effects of smoke (possibly due to a genetic predisposition)) to smokers. They also looked at the effects of stopping smoking on lung function and the graph shown below, adapted from their original research, is often

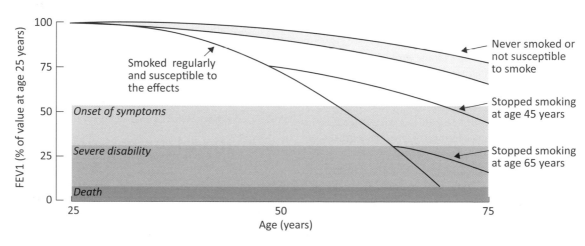

Fig. 13.3 Graph showing the effects of stopping smoking on lung function by age Reproduced with permission. Fletcher, C. and Peto, R. (1977)

used by health care practitioners to demonstrate to smokers that it is never too late to stop smoking.

Asthma

Asthma is defined by the presence of characteristic symptoms (of cough, wheeze and breathlessness) and by reversible airway narrowing and **airway hyper-responsiveness**.

Investigation and diagnosis of asthma is variable dependent upon age. For example babies and young children cannot be expected to perform peak flow measurements and diagnosis in the very young is often based upon family history, symptom monitoring and response to **bronchodilator therapy**. It is also important to realize that not all wheezy babies and toddlers have asthma they could just simply have smaller airways that may become inflamed as a result of viral infection (Chapman *et al.*, 2005). The most common feature of asthma in the very young is a persistent night time cough that disturbs their sleep or coughing severely during or immediately after running around (Levy and Pearce, 2004).

It is important to note that asthma can develop at any age and is not always present in childhood for those who will go on to develop it in adulthood (Levy and Pearce, 2004). Asthma is commonly part of the 'atopic triad' of asthma, hay fever and eczema and family or personal history of any of these conditions are significant when taking a history as part of the diagnostic, assessment process (Levy and Pearce, 2004). Smoking in itself does not cause asthma but tobacco smoke is a major airway irritant which does aggravate sensitive and often already inflamed asthmatic airways.

The role of the nurse in providing education and information is to ensure the recipient understands their underlying condition whether it be asthma or COPD. They need also to provide that information so that the patient understands the most likely cause of their long-term condition and what they can do to best manage or control that condition. Informed choice is only possible when the patient has sufficient knowledge. The measurement and recording of **peak expiratory flow rate** (a measurement of how many litres of air a person can blow out in approximately 1 second) and/or symptom diaries along with good inhaler technique can assist the person to manage their own condition along with support from a healthcare professional such as their practice nurse. Inhaler technique should be checked regularly to ensure that adequate technique is maintained and that the most appropriate device is used. Written self management plans developed between the patient and health care worker are strongly advocated (British Thoracic Society, Scottish Intercollegiate Guideline Network, 2008). National asthma campaign produces useful patient leaflets and online support including inhaler technique demonstrations which can be accessed by patients and healthcare professionals at **http://www.asthma.org.uk/**

Chronic Obstructive Pulmonary Disease (COPD)

Chronic obstructive pulmonary disease is a lung disease characterised by increased obstruction to airflow that does not change markedly over periods of several months (NICE Guideline 12. 2004). Most of the airways obstruction is permanent, although with some patients there may be some reversibility (opening up of the airways by the inhalation of bronchodilator medicines). COPD is a common clinical condition diagnosed most commonly in cigarette smokers but also in some non-smokers where occupational factors, atmospheric pollutants or inherited tendencies may be responsible for the disease.

COPD is an umbrella term for one or more of the following Illnesses: Emphysema (loss of support to the walls of the alveoli due to breakdown of the alveolar supports which can make the alveoli large and floppy with reduced capacity for exchanging gasses), Chronic bronchitis (over production of mucus, often with inflammation of the airways) and also some element of bronchospasm caused either by an asthmatic component or narrowing of the airways due to inflammation (wheezy bronchitis).

People with COPD have injury and destruction of the airways and alveoli and supporting tissues. A notable feature of the disease is that the damage seen in people with COPD is variably distributed throughout the lungs, which means that not all people with COPD have the same symptoms. The typical symptoms of COPD are those of a cough with sputum production, wheeze and most importantly breathlessness (dyspnoea). There is a range of clinical presentations from almost pure obstruction, causing breathlessness and hyper inflation of the chest with little sputum production (emphysema) to chronic mucous hyper-secretion (chronic bronchitis).

Since COPD is a **fixed obstructive airway disease** and asthma is a **reversible condition**, one might imagine that it would be easy to distinguish between the two conditions. However it is possible to have both conditions simultaneously and also for chronically under treated asthma to become fixed airway disease (ineffective treatment leads to chronic inflammation which in turn leads to the deposition of elastin fibres which 'fix' the airways in a constricted state, thereby stopping bronchodilator medicines from working).

On the other hand, in some chronic bronchitis patients the **FEV1** (forced expiratory volume in 1 second; the volume of air that can be forcibly expelled in 1 second) may be slightly improved with bronchodilators or steroids, suggesting that they have a degree of asthma. A low FEV1 indicates a reduced ability to expel air. A low FEV1 combined with a long exhalation time and high volume of air expelled (**FVC**— forced vital capacity) is an indicator of COPD.

167

Cough

Smokers often have a productive cough and an impairment of **ciliary** activity. If smoking cessation occurs the **cilia** regenerate very quickly with subsequent rapid reinstitution of the **mucociliary escalator**.

It is important that individuals trying to stop smoking are informed of this pathological process since it may result in increased sputum expectoration initially. This could be misinterpreted by the individual, as a worsening of their respiratory condition, some of whom may fall back into the trap of smoking to either reduce coughing or stimulate chest clearance.

In cases where chronic cough and thick mucous make expectoration difficult (therefore tiring, uncomfortable and/or socially embarrassing) an active cycle of breathing can be taught by a physiotherapist. This is a method of deep breathing, breath holding and huffing to aid chest clearance with less distress and physical exertion than constant coughing. Advice about increased fluid intake (to thin secretions) followed by a trial of **mucolytics** which can aid expectoration by breaking down the proteins in mucous can help. It is usual to give a trial of **mucolytics** before committing a patient to long-term medication as **mucolytics** are not effective for everyone.

Smokers have an increased rate of post-operative respiratory complications caused by increased secretion of mucus, impaired mucus clearance and small airway narrowing.

Stopping smoking

A person's decision to smoke is the result of a complex interaction of factors that vary from one individual to another. In the same way, reduction of tobacco use requires a comprehensive, multifaceted strategy that includes:

- Prevention (helping to prevent non-smokers from starting),
- Cessation (helping current smokers to stop smoking and preventing relapse),
- Protection (protecting non-smokers from second hand smoke and other harmful effects of tobacco),

Prevention

Prevention is the most important strategy of the three; being a non-smoker is a vital element of a healthy active life (DH, 2004). For those who already smoke, stopping smoking is the single most effective thing they can do to enhance the quality and length of their lives (Fletcher and Peto, 1977).

Recent Department of Health Policy 'A smoke-free future: A comprehensive tobacco control strategy for England' sets out targets of reducing smoking, preventing smoking and tobacco control within England (DH, 2010).

Most smokers are not happy with their habit and the majority, like Michael in our example, would like to stop (Office for National Statistics, 2008). But relapse rate is very high because of the addictive nature of tobacco and the possible social pressures on the smoker (Office for National Statistics, 2008). In most smoking cessation programmes, a success rate of between 15% and 20% is considered a positive outcome (NICE, 2006). Most smokers attempt to stop several times before they finally succeed (NICE, 2006).

Case Study 13.3: Michael (cont. from pp. 163)

On further investigation it is discovered Michael has COPD and that this is made worse by his smoking. This makes him more determined to stop smoking and he is referred to a NHS Stop Smoking Service for counselling.

Activity box

Make a list of the main signs and symptoms of COPD.

List some reasons why being diagnosed with COPD may make Michael more likely to want to give up smoking.

Smoking cessation

Nicotine is a highly addictive substance — more so than heroin and similarly is not simply pharmacologically addictive, but also socially, culturally, psychologically and economically addictive (Royal College of Physicians, 2000). People are more likely to smoke if they are socialised in a culture where smoking is an accepted norm. They may find smoking cessation more difficult if their family and friends smoke. A cessation intervention needs to consider ways in smokers could overcome these pressures.

The decision to stop smoking, like the decision to engage in any health related behaviour, is a complex process that is subject to several influences. Central to this decision are health beliefs, which are the individual's perception of what being healthy is, and the behaviour needed to maintain that health. Smokers may not, for example, believe that smoking is unhealthy. Most people will have encountered the smoker who denies the ill effects of smoking, and who describes the 90 year old person who has smoked for life and is unaffected. Many if not most of those who smoke know that it is extremely bad for their health and actually wish to stop smoking. Smoking cessation is most successful if the individual decides that they should stop and then takes the next step of either stopping or seeking help to stop NICE, 2006). The NHS smokefree campaign offers free Quit Kits to anyone who contacts them by telephone or email and also has a high profile media campaign to promote smoking cessation with support. Information and resources are available at www.http://smokefree.nhs.uk/.

Several factors may influence the smoker's decision to stop smoking. Health belief models such as those described in Chapter 3 in this book describe some of the influencing factors. These include costs versus benefits or changing established behaviour. The perceived risks of stopping smoking e.g. fear of weight gain or increased anxiety may deter a person from trying to stop smoking. The benefits of smoking cessation may be clear to an individual smoker (in terms of improved health or money saved), but what are the costs (being unable to go out socially with friends who still smoke, uncertainty about level of support from spouse, peer acceptance and difficulty with social interaction). The smoker may decide that the costs of smoking cessation outweigh the benefits.

Other factors include perceived **self-efficiency**, or the individual's perception of their ability to stop smoking. Theoretically, if an individual believes that they are able to stop smoking they are more likely to try. Also if all health care professionals routinely carry out the brief interventions as described by NICE (2006) (see Box 13.3) then more people may be prompted to consider stopping.

The factors affecting an individual's perception of their ability to give up smoking may be influenced by allowing them to express their feelings, anxieties, beliefs and reservations, and by enabling them to explore various solutions. This process may be enhanced by the support of people from similar backgrounds, for example during a group cessation intervention or may be better carried out on a more personal one to one basis to allow for an individually tailored approach.

For many patients, as discussed in Chapter 3 which looks at the theoretical models of behavioural change, the key element in successfully stopping smoking is motivation. For some, it may require explicit advice from a health professional or a severe smoking related/associated illness such as pneumonia to trigger the will to stop. Even three minutes cessation intervention can increase the chances of giving up long-term. When a more intensive approach is adopted, the chances of success are even greater (Hajek *et al.*, 2009).

Everyone who smokes should be given adequate information to allow an informed decision about stopping smoking. People who are not ready to stop should be asked to consider the possibility and encouraged to seek help in the future. If an individual who smokes presents with a smoking related illness, the cessation advice may be linked to their medical condition (NICE, 2006).

Nurses in primary and community care should identify those patients who wish to give up smoking and refer them to either their own support groups/clinics, GP surgery or an intensive support service (for example, NHS Stop Smoking Services). Those who are unwilling or unable to accept referral, but still want to stop, should be offered pharmacotherapy or interventions by practitioners with suitable training. The smoking status of those who are not ready to stop should be recorded and reviewed with the individual once a year, where possible (NICE, 2006).

Smoking cessation counselling is widely recognized as an effective clinical practice. Even a brief intervention by a nurse or other health professional significantly increases the cessation rates (NICE, 2006). A smoker's likelihood of stopping increases when he or she hears the message from a number of health care providers from a variety of disciplines. Health professionals are perhaps the country's most credible source of health information. Many people will consult a health professional at least once a year, often at teachable moments when they may by more motivated than usual to change their behaviour e.g. when they have a chest infection or other potentially smoking related health problem (NICE, 2006). Health professionals can tailor their messages to individuals and work with them on a one to one basis.

Box 13.3 Brief interventions in health and community care

Brief interventions involve opportunistic advice, discussion, negotiation or encouragement. They are commonly used in many areas of health promotion and are delivered by a range of primary and community care professionals.

For smoking cessation, brief interventions typically take between five and ten minutes and may include one or more of the following (NICE, 2006):

- Simple opportunistic advice to stop.
- An assessment of the patient's commitment to stop.
- An offer of pharmacotherapy and/or behavioural support.
- Provision of self-help material and referral to more intensive support such as NHS Stop Smoking Services.
- Referral to voluntary organizations such as ASH (Action on Smoking and Health) or websites for the more independent person.

Case Study 13.4: Michael (cont. from pp. 168)

Michael was spurred on to consult his practice nurse in a number of ways: his inability to keep up when walking with his peers, advertisements on television, concern for his health and his family. It has taken him a long time to seek help for his concerns and support from his wife.

Activity box

What could Michael do to increase his chances of stopping smoking? i.e. list his reasons for stopping, seek support from his wife, family and friends as well as help from an appropriate health care professional. List the benefits of stopping smoking to himself and those around him. Plan personal rewards for his success.

During a ten minute interaction with a smoker, the following can be achieved:

- Set a date to stop, stop completely on that day.
- Review past experience — what helped, what hindered.
- Agree that the client tell their family and friends and enlist their support.
- Plan what you are going to do about alcohol.
- Try nicotine replacement therapy. Clients may ask about the effectiveness of alternative therapies such as acupuncture and hypnotherapy. There is little evidence of their efficacy over and above the placebo effect. It may be that the attention received during these interactions is producing an attention placebo effect. However attention placebo is effective for some and smokers should not be discouraged from seeking these interventions from an informed perspective.

Smoking cessation advice should be available in community, primary and secondary care settings for everyone who smokes. Local policy makers and commissioners should target hard to reach and deprived communities including such groups as prisoners and mental health service users, paying particular attention to their needs.

Nicotine replacement therapy

Nicotine replacement therapy is now considered a major factor in any smoking cessation programme. Those who advocate its use it state that it doubles the short-term success rates of smoking cessation (NICE, 2006).

Nicotine replacement therapy works by swapping the very high concentrations of nicotine received by smokers form cigarettes, for lower doses delivered more slowly, helping to reduce the cravings and withdrawal symptoms. The choice of Nicotine Replacement Therapy (NRT) will depend upon the patient's needs, their tolerance and the cost. Some people miss handling cigarettes so an inhalator may be best. Others want to avoid cravings so a patch or gum could be the right option. Some smokers want to be able to choose when to give themselves nicotine. The lozenge and nasal spray offer that instant control. Many smokers who do not manage to stop smoking using one type of NRT often find success simply by

trying another. The different tools used in NRT and smoking cessation pharmacology are outlined below.

Patches

Patches are easy to use and easily hidden under clothing. They deliver a steady dose of nicotine into the blood stream through the skin. It takes about four to eight hours to reach peak level depending on the patch used — some types are for 24 hour use and will deliver a steady dose, whilst others should be applied first thing every morning and removed before retiring to bed. Patches should always be applied to a dry, hairless area of skin on the front or side of the chest, upper arm or hip. Sites should be rotated to avoid irritation of the skin.

Gum

The taste of NRT gum can be unpleasant at first but most people get used to it within a week or so. The benefit of stopping smoking using gum is that it allows the patient to control their nicotine dose. It is important to remember that NRT gum is not like ordinary chewing gum. There is a technique that the patient will need to use to get the most out of the gum because any nicotine that is swallowed is wasted. The idea is to chew the gum gently until the flavour is released. The gum is then "parked" in the cheek so that the nicotine is absorbed through the lining of the mouth. People generally use 10 to 15 pieces of gum each day for the first three months and then reduce the number of pieces. If the person starts with the full strength 4mg gum, they can change to the low strength 2mg gum during the reduction stage.

Inhalator

An inhalator suits people who need something to do with their hands when they give up smoking. The inhalator is a plastic mouthpiece with a replaceable nicotine cartridge inside, which the person sucks on like a cigarette. It is important not to expect the inhalator to be like a cigarette — it won't give a 'hit' that would normally be expected with a cigarette. But it will help with cravings by releasing nicotine which is absorbed through the lining of the mouth.

Nasal spray

The nasal spray is the strongest form of NRT available and is absorbed faster than other forms of NRT. This means it can be more beneficial for heavy smokers who find they still experience cravings even with gums or patches. The nasal spray is a small bottle of nicotine solution. It needs a bit of practice to use it properly. Some people find the spray irritates the nose.

Microtab

This is a small white tablet which is placed under the tongue (it is not chewed or swallowed). As it dissolves the nicotine is absorbed through the lining of the mouth.

Lozenge

There are 2mg and 4mg strengths. The stronger one is for people who normally smoke within 30 minutes of waking in the morning. One lozenge is taken every hour or two for the first six weeks of stopping smoking and then gradually reduced each day over the next six weeks.

Varenicline (Champix)

This is a relatively new medicine (launched in 2006) approved for use by NICE as a prescription only medicine for those who want to stop smoking and should usually be prescribed as part of a programme of behavioural support (NICE, 2007). It has side effects which are mainly gastro intestinal but it should be used with caution by people with a history of depression or suicidal tendencies and it should be discontinued if depression or suicidal thoughts develop (BNF, 2009).

Bupropion (Zyban)

This is another relatively new drug which is specifically for use in smoking cessation. It has more cautions and side effects than Varenicline including lowering the threshold for seizures. It should be used as described in the **BNF** for a fixed term prescription as part of a supported cessation programme. It does not have the same associated increased risk of suicide as Varenicline but can have psychological side effects such as depression (BNaFo, 2009).

Case Study 13.5: Michael (cont. from pp. 169)

Michael has stopped smoking for two weeks now and is experiencing a number of withdrawal symptoms. His wife reports that he is increasingly irritable and bad tempered. At times he feels light headed and has trouble concentrating at work. Michael is worried about putting on weight as he is now eating more.

Activity box

Write down the reasons why you think Michael is now displaying the behavioural characteristics above. Revisit the discussion on the addictive nature of nicotine.

Can you think of some ways in which his symptoms could be alleviated? Revisit nicotine replacement therapy and support from health care workers, peers and family.

What do you think is the role of the nurse in helping Michael through this difficult time? Revisit the role of the nurse or health professional in supporting people to stop smoking.

Withdrawal symptoms are the physical and mental changes that occur following interruption or termination of use (of any addictive substance). They are normally temporary and are a product of the physical or psychological adaptation to long-term use, requiring a period of readjustment when the drug is no longer used.

Protection

The British and Scottish governments along with the Welsh assembly and Eire have been active in recent years in the development of policies, funding cessation programmes and setting cessation targets. The aim of these are to protect the public from the harmful effects of smoking, to reduce the number of people starting to smoke, to aid and encourage smoking cessation and to promote healthier lifestyles. In July 2007, legislation was introduced whereby virtually all enclosed public places and workplaces in England became smoke free (this legislation was introduced about one year earlier in Scotland and even earlier in Eire). This means that it is now illegal to smoke inside almost all enclosed public spaces including pubs, bars, nightclubs, cafés and restaurants, lunch rooms, membership clubs and shopping centres. The smoke free law was introduced to protect employees and the public from the harmful effects of passive smoking (second-hand smoke). There are exceptions to the legislation which bans smoking in public places; most notably these include prisons and mental health institutions where it would be unreasonable to expect smokers to go outside.

Under the smoke free law, smoking inside, at work, including in smoking rooms is prohibited. Public transport, and work vehicles, that are used by more than one person are also smoke free. 'No smoking' signs are mandatory in all smoke free premises and vehicles. The UK government was considering a ban on smoking in cars particularly if children under the age of 18 are also in the car. This legislation is already in place in America, Canada and South Africa. It is now apparently no longer under consideration for the UK although campaigners from ASH and other groups would like it to be.

Anyone who smokes in a smoke free place within the UK can face an on the spot fine of £50 (or up to £200 if the matter goes to court). Anyone in charge of smoke free premises, or vehicles, can face fines for two separate offences: failing to prevent smoking in a smoke free place and failing to display 'no smoking' signs.

Legal age for purchase of tobacco

From the October 2007 it became illegal to sell tobacco to anyone under the age of 18 in England and Wales. The age limit was previously 16. This includes banning the sale of cigars, rolling tobacco, rolling papers and cigarettes from vending machines. Strict penalties can be incurred by those found selling tobacco to under 18s. This brings the age restriction in line with the purchase of alcohol. Scotland will follow suit in the near future, by raising the age limit to 18.

The reason for the age change is to try and deter young people from taking up smoking. Early onset of smoking is associated with addiction in later life (Goddard, 2006).

Tobacco packaging and legislation

For some years there has been a legal obligation for tobacco companies to print a health warning on cigarette packets. The legislation includes the requirement for a strongly worded warning message to cover 30% of the front of the pack and 40% of the back of the pack (ASH, 2009) printed in black on a plain white background. Point of sale advertising is now limited to one A5 size poster which must contain a health warning. It is no longer permissible to encourage smoking via rewards such as collecting coupons to exchange for goods. The factors that motivate people to smoke are complex and most people are aware of the risks to their health. However, despite this increased awareness, young people continue to start smoking (Information for Health and Social Care, 2008).

Box 13.4 Targets

In December 1998 the Government published **Smoking Kills** —a white paper on tobacco, which included targets for reducing the prevalence of cigarette smoking amongst adults in England. In 2000 further targets set out in the NHS Cancer plan:

- to reduce smoking rates among manual groups from 32% in 1998 to 26% by 2010,

- to reduce adult smoking prevalence from 28% in 1996 to 24% by 2010,

DH, 2000

Smoking was a priority area in the Choosing Health white paper 2004 and the Delivery Plan in 2005, which set out comprehensive proposals for action. In July 2004 the Government set a new target:

- to reduce the overall proportion of cigarette smokers in England from 26% in 2002 to 21% by 2010 — with a

reduction from 31 to 26% or less among routine and manual groups.

DH, 2004

In relation to young people the 2004 target was:

- to reduce the number of children aged 11–15 who smoke regularly, (defined as usually smoking at least one cigarette a week) from a baseline of 13% in 1996 to 11% by 2005 and 9% by 2010.

DH, 2004

Taxation policy

In addition to public policy on advertising it has been demonstrated that increasing the cost of smoking can result in some people stopping (Action on Smoking and Health, 2008). Taxation policy is therefore an important factor in stimulating smoking cessation. There is concern however that in some sectors especially lower social groups, smoking persists. Higher taxation may therefore be punitive and lead to other forms of privation (Saad, 2009).

Summary

The use of tobacco is still widespread within the developed world and is becoming an increasing problem within the developing world (WHO, 2009). Tobacco is recognized to be a highly addictive substance (Yeaman, 1963) which fosters dependence on both a physical and psychological level to the extent that in 1980 the US Tobacco Institute acknowledged 'We can't defend continued smoking as 'free choice' if the person was 'addicted' (Tobacco Institute, 1980).

The World Health Organization is leading on implementing smoke free environments (WHO, 2009) and tobacco control measures including taxation. Many countries are developing legislation and health promotion campaigns to reduce tobacco consumption, with varying degrees of success. The World Health Organization along with other pressure groups are attempting to control the production and sales methods of the biggest tobacco companies who tie farmers in the developing world into punitive contracts which sees them cultivating tobacco for a minimal return instead of growing food crops. This legislation takes time to be developed and implemented and in poorer countries may not be immediately seen as beneficial (large tobacco companies tend to have the processing plants in the developing world and often include schools and medical facilities to encourage favourable contracts and support from the local people and government).

The use of tobacco is a global issue and although some success in reducing smoking has occurred within the developed world it is possible that the industry has moved its focus to a new developing market.

Smoking is not just directly dangerous to the individual smoker's health it can also impact upon other aspects of the smoker's life including the financial (cost of tobacco), impacting upon the health of those closest to them, their ability to work, psychological dependency and addiction.

 # Online Resource Centre

For more information on smoking visit the Online Resource Centre — http://www.oxfordtextbooks.co.uk/orc/linsley/.

Further reading

http://www.asthma.org.uk/
www.http://smokefree.nhs.uk/
http://www.ash.org.uk/

Action on Smoking and Health (2001). *What goes in? What comes out? Cigarette and smoke composition*. London: ASH.

Action on Smoking and Health (2006). *Tobacco advertising and promotion*. London: ASH.

Action on Smoking and Health (2008). *Beyond Smoking Kills: Protecting children, reducing inequalities*. ISBN 978–1–872428–79–6. London: ASH.

Action on Smoking and Health (2009). *Tobacco policy and the European Unionoke chemistry analysis*. http://www.bat-science.com/groupms/sites/BAT_7AWFH3 (accessed 20/04/10). London: ASH.

British National Formulary (2009). *BNF 58*. London BMJ Publishing Group Ltd.

British Thoracic Society & Scottish Intercollegiate Guideline Network. (2008). *British Guidelines on the Management of Asthma*. London & Edinburgh:.BTS.

Chapman, S., Robinson, G., Stradling, J. & West, S. (2005). *Oxford handbook of respiratory medicine*. Oxford: Oxford University Press.

Department of Health (1988). *Smoking kills: a white paper on tobacco*. London: DH.

Department of Health (2000). *The NHS Cancer Plan— A plan for investment. A plan for reform*. London: DH.

Department of Health (2004). *Choosing Health: Making healthy choices easier*. London: DH.

Department of Health (2005). *Cigarette Smoking*. General Household Survey summary findings. GHS 2004/05. London: DH.

Department of Health (2005). *Tackling health inequalities: Status report on the Programme for Action*. London: DH.

Department of Health (2010). Λ smokefree future—Λ comprehensive tobacco control strategy for England. London: DH

Edwards, R. (2004). The problem of tobacco smoking. *British Medical Journal*. 328: 217.

European Health for All database (HFA-DB) (2010). European Health for All Database. Copenhagen: WHO Regional Office for Europe.

Fletcher, C. & Peto, R. (1977). The natural history of chronic airflow obstruction. *British Medical Journal* 1:1645–1648 .

Fuller, E. *et al*. (2004). *Smoking, drinking and drug use among young people in England in 2004*. A survey carried out on behalf of the NHS Health and Social Care Information Center by the National Center for Social Research and the National Foundation for Educational Research.

Gilbert, D. & Spielberger, C. (1986). Effects of smoking on heart rate, anxiety, and feelings of success during social interaction. *Journal of Behavioral medicine* 10:(6) 629–638.

Goddard, E. (2006). *General household survey: Smoking and Drinking among adults*. London: Office for National Statistics.

Hajek, P., Stead, L. F., West, R., Jarvis, M., & Lancaster, T. (2009). *Relapse prevention interventions for smoking cessation*. London: Cochrane Database of Systemic Reviews.

Information Centre for Health and Social Care. (2008). *Drug use, smoking and drinking among young people in England in 2008*. www.ic.nhs.uk

Lader, D. & Goddard, E. (2005). *Smoking-related Behavior and Attitudes, 2004*. A report on research using the ONS Omnibus Survey produced by the Office for National Statistics on behalf of the Department of Health. ISBN 1 85774 603 1.

Lantz, P. M. (2003) Smoking on the rise among young adults: implications for research and policy. *Tobacco Control 12:i60-i70* London: BMJ Group.

Levy, M. & Pearce, L. (2004). *Asthma. Rapid Reference*. London: Mosby.

National Institute for Health and Clinical Excellence (2004). *Chronic Obstructive Pulmonary Disease. Management of Chronic Obstructive Pulmonary Disease in adults in primary and secondary care. Clinical Guideline 12*. London: NICE.

National Institute for Health and Clinical Excellence (2006). *Brief interventions and referral for smoking cessation in primary care and other settings*. London: NICE.

Office for National Statistics (2007). *General Household Survey*. www.statistics.gov.uk/ghs

Office for National Statistics (2007). *Smoking related behavior and attitudes* London: ONS.

Perkins, K. (1993). Weight gain following smoking cessation. *Journal of Consulting Clinical Psychology*. 61(5): 768–777.

Peto, R. *et al*. (2000) *1950–2000. Mortality from smoking in developed countries* (second edn.). Oxford: Oxford University Press.

Royal College of Physicians (1991). *Smoking and the Young*. London: http://www.roycastle.org/quit/health.htm

Royal College of Physicians (2000) . *Nicotine addiction in Britain. A report of the Tobacco Advisory Group of the Royal Collage of Physicians*. London: RCP.

Saad, I. (2009). *Gallup poll*. NY: Gallup.

Scottish Office for National Statistics (2007) *Scottish Schools Adolescent Lifestyle and Substance Use Survey (SALSUS) 2006 National Report* Edinburgh: SALSUS.

Shahab, L., Jarvis, M. J., Britton, J. & West, R. (2006). Prevalence, diagnosis and relation to tobacco dependence of chronic obstructive pulmonary disease in nationally representative population sample. *Thorax* 61:1043–1047. http://smokefree.nhs.uk/

Steele, C. (1993). *Quit smoking with the nicotine phaseout programme*. Bromsgrove: Swift Publisers.

Thorax, (1998) *Smoking cessation guidelines and their cost effectiveness.* Thorax 53(5), 2: S11-S16.

Tobacco Institute (1980). Minnisota trial exhibit 14,303. Cited In: ASH. *Essential information on Nicotine and Addiction.* London: ASH.

United States Environmental Protection Agency (1992). Respiratory health effects of passive smoking. EPA/600/6–90/006F. NY: EPA

World Health Organization (2009). WHO Report on the global tobacco epidemic: implementing smoke free environments. Geneva: WHO.

Yeaman, A., Brown, & Williamson (1963) memo 1802.05, 17/7/63. Cited In: *ASH essential information on Nicotine and Addiction.* London:ASH.

Chapter 14
Tackling health inequalities

Roslyn Kane and Ruth Reilly

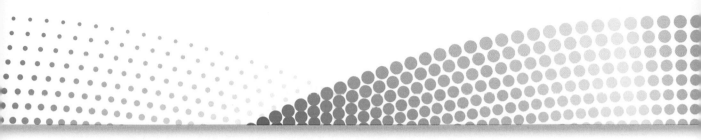

Introduction

Globally, health has been steadily improving: on the whole, people are healthier, wealthier and living longer today than they did thirty years ago (WHO, 2008). However these improvements are not equally distributed: health status varies greatly *between* countries and there is now extensive evidence of considerable and often growing health inequalities *within* countries both by geographical location and by socioeconomic group (WHO, 2008).

Evans (2007) explains that: 'In the UK despite the creation of the welfare state and the virtual abolition of absolute poverty, although the health of the poorest has improved over time this has not occurred at such a quick rate as the health of the richest thus the gap between rich and poor has widened'.

The issue of health inequalities is much more significant in some countries than in others. For example inequalities are markedly smaller in absolute terms in Sweden which has for many years pursued equality orientated social policies, than in the UK, suggesting that social policy can make a difference (Evans, 2007).

Improving the health of the poor and reducing health inequalities has become the central goal of many international organizations including the World Bank and the World Health Organization (McKee and Pomerleau, 2005). This is also evident in the domestic policies of many countries. In the UK there is much interest and debate on the reasons behind inequalities in health. Policy makers, academics, charities and campaigning organizations have differing opinions on what causes health inequality. However all generally agree that health inequality should be reduced, if not eradicated, but not everyone is in full agreement about just how this can be achieved.

By the end of this chapter you should be able to: describe meaning of health inequality; discuss the historical context to the health inequalities debate; present some of the current debates about the underlying cases of health inequalities; have some insight into the measurement of health inequalities; describe some initiatives to tackle health inequalities and understand some ways in which nurses can recognize and respond to health inequality in their personal practice.

The meaning of health inequalities

Health inequalities can be defined as differences in health status or in the distribution of health determinants between different population groups (HDA, 2003), for example, differences in mortality rates between people from different social classes (WHO, 2009). Much has now been published about inequalities in health between people from different populations and as the body of research continues to expand, studies have also been conducted to investigate health inequalities between other subgroups of populations for example inequalities in health status between men and women or between people of different age or ethnic groups. Many of these factors are linked and sometimes it is difficult for researchers and policy makers to tease out whether, for example, it is the area in which someone lives or the socio-economic group which they are from, which has the greatest impact on their health.

Activity box

Using consistent terminology is very important. Take a look at the following terms. Write down your definition of each, spelling out the key differences between each.

- Health inequalities,
- Health variations,
- Health disparities,
- Health inequities;

Discussion points

The term **health inequalities** is used to refer to a broad range of differences between different population groups (for example countries, regions, socio-economic groups, ethnic groups). It generally reflects population differences in circumstances and behaviours that are in most cases socially determined (Leon *et al.* 2001).

During the 1980s and early 1990s health inequalities were not very high on the political agenda in the UK. However with the ever increasing evidence of the impact of socio-economic status on health, the then conservative government conceded that there were variations in health across the population. The term **health variations** was used in political rhetoric during this period. However it has now fallen out of use in academic circles, with the recognition that there are actually inequalities, rather than simply variations, to be addressed.

Health disparities is a term which came to prominence in the USA for similar reasons to the emergence of the term health variations in the UK i.e. that it was generally felt to be less a controversial term than 'health inequalities'.

The term **health inequities** represents unfair inequalities that, at least in theory, could be addressed. Evans (2007) argues that this is not always explicit in the literature. Inequities are variations, which are perceived to be *unfair*. On average, younger people experience better health than older people but these differences are not usually regarded as unfair. So the concept of health inequity is distinct from inequality in that it has a moral and ethical dimension. Health inequities can be seen as resulting from avoidable and unjust differentials in health status (HDA, 2003; McKee and Pomerleau, 2005).

Activity box

Take some time to consider the points below. Spend a few moments on each one, considering which, if any, you think put people at risk of poor health. Write down your thoughts before consulting the points of discussion below.

1. Having to pay for medication or health care,
2. Not having enough money to do PE or go on a school trip,
3. Being of employment age but not in paid employment,
4. Having a special educational need,
5. Living in an economically deprived area.

Discussion points

Many recent studies highlight the above as indicators of likely health inequality.

1. Studies have shown that many economically poorer people have to decide whether they can afford to collect a prescription or to take time off work when ill, as they will lose money. Statutory sick pay will usually not fully compensate for their loss of earnings.
2. A report from the Child Poverty Action Group (CPAG) (Preston, 2008) reviewed a number of studies, which showed that incomes affected parents' choice of school for their children. Once at school children from poorer households cannot always afford a PE kit and may avoid school on those days and children of parents on low income are less likely to be able to find extra money for the school trips (Preston, 2008).
3. Inadequate income, arising primarily from worklessness, and inadequate wages and benefit is the primary cause of poverty (JRF, 2007). Furthermore, many who are out of work are those with disability or mental health or behavioural problems (JRF, 2007) and being in work is no guarantee of being out of poverty. Other barriers to work include caring responsibilities and discrimination of all types.
4. Having a special educational need clearly limits the access to highly paid employment and as we have just seen employment on its own does not mean and end to poverty. A recent MENCAP report (2007) identified six case studies, which demonstrated just how learning disabled individuals are affected by health inequality.
5. The identification of poor health status in people living in geographical areas of deprivation is now well established.

The historical context to the health inequalities debate

Research on inequalities in health has a long history and much of the work has been conducted in the UK. Many academics and policy makers have dedicated their careers to trying to inform the debate on both the underlying causes of health inequalities and on the best ways to minimize the effect of social and economic inequalities on health status. The evidence for the existence of inequalities in health has been observed and reported in the UK since the work of William Farr on vital statistics in 1837 (Davey Smith, *et al.* 2001). Indeed, as far back as 1860 mortality data were being used to document differences in mortality between geographical areas (McKee and Pomerleau, 2005). A major step in understanding inequalities came in 1911 with the introduction of questions on occupation into the British census, which allowed statistical analysis of mortality by specific occupational groups.

However, a major turning point in Britain was the birth of the 'Welfare State'. At the height of the Second World War, the coalition government commissioned Lord Beveridge to look at the problems affecting Britain. The commission reported in 1942 and the recommendations became the blue print for social justice and welfare provision. The **Beveridge Report** was perhaps the most influential of all the twentieth century inquiries and Lord Beveridge became known as 'the father of the welfare state.'

Beveridge described five so-called 'giants' terrorising the nation and although the language has changed, the nature of the health inequalities debate remains as we continue to deal with the same five issues.

Fig. 14.1 appeared in the Daily Herald newspaper at the time of the release of the Beveridge Report.

Activity box

Can you suggest some equivalent problems in today's society that would equate to the five giants Beveridge named?

- Want,
- Ignorance,
- Disease,
- Squalor,
- Idleness.

Write a few sentences about each.

Post modernist sociologists have suggested that two more giants should also be added to the list, do you have any ideas what they might be?

Discussion points

1. **Want** can be interpreted as living on a low income and not being able to afford to do the things discussed earlier indeed living in twentieth-century poverty.

2. **Ignorance** would now be seen as a lack of education and or leaving school without qualifications. This problem has not gone away; the most deprived in society tend to leave school with the poorest results at GCSE (*Hirsch,* 2007). This in turn means future employment opportunities are often limited to jobs paying the minimum wage.

3. **Disease** included many of the infectious diseases prevalent in the 1940's which are now of less importance, others have emerged. Chronic diseases like coronary heart disease, lung cancer and liver disease continue to affect a sizeable population have a strong socio-economic gradient

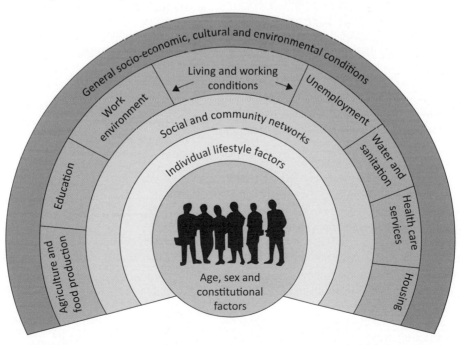

Fig. 14.1 Dahgren and Whitehead 'rainbow' showing the many social, environmental, cultural, and biological influences on health. Reproduced with permission. Dahgren, G. and Whitehead, M. (1998).

177

with those in the lowest earning groups being worst affected (Macintyre, 2007).

4. **Squalor** is rarely used today but the issues of poor housing and homelessness still affect too many people and have very serious implications for health and well-being .

5. **Idleness related to employment ethic**. Whilst the term unemployment is now used and has less stigma than the term idleness both are often seen to infer they are lifestyle choices. This intractable issue is still having a significant and adverse impact on both physical and mental health.

Sexism and racism have been proposed by post modernist sociologists as two additional 'giants' affecting health status. A growing body of evidence indicates differentials in both socio-economic status and in health, by gender and ethnicity.

Although the post war social agenda improved the health of the British nation it did not solve all of the problems. There remained an uneven distribution of health with those from the more affluent sections of society achieving better health status than those from poorer groups. There was growing academic and social concern for an explanation as to why this health gap had continued, even following the introduction of free health provision for all. A similar situation was emerging across Europe, where despite booming economies and the development of social support strategies, evidence of health inequalities was also apparent.

This concern led to the next watershed investigation into the causes of inequalities in health in the UK, commissioned by the then Labour Government. The Department of Health and Social Security, publish the **Black Report** in 1980. An expert committee under the chairmanship of Sir Douglas Black examined health inequality in depth as a discrete subject. This report turned out to be a political 'hot potato' with extremely controversial recommendations. Originally commissioned by a Labour minister in 1977 it was delivered to a Conservative government in April 1980. The findings highlighted that although overall health had improved since the introduction of the welfare state, health inequalities were not narrowing in the UK.

The findings of the report did not make easy reading for the new conservative administration and only 260 copies were made available. There was continual media speculation that the Conservative government had tried to bury the unpalatable findings by publishing the report on a Bank holiday when parliament was not sitting!

The box below highlights some of the key findings of the **Black Report**. Take some time to think about the significance of these findings for inequalities in health and why they may have been politically controversial.

Many of the findings of the **Black Report** indicated that the causes of ill health are often determined by the socio-economic environment in which people live. This means individuals are

---

> **Box 14.1** Key findings of the Black Report
>
> • Health facilities and services are geared to the middle class consumer.
>
> • People from higher social groups have more medical checks and access health care more frequently than those from lower groups.
>
> • People whose health was at greatest risk are those with the lowest income and have the worst living conditions.
>
> • The main cause of health inequalities is poverty, and that it is living standards rather than health care services which determines the overall state of the nation's health.
>
> • Cultural and personal lifestyle play an important contributory role.
>
> • Financial, educational and employment opportunities are needed if health is to be improved.

---

not to blame for their ill health but that political solutions are required. Social and economic policies were needed if the recommendations of the **Black Report** were to be fully implemented.

However, among some of the possible explanations for inequalities in health from the **Black Report**, were the observation that individual personal behaviour may sometimes play a part. Black argued that:

'Health inequalities are [sometimes] the result of people engaging in health damaging behaviours and those in the lowest social classes are most likely to exhibit such behaviours' Cited In: Earle and O'Donnell, 2007:71

Later, in 1987, the British government published **Promoting Better Health** which emphasized the importance of behavioural change at the individual level, urging members of the public to take greater responsibility for their own health.

Activity box

Take time to consider the implications of the government arguing that people must take responsibility for their own health.

Can you think of any circumstances where people are unable to do this?

What are the limitations to individual people trying to change their health behaviour?

Discussion points

Placing too much emphasis on the actions and behaviours of individual people, has the danger of people being blamed for their own ill health. This concept is known as victim blaming. The determinants of ill health are much more complicated than simply the action of individual people. Individual choices about lifestyle are influenced by a range of social, economic, environmental and cultural factors and it is argued that significant improvements in public health are not likely to occur unless policies fully acknowledge this (Baggott, 2000). This action to reduce inequality must operate at the structural as well as at the individual level —addressing change through wider socio-economic reform.

The **Black Report** recommendations that, in order to reduce health inequalities resources should be targeted at those in most need, necessitating increased public expenditure and taxation, did not match the political ideology of the day. However concern expressed by many politicians, academics and health professionals ensured the issues raised by the **Black Report** did not go away. There was continued debate in and out of Parliament on the accuracy of the findings of the **Black Report** with challenges to the accuracy of the statistical evidence, and even more debate on what could be done to reduce health inequality.

In 1987, the findings of the **Black Report** were confirmed and expanded in **The Health Divide**, (Whitehead, 1987), which reviewed the evidence and concluded that the issues were unresolved and had indeed worsened. This report suffered much the same fate as its predecessor: publication was limited and results were disputed with a furore breaking out in both houses of parliament and in the press. Ironically this had the effect of raising its profile even higher.

By the 1990s, the growing body of research was pointing to the very strong influence of the environment in which people live, on their health-related behaviour and subsequently on their health status. The now seminal work by Dahlgren and Whitehead in 1991 described how the general socio-economic, cultural and environmental environment in which people live influence a number of other mechanisms (such as level of education, living conditions, housing, employment etc all of which in-turn influence of health-related behaviour). Fig. 14.2 illustrates this.

On a global level, the publication of the **Ottawa Charter for Health Promotion** by WHO in 1986 had also recognized that if health is to be improved action is needed as at number of different levels. The Charter did recognize the need for the development of personal skills to facilitate change at the individual level, but also emphasized the importance of the development of healthy public policy, supportive environments, community action and the reorientation of health services (WHO, 1986).

In the UK, progress was being made with the publication of The Health of the Nation (HOTN) — a strategy for health in England by the conservative government in 1992, which aimed to ensure that health would be tackled from a number of different levels. It was however, heavily criticized for not sufficiently emphasizing the influence of structural factors and failure to acknowledge the impact of social, economic and environmental factors (Baggott, 2000; Earle and O'Donnell, 2007) and for its largely disease based model of health in terms of both its direction and the targets set (Hunter, 2007). Some argued that the targets and activities should focus on the factors that led to ill health (smoking, poverty, poor housing) rather than on the diseases that resulted (Holland and Stewart, 1998). Hunter (2007) argues that the HOTN was remarkable not only for being the first strategy of its kind but for being produced by a Conservative government not renowned for its commitment to the broader health agenda and a government which did not subscribe to the notion of health inequalities or believe that poverty might have something to do with the widening health gap between social groups (Hunter, 2007).

The political see-saw continued with disputes between all parties on both the cause of health inequalities and the best way to address them. In 1997 the newly elected Labour government commissioned an inquiry, chaired by Sir Donald

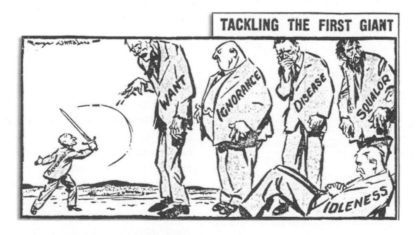

Fig. 14.2 Tackling inequalities: the five giants cartoon.

Acheson, who further reviewed the evidence on health inequalities in England in order to identify areas for policy development.

The **Acheson Report** (published in 1998), which drew on the framework suggested by Dahlgren and Whitehead in 1991, it is argued (McKee and Pomerleau, 2005), did more than any previous commission, both in Britain and elsewhere: it based its recommendations on scientific evidence and the wide scope of the inquiry provided evidence on mechanisms of inequalities and the underlying influences on health. In total the report made thirty-nine recommendations for action and it noted that the number of people living below the poverty line had increased in the UK during the 1980s and that the gains in health among the highest social class had not been replicated in the lower social groups. It found that the health gap in the UK had been widening since the 1970s. By the early 1990s mortality amongst unskilled workers was three times higher than for those in professional occupations (McKee and Pomerleau, 2005).

The **Black Report** (1980) and the **Health Divide** (1987) established the issue of health inequalities within policy discourse but, it is argued, were unable to drive the policy agenda (Marmot, 2009). Marmot argues that is was the publication of the **Acheson Report** in 1998 which really provided the catalyst for concerted action.

In 1999 the government in England published the **white paper Saving Lives: Our Healthier Nation** (DH, 1999a), which identified broad priority areas and new targets for health improvement and expressed the government's commitment to reducing health inequalities. This work was further developed in **Reducing Health Inequalities: An Action Report** (DH, 1999b), **The NHS Plan** (DH, 2000) and in **Tackling Health Inequalities: A Programme for Action** (DH, 2003a) which set out the national strategy to tackle health inequalities in England over the following three years. Then in 2004 the publication of **Choosing Health: Making Healthier Choices Easier** (DH, 2004) which although recognizing the impact of social, environmental, economic and cultural influences on health, focused on reducing and preventing unhealthy lifestyles.

A further significant move of the New Labour government in 1997 was the adoption of the concept of social exclusion and the establishment of the Social Exclusion Unit (SEU) and for the first time the post of Minister for Public Health.

Developments around the UK

Public health policies have often varied between different parts of the UK and this is likely to be increasingly so in the future. Political devolution to Wales, Scotland and Northern Ireland in 2000 meant that political leadership and health policy became devolved responsibilities (Hunter, 2007). Baggott (2000; 2007) has set out key developments in health policy across the different parts of the UK. Whilst it is not possible to cover these in great detail this work is strongly recommended for further

> **Box 14.2** Main policy initiatives from Wales, Scotland and Northern Ireland
>
> Welsh health policy has prioritized public health, health inequalities and health promotion to a far greater extent than England (Baggott, 2007). Wales was first in the UK to launch a public health strategy when in 1989 the Welsh Office published 'Strategic intent and direction for the NHS in Wales' (Welsh Office NHS Directorate, 1989). It set out ten priority areas: cancer, maternal and child health, mental handicap, mental distress and illness, injury, emotional health, respiratory illness, cardiovascular disease, a healthy environment, and physical disability/discomfort (Baggott, 2000). Baggott (2000:69) describes how (although ultimately unsuccessful) protocols in each of the above areas were to highlight priorities for investment and plans were introduced to involve local authorities, the voluntary sector and service users in the development of local health strategies. Later, in 1998, a revised health strategy and strategic framework, which focussed on the economic and social context of health, were published by the Welsh Assembly. Key recent developments include the abolition of prescription charges for people under 25 and costs frozen for those who have to pay. People under 25 and over 60 also receive free dental checks in Wales (Baggott, 2007).
>
> In Scotland, in 1975 Sir John Brotherston, Chief Medical Officer (CMO) in Scotland, reviewed mounting evidence for continuing and increasing inequalities in health, despite the introduction on the NHS and Welfare State. It is now recognized that the problem of health inequalities is particularly serious in Scotland. Studies have shown that health and life expectancy — especially for women — compare unfavourably to the rest of the UK and most Northern and Western European countries (Barry and Yuill, 2008; Hanlon et al., 2001; Leon et al., 2001). Health inequalities between socio-economic groups in Scotland have increased over recent decades (Shaw et al., 2003).
>
> Early health policy in Scotland placed a much greater emphasis on health promotion than England (at least until the publication of *Choosing Health* in 2004 (Baggott, 2007). Specifically Scotland was ahead of England in adopting a strategy on health inequalities as well as programmes promoting healthy eating, exercise and the introduction of a smoking ban (Baggott, 2007: Chapter 9). In 1999 **'Towards a Healthier Scotland: a white paper on Health'** was published. It called for a coherent attack on health inequalities, a special focus on improving children and young people's health, and major initiatives to drive down cancer and heart disease rates. Baggott (2000) argues that the Scottish strategy included a stronger desire to tackling health inequality than was seen in its English counterpart.

Later, in 2003, The Scottish Executive published *'Inequalities in Health: Report of measuring inequalities in health Working Group'* which recommended against setting targets for the reduction of inequalities, but proposed twenty three indicators by which progress could be measured (SE, 2003a). Also in 2003 **'Improving Health in Scotland: the Challenge'** endorsed previous commitments to tackling health inequalities as an overarching aim of the health improvement agenda (SE, 2003b).

In October 2007 the first meeting of a task force to tackle health inequalities was set up and in 2008 it produced its first report: *Equally Well: Report of the Ministerial Task Force on Health Inequalities*, which emphasized the need for a cross-government approach. Other key developments include free long-term personal care for the elderly in Scotland and free eye and dental checks for everyone since 2007 (Baggott, 2007).

In Northern Ireland, two key documents were published in the late 1990s outlining its public health strategy: **Well into 2000: A Positive Agenda for Health and Well being** (NI Dept of Health and Social Services, 1997a) placed an emphasis on tackling health inequalities. It endorsed regional targets for public health which had earlier been outlined in **Health and Well being : Into the Next Millennium** published by the NI Dept of Health and Social Services 1997 (DHSS, 1997b). These targets included smoking, breastfeeding, physical activity, sexual health, immunization, the needs of elderly people, stillbirth, child hospitalization, child protection and learning disability alongside targets for accidents, cancer and circulatory disease (see Baggott, 2000:70). Public health interventions are specifically linked to wider social welfare programmes such as Targeting Social Need and Promoting Social Inclusion (Baggott, 2007). The Northern Ireland Public health strategy set out in *Investing for Health* (DHSSPS, 2002) emphasized stronger partnership working and joint planning arrangements between the NHS and local government. The strategy also set targets for reducing health inequalities and introduced Health Action Zones (which remained until 2008).

reading. Box 14.2 however highlights some of the main policy initiatives from Wales, Scotland and Northern Ireland.

Current debates about the underlying cases of health inequalities

The current debate is dominated by two in many ways rival and competing theories that seek to explain social inequalities in health. The two schools of thought: *the psycho-social* and *the neo-material* are presented very succinctly by Barry and Yuill (2008) and by Earle and O'Donnell (2007) and both of these texts are recommended for further reading. In brief:

The psycho-social perspective

In brief this refers to explanations of health inequality that emphasizes the negative emotional experiences of living in an unequal society and the impact on health of the feelings of stress, shame and powerlessness that this brings (Barry and Yuill, 2008). Psycho-social arguments focus on the way in which contemporary conditions of life produce social stresses that affect social groups unevenly, and on how members of these groups have uneven access to material and personal resources to manage these stresses (Earle and O'Donnell, 2007). These stresses affect both mental and physical well being through changes to the cardiovascular, endocrine and immune systems (Earle and O'Donnell, 2007).

Probably the two leading academics supporting this argument are Professor Richard Wilkinson and Professor Sir Michael Marmot. Wilkinson's groundbreaking work in 1996 showed that in affluent societies it is relative rather than average income that affects health (Wilkinson, 1996). He argues that the greater inequity in a given society, the less social cohesion it has and therefore the more insecurity and isolation experienced by the most disadvantaged groups. This results in greater levels of chronic stress, which in turn ultimately impacts on health status.

Marmot's Whitehall study (described below) demonstrated poorer health status among more junior civil servants compared with those more senior, suggesting that social hierarchies can have adverse effect on health (Marmot, 1986) and the association between stress created by inequality and health in the workplace (Bosma *et al.*, 1997; Martikainen, 1999). This evidence supports argument such as health inequalities being caused by the effects of chronic stress on the individual due to their perceived lack of control associated with their place at the bottom of an unequal social class hierarchy.

Oakley and Rajan (1991) investigated social class and social support in relation to young pregnant women and showed that women who had supportive relationships with others gave birth to heavier, healthier babies indicating another positive advantage of strong social cohesion to health outcomes.

The neo-material perspective

The psycho-social stance has been heavily criticized by academics proposing a neo-material explanation, probably most notably Professor George Davey Smith and Professor John Lynch.

They argue that it ignores material factors such as educational disadvantage, poor housing, employment opportunities and income and argue that Wilkinson fails to address or explain why inequality exists in the first place (Lynch *et al.*, 2000).

Shaw *et al.* (2003) argue that there are many ways in which differentials in life chances can be explained by material factors but probably the most important are those which relate to income and employment.

Neo-materialist explanations refer to explanations of health inequality that emphasize unequal distribution of resources such as housing, income and access to education (Barry and Yuill, 2008). They focus on the way in which adverse socio-economic and psycho-social environments and the health damaging mechanisms associated with them are products of material and social formations which produce unequal distribution of personal income and wealth which in turn leads to unequal access to food, transport, housing health care and education as well as unequal consumption of a healthy lifestyle (Earle and O'Donnell, 2007). Proponents of the neo-materialist approach argue that structural change is needed to address underlying inequalities in society, rather than interventions which are targeted at individual or communities whose ability to institute changes in their lifestyles may be hampered by their immediate circumstances. Such individualized approaches are in danger of leading to **victim blaming**.

Lifecourse explanations

A further school of thought is offered by lifecourse explanations which consider how the health effects of adverse socio-economic circumstances accumulate throughout the lifecourse (Earle and O'Donnell 2007). They explain how it is the *accumulation* of material deprivation *throughout* the lifecourse that causes the damage. Barker (1989) argued that the effect of adverse conditions begins at conception and this work led to the concept of foetal programming which suggests that maternal poverty can affect the development of the foetus (Earle and O'Donnell, 2007).

The Foetal Origins theory suggests that major causes of chronic conditions such as hypertension, high cholesterol, CHD and type 2 Diabetes are hardwired in utero in underweight babies in the second and third trimester and within the first year of life. Material and social disadvantage in adults can thus be reflected in the low birth weight and poorer health of their children (Earle and O'Donnell 2007). Poverty during childhood has also been shown to be related to both adult health and socio-economic status and the effects have been shown to be the strongest in people who are born into, grow up and remain in disadvantaged material circumstances (van de Mheen *et al.*, 1998, cited in Earle and O'Donnell, 2007). It is theory and evidence such as this that has been influential in the development of policies which aim to break this cycle of poverty to, in the long-term improve health, such as those which give a high priority to the health of families with children and to improving the living standards of poor households.

The measurement of health inequalities

There are different ways of examining inequalities in health status across populations. Indicators of health may be compared between people from different socio-economic groups, to explore whether those from higher socio-economic groups are generally healthier than those from lower socio-economic groups. Alternatively differences between the health status of people living in different geographical locations (less deprived compared with more deprived areas) can be compared as can those between different ethnic or gender groups, and so on.

The data used to analyse these differences can be accessed from a range of sources. Historical data is available through national sources. Governments have always needed information about populations. In Britain, William the Conqueror was the first ruler to understand the value of demographics and commissioned the Doomsday Book in 1085. Much later, following the industrial revolution, amidst fears that Britain's growing population would outstrip the country's supply of food, the first census of the population was conducted. The first UK census was carried out in 1801 and since then has been held at regular ten-yearly (decennial) intervals. The only exception to this was in 1941, the Census being abandoned due to World War II.

In England and Wales the census is coordinated and conducted by the Office for National Statistics (ONS: **www.ons.gov.uk**) and in Scotland by the General Register Office for Scotland (GROS: **http://www.gro-scotland.gov.uk/**) and by the Northern Ireland Statistics and Research Agency (NISRA: **http://www.nisra.gov.uk/**) in Northern Ireland.

Statistical information is made available in published reports and directly on the above websites, however full public access to the census returns is restricted under the terms of the 100-year rule; the most recent returns made available to researchers are those of the 1911 Census for England and Wales. The Scottish 1911 census will be available in 2011.

Although many researchers set up their own studies data collected by others is also useful in the analysis of health inequalities. Probably the two most notable studies and the Whitehall study (I and II) managed by Professor Sir Michael Marmot at University College London, and the Longitudinal study, run by the ONS.

The original Whitehall Study investigated social determinants of health, specifically the cardio-respiratory disease prevalence and mortality rates among British male civil servants between the ages of 20 and 64. The initial study, the Whitehall I Study, was conducted over a period of ten years, beginning in 1967. A second phase, the Whitehall II Study, examined the health of 10,308 civil servants aged 35 to 55, of whom two thirds were men and one third women. A long-term follow-up of study subjects from the first two phases is ongoing and data from the study are published regularly by the research team.

The Whitehall study has shown employment grade within the civil service to be a powerful predictor of death rate and within each employment group, car ownership further predicts mortality risk. This shows that more refined measures of socio-economic position can lead to more precise predictions of differentials in health outcome.

The ONS Longitudinal Study (LS) was set up in the 1970s to meet the need for better data on mortality and fertility. It contains data for one of the population of England and Wales. Information from the 1971, 1981, 1991 and 2001 censuses has been linked together, along with information on events such as births, deaths and cancer registrations. At each census, data on more than 500,000 sample members are included.

Studies that make the fullest use of LS data are those that link social, occupational and demographic information at successive censuses to data on vital events. Examples include studies of mortality, cancer incidence and survival, and fertility patterns. Further information can be found at: http://www.statistics.gov.uk/services/Longitudinal.asp

Data from the LS study has been used to demonstrate the independent and combined influence of a number of variables indicative of socio-economic status (occupation, education, income, assets, wealth and characteristics of residential area — all of which demonstrated the same general associations with health outcome (Shaw *et al.*, 2003).

Other notable studies include:

The 1958 birth cohort study

This involved all children born in England, Wales and Scotland during one week in 1958. Follow-up surveys were conducted when the children reached ages 7, 11, 16, 23 and 33 with over 10,000 participants being studied at each phase (Shaw *et al.*, 2003). This large scale study provides data for detailed investigation of the development of inequalities in health throughout childhood and into adulthood and has been used to illustrate the influence of lifetime social circumstances on morbidity and striking differentials in health status between social class groups (Power *et al.*, 1999: cited in Shaw *et al.*, 2003).

The collaborative study

This study followed of nearly 6000 men aged 35–64 in the West of Scotland over 20 years and demonstrated that the risk of dying is also influenced by the cumulative effect of social circumstances across the lifespan (Davey Smith *et al.*, 1997, cited in Shaw *et al.*, 2003). This study showed that the risk of dying was related to the social circumstances of the participants in early life (occupational social class of their father being used as a proxy measure), social circumstances in early adulthood and those at the time of entering the study. The authors constructed an index of lifetime social circumstances and argued that the risk of dying in later adulthood is influenced by social circumstances acting in childhood and then

> **Box 14.3** Initiatives in place to address the issue of inequalities in health
>
> - Health Action Zones,
> - Healthy living centres,
> - Sure Start programme,
> - The Healthy Schools Programme,
> - Connexions service,
> - The National Minimum Wage Act 1998,
> - Working tax credit,
> - New Deal programmes,
> - National strategy for neighbourhood renewal,
> - Strategy to reduce the number of people sleeping rough,
> - Establishing drug action teams,

throughout adult life. Findings such as these have led to calls for investigations into the causes of health inequalities to take a broad perspective to include the analysis of influences across the lifecourse rather than simply an analysis of the impact of adult social circumstances on health (Shaw *et al.*, 2003).

Initiatives to tackle health inequalities

So far this chapter has looked at activity and commitment at policy level. Let's now examine how this may translate into action. Box 14.3 below highlights some of the main initiatives, which have emerged in attempts to address the issue of inequalities in health. Take some time to research each. Consider how they might make a difference to inequalities in health across the country.

> **Box 14.4** NGOs working on reducing health inequalities
>
> **The Child Poverty Action Group** is a campaigning charity for children it constantly monitors and works to improve children's lives and has proposed a number of strategies to tackle issues for children. http://www.cpag.org.uk
>
> **The Joseph Rowntree Foundation** is social research organization which undertakes research and projects to reduce the effects of poverty and social exclusion http://www.jrf.org.uk/

MENCAP works to raise the issue of health discrimination for those with a learning disability. through their 'Treat me right' and 'Death by Indifference' campaigns http://www.mencap.org.uk/ This work has led to national health initiatives to provide annual health checks for all those registered as having a learning disabled with GP practices which results in very individual having a health action plan.

The Community Development Exchange (CDX) is the UK-wide membership organization for community development. CDX works to ensure that community development is recognized and supported as a powerful way of tackling inequality and achieving social justice: http://www.cdx.org.uk/.

The Tudor Trust is an independent grant making trust which supports organizations working across the UK addressing the social, emotional and financial needs of people at the margins of society. All their work has the potential to positively influence health: http://www.tudortrust.org.uk/

The Queens Nursing Institute is a charity dedicated to the improvement of patient care by supporting community nurses. http://www.qni.org.uk/ Examples of nurses working innovatively to reduce health inequality can be found at: http://www.qni.org.uk/project-funding/funded-projects.html

The above all constitute initiatives by government. However other agencies are also central to the effort to tackle inequalities in health. The box below illustrates some examples of other organizations which are particularly active in contributing to the agenda. Non-Government Organizations (NGO's), organizations which campaign, research or provide services that are either not funded or partially provided from central taxation play a particularly important role. They are often registered charities and work toward meeting the harder to tackle issues or supporting underrepresented groups and small local projects.

The following organizations are a few of those NGOs working either directly or indirectly for the reduction of health inequalities.

Are there any solutions to the problems?

A huge body of literature now exists on the problems of health inequalities and on trying to explain the phenomenon, but the lack of information on just what to do about it and how to evaluate health promotion interventions in this area has

recently been noted (Evans, 2007; Asthana and Halliday, 2006). Crucial to all interventions however is the production of evidence on the extent of their effectiveness. Evaluation of public health interventions is covered in detail in Chapter 12 of this book.

Action to address health inequalities can take place at a number of different levels. Policies can be implemented to address the underlying root causes of ill health with for example actions to eliminate poverty, homelessness, unemployment and so on. Alternatively we can work closely with smaller communities to try and help with their more immediate problems.

Interventions to reduce health inequalities or often categorized as being either 'upstream' (tackling the fundamental causes of inequality though national, social and economic policy) or 'downstream' working directly with individuals or communities to tackle their immediate socio-economic or health problems.

This has been effectively illustrated with the following scenario:

You will often hear about health workers being equated to lifesavers standing beside a fast flowing river. Every so often a drowning person is swept alongside. The lifesaver dives in to the rescue, retrieves the 'patient' and resuscitates them. Just as they have finished, another casualty appears alongside. So busy and involved are the lifesavers in all of this rescue work that they have no time to walk upstream and see why it is that so many people are falling in the river. What is necessary, it is argued, is to refocus upstream and what is needed generally amongst health workers is more 'upstream thinking'.

Ashton and Seymour, 1988:vii

Davies and Macdowall (2006) use this parable to explain that interventions made at the upstream level i.e. in terms of prevention, will be most effective in producing a health gain.

A second important distinction between approaches is whether they are universal (ensuring everyone receives the same standard of service) or selectivist (a means tested approach which targets benefits and services to those with greatest need) Evans (2007). The terminology 'population level' versus 'targeted' approaches is also often used in this context.

Leading academics in this field (Davey Smith, et al. 1999) argue that the solution to health inequalities is an upstream and universalist approach:

'There is one central and fundamental policy that should be pursued' the reduction of income equality and consequently the elimination of poverty. Ending poverty is key to ending inequalities in health'

Davey Smith, et al. 1999, cited in Evans, 2007:163

Indeed this approach is supported elsewhere. Mitchell et al. (2000) conducted comprehensive statistical modelling of every parliamentary constituency in Britain to test the potential impact on health inequalities of a number of different social policy scenarios and concluded that strategic economic policies, such as those which help to achieve full employment, had the greatest potential in narrowing the inequalities gap.

Macintyre (2007) provides a very useful summary of policy principles, derived from the evidence about what works best and concludes that whilst structural policies addressing inequalities in, for example, education, income and employment are of extreme importance and should be prioritized, more 'downstream' targeted approaches are also needed.

She argues that:

'Interventions at the higher, more regulatory or structural, levels (Clean Air Acts, seat belt legislation, food supplementation, banning smoking in public places) appear to do more to reduce health inequalities than information based approaches (e.g. nutrition labelling, anti-smoking adverts, drink driving campaigns, etc.). This is because more advantaged groups in society find it easier, because of better access to resources such as time, finance, and coping skills, to avail themselves of health promotion advice (e.g. to give up smoking, improve diet, use fluoride toothpaste etc.) and preventive services (e.g. immunization, dental check ups and cervical screening). Disadvantaged groups tend to be harder to reach, and find it harder to change behaviour'.
Macintyre, 2007

Evans (2007) also highlights a problem with the tackling health inequalities only through national macro-economic policy: what role does this leave for the public health practitioner working at the community? Indeed it is well recognized that most of the major drivers of the distribution of health in the population lie outside the NHS (Macintyre, 2007).

Given that it is unethical to do nothing, Evans suggests five key options for public health practitioners, including nurses: lobbying, partnership working, community development, promoting healthy behaviours and improving access to healthcare (Evans, 2007:164).

How can nurses recognize and respond to health inequalities in their personal practice and influence policy?

As discussed above, health is rarely evenly spread throughout any population. As a general rule, poor people tend, on average to be less healthy than richer people. Working towards

reducing these inequalities in health is not only a major challenge to politicians but also to health professionals. Indeed, it is argued (Evans, 2007) that action to address health inequalities should involve *every* public health worker from those working at a national level of government to those working at local level: social workers, community workers, nurses, environmental health practitioners, GPs and so on. Interventions to try and reduce health inequalities operate at a range of levels from changes in national policy right through to one-to-one interventions between nurses and individual patients.

A number of key publications in the UK recently have discussed the changing role of nursing and the activities of nurses. These are discussed more fully in Chapter 4 of this book. In relation to inequalities in health, nurses are no longer only expected to contribute to the agenda, but to lead on initiatives that make real improvements to people's lives (DH, 1999c: DH, 2002: DH, 2003b; Wanless, 2004). This work demands very different skills to those of the more conventional clinical side of nursing (Dion, 2008).

This section looks at the influence of nurses in reducing health inequalities from two levels: individual practice and influencing policy and strategy.

Individual practice

Two important questions re:

1. The role of the nurse at the individual level
2. What can individual nurses do to reduce health inequalities in their daily work?

Activity box

Take some time out to think about how as a student and as a qualified nurse you can play your part in reducing health inequalities in your professional practice.

Discussion points

You could consider some of the following:

- Search for the unmet health needs of all service users in your student clinical placements.
- Think about explanations for causes of poor health of the patients in your care.
- Recognize personal, local, environmental, national and international health inequality problems or issues.
- Recognize the need for nursing involvement and action in day to day practice.

Box 14.5 Social capital

The concept of **social capital** has become increasingly important for public health practitioners (Gibson, 2007). Robert Putman, an American political scientist has arguably been the most influential in bringing the concept to prominence (Gibson, 2007) and he is regarded as a key inspiration behind the use of the term in research into the causes of health inequality in the UK (Wilkinson, 1996, cited in Gibson, 2007). He defines it as:

'features of social life such as networks, norms and social trust that facilitate coordination and cooperation for mutual benefit'
Putman, 1993:85, cited in Gibson, 2007:247

Putman argues that social capital has a direct effect on health (Putman, 2000) (and indeed the links between social capital and health have come to increasing prominence in the literature (Gibson, 2007)), and as such, argues that efforts to improve health should include initiatives to improve social capital.

It is argued (Heller *et al.*, 2007) that it is important for those involved in promoting public health to have a real commitment to reducing inequalities within their own practice and to have an informed understanding of the nature and extent of poverty within their own locality. Heller *et al.* (2007) capture the role of the public health worker in this context very succinctly:

'...public health workers will be better able to create 'helping relationships' that do not blame the victims of poverty but assist individuals, households and communities in a realistic way to break out of a cycle of poverty'
Heller *et al.*, 2007:181

It is likely for example that nurses may become involved in initiatives aimed at promoting social cohesion — community development initiatives or those which aim to ensure people are received all sources of income to which they are entitled, through for example welfare benefit screening and signposting to services and information sources.

- Keep up to date with current trends and policy documents.
- Get involved, professional representation groups e.g. the Royal College of Nursing (RCN), The Queens Nursing Institute (QNI), the Community Practitioners' and Health Visitors' Association (CPHVA), the Child Poverty Action Group (CPAG), the Save the Children Fund.
- Take part in local and national professional consultations such as those led by the Nursing and Midwifery Council or the Department of Health.

- Participate in local community action and local research projects.
- Implement research findings into personal practice participation.
- Try to understand the underlying social/economic and environmental causes of poor health of the patients in your care.

Understanding risk behaviour

Arguably one of the most important things a nurse can do, when working with individual patients, is to understand the complex ways in which a person's individual background and social circumstances influences their health behaviour. If for example, a nurse is caring for a patient with a smoking related illness, and it has been recommended that the patient stop or at least reduce the number of cigarettes smoked per day, in order for the nurse to support the patient through this process it is essential that s/he has some understanding of why the patient smokes (even perhaps when they have a good understanding of how detrimental it is to their health). The nurse therefore needs to have an understanding of the epidemiology of smoking — why it is more common among some population groups. Has the patient been brought up in a cultural environment where smoking is considered the norm? Was there peer pressure to take up smoking as a young person? Does the person smoke as a coping mechanism because they find smoking helps them to deal with stressful situations etc. The nurse must have a strong understanding of the importance of the socio-economic cultural and environmental influences on health before he can begin to help the patient address these behaviours.

Case Study 14.1: Nursing interventions by the Queen's Nursing Institute which address inequalities in health

Homeless Health Initiative

The Queen's nursing Institute's Homeless Health Initiative, funded by the Big Lottery Fund for 3 years, supported nurses working with people lacking a secure home e.g. people living on the streets, in B&Bs, hostels, refuges, or in temporary housing. The support given by the project to community nurses working with homeless people included:

- Professional development opportunities relating to homelessness and health,
- Resources and guidance on health care with homeless people,
- Peer support and networking,
- Information sharing and regular updates.

Following the recommendations of the Acheson Report, working with families and children became a priority and a means to tackle health inequalities.

Active case management project

The Queen's Nursing Institute puts community nursing at the forefront of patient care and has set up an innovation fund which supports local small-scale projects through which nurses tackle some of the most challenging health issues by addressing the health inequalities.

One example is the active case management project in Belfast, Northern Ireland, which, (using a relatively small grant of £7290) aimed to actively find patients in local communities whom it was felt would benefit from referrals to a range of nursing services to reduce their risk of developing chronic illness.

Health events were held in pubs and clubs in Belfast during which 351 people were screened. 115 people were found to have risk factors for respiratory or cardiac disease, diabetes and hypertensive conditions. All participants were referred for further investigation to try and prevent the development of disease.

Colin the Cabbie

In Liverpool, England, another project which was known as Colin the Cabbie was developed on the recognition that those in most need often do not access health promotion and public health screening initiatives. It aimed to encourage men to be healthier by giving them information on diet, physical activity and stopping smoking. Taxi drivers working in the Sefton area of the city were specifically targeted with health promotion materials and eight were trained as peer mentors to offer advice and a social supportive network to other drivers, and to the general public.

Discussion points

- What do these three initiatives have in common?
- Can you think of the reasons why homeless people, people in pubs and taxi drivers were chosen as the target groups?
- Do these initiatives link to the targets for tackling health inequalities?

The practitioners chose groups of people who, through the traditional approach, may not otherwise have come into direct contact with health professionals.

Nurses identified a health issue not being met effectively by local or national schemes.

Not only did they link to national strategies they provided care to those who otherwise might have missed out and whose health might have suffered.

Reducing inequalities in health through strategic nursing interventions: nurses influencing policy

Nurses are regularly invited to participate in national consultation events through for example the Nursing and Midwifery Council in the UK. The Royal College of Nursing is also very proactive in getting the voice of nurses heard and it is very easy to sign up to participate in events and consultations online.

The Queens Nursing Institute (QNI) is also committed to giving community nurses a voice on national policy. The QNI works to influence government policy on changes to NHS organizations, primary care, nursing education and issues such as services for homeless people and reducing health inequalities. By contributing to stakeholder meetings, responding to national consultations, taking up issues raised by local projects where it appears they may have wider significance, and providing examples and information to policymakers.

In 2009 the QNI launched the Community Nurse Forum which enables community nurses to make their contribution to key debates in primary care via email or forum meetings, putting their expert front line views to policymakers. Nurses interested can simply register online (www.qniforum.org.uk) to receive regular updates and to take part in the consultation process in a range of national policies.

Summary

In this chapter you have been introduced to the concept of health inequalities and its development as a growing academic discipline and importance as a policy and health care priority. Some argue that the previous British Labour government did more than any other European government to reduce inequalities in health and that the U.K.'s experience has lessons for other governments (Exworthy et al., 2003). However, most agree that there are some signs of progress still more needs to be done in order to have a real impact.

As detailed in Chapter 1, in England the agenda is currently being taken forward by Professor Sir Michael Marmot, whom the government has asked to advise the Secretary of State for Health on the future development of a health inequalities strategy post-2010.

There has for some time been a formal commitment to increasing the contribution nurses make to public health and tackling inequalities, but it is only now that it is starting to gain momentum. As nurses we must realize that health care is not just about the delivery of care to the sick. It is also about recognizing that health enhancing activities should be available to all regardless of income, geography, gender, ethnicity, ability or level of education. Furthermore, we need a firm understanding of the ways in which the socio-economic environment in which a person lives, in turn can influence their behaviour and ultimately their health status.

 ## Online Resource Centre

For more information on health inequalities visit the Online Resource Centre –
http://www.oxfordtextbooks.co.uk/orc/linsley/

Further reading

http://www.povertyinformation.org/
http://www.cpag.org.uk/
http://www.jrf.org.uk/
http://www.qni.org.uk/
http://www.cabinetoffice.gov.uk/social_exclusion_task_force.aspx
http://wales.gov.uk/splash;jsessionid=pTCpLfJps27cgrJqMYxrfl MpTSZ15gQsqdx1XJnwlghg21jyRhlC!2138048893?orig=/
http://www.scotland.gov.uk/Home
http://www.dh.gov.uk/en/index.htm

Acheson, D. (1998). *Independent Inquiry into Inequalities in Health Report*. London: The Stationery Office.

Ashton, J. & Seymour, H., (1988). *The New Public Health: The Liverpool experience*. Milton Keynes: Open University Press.

Asthana, S. and Halliday, J. (2006). *What works in tackling health inequalities? Pathways, Policies and Practice through the lifecourse*. Bristol: The Policy Press.

Baggott, R. (2000). *Public Health Policy and Politics*. New York: Palgrave Macmillan

Baggott, R. (2007). Health policy in other parts of the UK. Chapter 9 in: Baggott, R, *Understanding health policy*. Bristol: The Policy Press.

Barker, D.J.P. (1989). Growth in utero, blood pressure in childhood and adult life and mortality from cardiovascular disease. *British Medical Journal* (298) 564–7.

Barry, A. and Yuill, C. (2008). *Understanding the Sociology of Health. An introduction*. Second Edition. London: Sage Publications.

Black, D., Morris J., Smith C., & Townsend P. (1980). *Inequalities in health: report of a working party*. London: Department of Health and Social Security.

Bosma, H., Marmot, M., Hemingway, H., Nicholson, A. C., Brunner, E., Stansfield, S. A. (1997). Low job control and risk of coronary heart disease in Whitehall II (prospective cohort) study. *British Medical Journal*. 214:558–65.

Dahlgren, G. & Whitehead, M. (1991). *Policies and Strategies to Promote Social Equity in Health*. Stockholm: Institute for Futures Studies.

Dahlgren, G. and Whitehead, M.(1998). *Health Inequalities*, London: Her Majesty's Stationery Office.

Davey Smith, G., Dorling, D., Gordon, D. and Shaw, M. (1999). The widening health gap: what are the solutions? *Critical Public Health*. 9(2):151–170.

Davey Smith, G., Dorling, D. and Shaw, M. (2001). *Poverty, Inequality and health in Britain: A Reader*: Bristol: Policy Press.

Davey Smith, G., Hart, C., Blane, D., Gillis, C. & Hawthorne, V. (1997). Lifetime socioeconomic position and mortality: prospective observational study. *British Medical Journal* 314:547–52.

Davies, M. & Macdowall, W. (2006). *Health promotion theory*. Maindenhead: Open University Press.

Department of Health (1992). *The Health of the Nation — a strategy for health in England*. London: HMSO.

Department of Health and Social Services (1997a). *Well into 2000. A positive agenda for health and well being*. London: DHSS.

Department of Health and Social Services (1997b). *Health and well being into the next millennium. Regional strategy for health and social well being 1997–2002*. London: DHSS.

Department of Health (1999a). *Saving lives: Our Healthier Nation*. London: The Stationery Office.

Department of Health (1999b). *Reducing health inequalities an action report*. Department of Health. London: The Stationery Office.

Department of Health (1999c). *Making a difference: strengthening the nursing, midwifery and health visiting contribution to health and healthcare*. London: DH.

Department of Health (2000). *The NHS Plan: A plan for investment, a plan for reform*. London: DH.

Department of Health (2002). *Shifting the balance of power: next steps*. London: DH.

Department of Health (2003a). *Tackling health inequalities: A programme for action*. London: The Stationery Office.

Department of Health (2003b). *Public Health in England*. London: The Stationery Office.

Department of Health (2004). *Choosing Health: Making healthy choices easier*. London: The Stationery Office.

Department of Health, Social Security & Public Services (2002). *Investing for Health*. Belfast: DHSSPNI

Dion, X. (2008). Developing Programmes, Services and Reducing Inequalities. Chapter 14 in: Coles, L. and Porter, E. (eds.) *Public Health Skills: A practical guide for nurses and public health practitioners*. Oxford: Blackwell Publishing: Oxford.

Earle, S. and O'Donnell, T. (2007). The factors that influence health. Chapter 3 in: Earle, S., Lloyd, C.E., Sidell, M. and Spurr, S. (eds.). *Theory and research in promoting public health*. London /Maindenhead: Sage PublicationsThe Open University.

Evans, D. (2007). New directions in tackling inequalities in health. Chapter 9 in: Orme, J., Powell J., Taylor, P. and Grey, M. (eds.). *Public Health for the 21st Century: New Perspectives on Policy, Participation and Practice*. Second edition. Berkshire: Open University Press.

Exworthy, M., Stuart, M., Blane, D. & Marmot, M. (2003). *Tackling health inequalities since the Acheson inquiry*. Published for the Joseph Rowntree Foundation. Bristal: Policy Press.

Gibson, A. (2007). Does Social Capital have a Role to Play in the Health of Communities? Chapter 28 in: Douglas, J., Earle, S., Handsley, S., Lloyd, C. & Spurr, S. (eds.) *A Reader in Promoting Public Health. Challenge and Controversy*. London: Sage Publications.

Hanlon, P., Walsh, D., Buchanan, D., Redpath, A., Bain, M., Brewster, D., Cahalmers, J., Muir, R., Samlls, M., Willis, J., & Wood, R. (2001) *Chasing the Scottish Effect: Why Scotland* needs a step-change in health if it is to catch up with the rest of Europe. Edinburgh: Public Health Institute of Scotland.

Health Development Agency (2003). Addressing inequalities through health impact assessment. *Learning from practice bulletin*. London: HDA.

Heller, T., Beaumont, K., Earle, S. & Douglas, J. (2007). Addressing Poverty and Health. Chapter 6 in: Lloyd, C., Handsley, S., Douglas, J., Earle, S., & Spurr, S. (eds.) *Policy and Practice in Promoting Public Health*. London: Sage Publications.

Hirsch D. (2007). Chicken and Egg: child poverty and education inequalities. CPAG Policy Briefing September 2007. London: Child Poverty Action Group.

Holland, W. W. and Stewart, S. (1998). *Public health: The vision and the challenge.* London: The Nuffield Trust.

Hunter, D. (2007). Public health: Historical context and current agenda. Chapter 2 in: Scriven, A. and Garmen, S. (eds.) *Public Health: Social context and action*. Berkshire: Open University Press.

Leon, D.A., Walt, G., Gilson, L. (2001). Recent advances: International perspectives on health inequalities and policy. *British Medical Journal*. 10(322):591–4.

Lynch, J., Davey Smith, G., Kaplan G, House, J. (2000). Income inequality and mortality: importance to health of individual income, psychosocial environment or material conditions. *British Medical Journal*. 320:1200–4.

Macintyre, S. (2007). *Inequalities in health in Scotland: what are they and what can we do about them?* Glasgow: MRC Social and Public Health Sciences Unit, Occasional Paper Number 17.

McKee, M. & Pomerleau, J. (2005). Inequalities in Health. Chapter 4 in: McKee M. & Pomerleau, J. (eds.) *Issues in Public Health*. Berkshire: Open University Press.Marmot, M. (1986). Social inequalities in mortality: the social environment. In: Wilkinson, R. (ed.) *Class and Health: Research and Longitudinal Data*. London: Tavistock.

Marmot M (2009) *Strategic Review of Health Inequalities in England post-2010*. Marmot Review: First Phase Report. June 2009

Martikainen P, Stansfield S, Hemingway H, Marmot M (1999). Determinants of socioeconomic differences in physical and mental functioning. *Social Science and Medicine*. 49:499–507

MENCAP (2007). *Death by Indifference. Following up the Treat me Right Report*. London: MENCAP.

Mitchell, R., Dorling, D. & Shaw, M. (2000). *Reducing health inequalities in Britain*. Published for the Joseph Rowntree Foundation. Bristol: The Policy Press.

Oakley, A. & Rajan, L. (1991). Social class and social support: the same or different? *Sociology* 25(1): 31–59.

Palmer, G., MacInnes, T. & Kenway, P. (2007). *Monitoring poverty and social exclusion 2007*. York: Joseph Rowntree Foundation.

Preston, G. (2008). *2 Skint 4 School: time to end the classroom divide*. London: Child Poverty Action Group.

Power, C., Manor, O., & Matthews, S. (1999). The duration and timing of exposure: effects of socioeconomic environment on adult health. *American Journal of Public Health*. 89 (7): 1059–65.

Putman, R. (1993). *Making Democracy Work: Civic Traditions in Modern Italy*. Princeton NJ: Princeton University Press.

Putman, R. (2000). *Bowling Alone: the Collapse and revival of American Community*. New York: Simon and Schuster.

Shaw, M., Dorling, D., Gordon, D. & Davey Smith, G. (2003). *The widening gap: Health Inequalities and Policy in Britain*. Bristol: The Policy Press

Whitehead, M. (1987). *The Health Divide: Inequalities in health in the 1980s*. London: The Health Education Council.

Wilkinson, R. (1996). *Unhealthy Societies: The Afflictions of Inequality*. London: Routledge.

World Health Organization (1986). *Ottawa Charter for Health Promotion*. Copenhagen: WHO Regional Office for Europe.

The Scottish Office (1998) *Working Together for a Healthier Scotland. A Consultation Document*. London: The Stationery Office.

The Scottish Executive (1999). *Towards a healthier Scotland: a white paper on health*. Edinburgh: The Stationery Office.

The Scottish Executive (2003a). *Inequalities in Health*. Edinburgh: Report of Measuring Inequalities in Health Working Group.

The Scottish Executive (2003b). *Improving Health in Scotland —The Challenge*. Edinburgh: The Scottish Executive.

The Scottish Government (2008). *Equally Well — The Report of the Ministerial Task Force on Health Inequalities*. Edinburgh: The Scottish Executive.

van de Mheen, H., Stronks, K., Mackenback, J.P. (1998). A life-course perspective on socio-economic inequalities in health: the influence of childhood socio-economic conditions and selection processes. *Sociology of Health and Illness*. 20(5) 754–77.

Wanless, D. (2004). *Securing Good Health for the Whole Population*. London: HMSO.

Welsh Health Planning Forum (1989). *Strategic intent & direction for the NHS in Wales*. Cardiff: Welsh Office NHS Directorate.

Wilkinson, R. (1996). *Unhealthy Societies: the Afflictions of Inequality*. London: Routledge.

World Health Organization (1986). *The Ottawa Charter for Health Promotion*. Geneva: WHO.

World Health Organization (2008). *The World Health Report 2008 — primary Health Care (Now More Than Ever)*. Geneva: WHO.

World Health Organization Glossary: http://www.who.int/hia/about/glos/en/index1.html.

Chapter 15
Tackling obesity

Alison Mostyn and Dilip Nathan

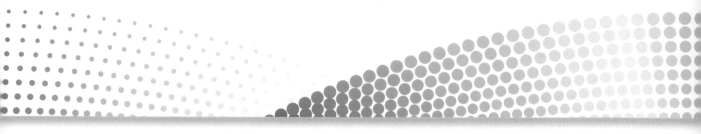

Introduction

The media appears to be obsessed with the 'obesity epidemic' sweeping the UK, but is there an evidence base to support such extensive coverage on television, radio and in newspapers and magazines? This chapter will investigate the assessment and definition of obesity, the current levels of overweight and obesity in adults and children in the UK and worldwide, causes and consequences of obesity, strategies and interventions to tackle obesity and whether these interventions are working.

Defining obesity

Before we can explore the causes and consequences of obesity, it is important to understand how obesity is measured and defined. Typically, body mass index (BMI) is used to determine if an individual is overweight or obese; BMI is calculated by dividing weight in kilograms by height squared in metres (kg/m^2).

Discussion points

Can you think of some occasions when a nurse will have the opportunity to make these measurements (height and weight), and calculate BMI?

Please see page 203 (role of the nurse section) for discussion points.

Sometimes a BMI chart is used to determine an individuals' BMI (Fig. 15.1). The National Institute for Health and Clinical

Excellence (NICE) has determined classifications using BMI (Table 15.1), a BMI greater than 30 is classed as obese (NICE, 2006).

However, there are some inherent problems with using BMI; BMI does not assess adiposity — that is, the amount of adipose tissue (fat) within the body and it is this fat which causes many of the health problems associated with obesity. If an individual is short and has a muscular physique; for example a professional rugby player who is 1.78m and 88kg would be classified as overweight using the NICE BMI benchmarks (NICE, 2006). Try plotting this individual on the BMI chart in Fig. 15.1. BMI is not an effective determinant of obesity in the elderly and also some ethnic minority groups. The link between BMI and mortality is weaker after 75 years of age and the 'normal' range for BMI may be extended in this age group (Stevens, 1998). Some Asian populations have a higher percentage body fat for a given weight compared to white Europeans; this may lead to underestimation of health risks in these groups (WHO expert consultation, 2004). As you will see later in the chapter, people from some minority ethnic groups are at a high risk of obesity.

Table 15.1 NICE guideline definitions of overweight and obesity

Classification	BMI (kg/m^2)
Healthy weight	18.5–24.9
Over weight	25–29.9
Obesity I	30–34.9
Obesity II	35–39.9
Obesity III	40 or more

NICE, 2006

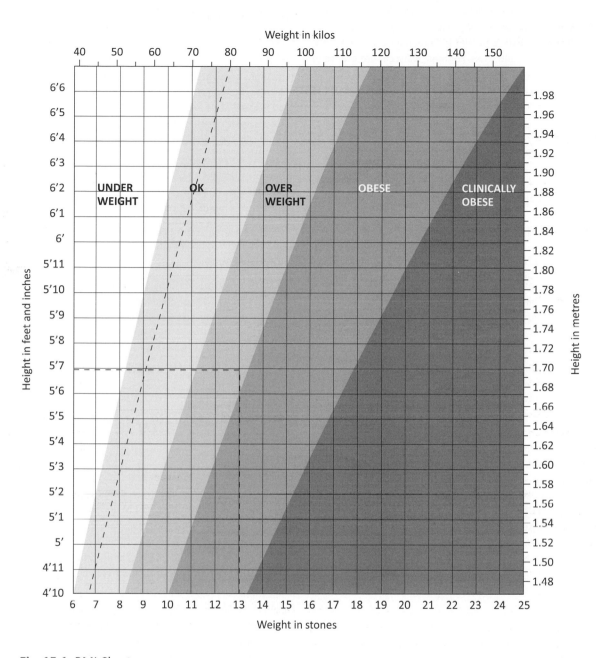

Fig. 15.1 BMI Chart.

Nursing Practice box

How to measure BMI

First measure height using a stadiometer; feet should be flat on the base and heels hard against the back of the stadiometer, the person being measured should be looking straight ahead while height is assessed. Secondly, measure their weight using approved calibrated scales.

The height and weight can then be used to calculate BMI with the equation:

$$BMI = kg/m^2$$

Have a go at calculating your own BMI.

Also consider http://www.healthforallchildren.co.uk/?SHOP=HFAC4&DO=USERPAGE&PAGE=calculator

Despite these flaws, BMI is the most widely used determinant of obesity in the UK. Waist circumference can also be used along with BMI to further identify individuals with low, high or very high health risks. For men, waist circumference of <94 cm is low, 94–102 cm is high and >102 cm is very high risk. For women, waist circumference of <80 cm is low, 80–88 cm is high and >88 cm is very high risk (NICE, 2006).

Activity box

Can you think of any reasons why measuring waist circumference might be unreliable?

Discussion points

The main problem with assessing waist circumference is inter-assessor variability — in layman's terms, I might measure a waist slightly differently to how you might measure a waist! The 'waist' can be a rather subjective area, particularly in obese individuals. Factors such as whether the clothing the client is wearing can also affect the measurement.

Determining whether a child is overweight or obese using BMI is more difficult as gender and age must also be taken into account. The Child Growth Foundation produced gender specific growth charts for BMI in 1990. These charts use data collected from many children to obtain 'standard' data, in this case, BMI is split into 100 'centiles'. If a child has a BMI on the 3rd centile, then for every 100 children of that age, 3% would be expected to have a lower BMI and 97 a higher BMI. A child with a BMI ≥91st centile is classified as overweight and ≥98th centile as obese. The International Obesity Taskforce has determined BMI benchmark points for overweight and obesity in children which take into account age and gender as well as ethnicity (Cole *et al.*, 2000).

Case Study 15.1: James

James aged 11 presents at the practice nurse with his mum. His mum is concerned about his weight. He is about to start secondary school and she feels name calling/bullying will be an issue. James weighs 70kg and is 150cm tall.

What information should the nurse gather during this initial consultation? What should s/he do with this information? i.e. How would it be recorded? How would it be used?

Do you think that health care professionals would be able to recognize childhood obesity easily?

Discussion points

- Provide the opportunity for James and his Mum to talk about bullying.
- Is James motivated to control his weight? See him on his own to discuss his perspectives? Is his self-esteem affected by his size? This is often a stronger motivating factor than future health risks. Is obesity actually beneficial to him— as physically big, can be selected for rugby?
- Can the nurse speak to the school nurse responsible for his current primary school and secondary school (what anti bullying measures can be implemented and essential mum is part of communication).
- Have they got previous weight/height measures to calculate the trend in his weight gain? This can be obtained from the school nurse.

A study of 80 professionals, including paediatric nurses, found that only 55% of children were correctly assessed in a visual test to determine healthy weight, overweight or obese. This suggests that regular measurements are crucial to determine obesity in childhood, not just a visual assessment or a reliance on 'gut feeling'.

The UK obesity 'epidemic'

The prevalence of overweight and obesity in adults and children in the UK has been increasing over the last 20 years. The main source of data on overweight and obesity comes from the Health Survey for England (HSE) 2006. The HSE is an annual review of surveys commissioned by the Department of Health which are designed to provide regular information on various aspects of the nation's health. The surveys began in 1991 and have covered the adult population aged 16 and over living in private households in England. Children were included in every year since 1995 (The Information Centre, 2008). According to the data from the HSE, in 2006 24% of adults (over 16 years of age) in England were classified as obese, this is an increase of 9% since 1993 (Figure 15.2). The Scottish Public Health Observatory (ScotPHO) published a report in 2007 outlining the rates of overweight and obesity using data collected from The Scottish Health Survey, this is a national sample survey carried out in 1995, 1998 and 2003. This data are somewhat older than the HSE information, but are still useful. ScotPHO data demonstrates that 22% of adults (16–64) are obese, an increase of 6% from 1995. These surveys demonstrate that 1 in 4/5 adults in Scotland and England are now obese.

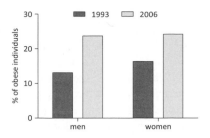

Fig. 15.2 Graph demonstrating the increase in obesity in England between 1993 and 2006. (The Health and Social Care Information Centre, 2008).

Children

In 2005, The National Child Measurement Programme (NCMP) was established as one element of the Government's work programme on childhood obesity. Every year, children in reception class (age 4–5) and year 6 (age 10–11) are weighed and measured in school, usually by the school nurse, to inform local planning and delivery of services for children and gather population-level surveillance data to allow analysis of trends in growth patterns and obesity (DH, 2008).

Some primary care trusts (PCTs) send the results of the measurement to parents, some PCTs require parents to ask for the results. These measurements are not compulsory and parents may opt their children out of the process. Health professionals had concerns that children who were overweight might be more likely to opt out of the measurement, thus skewing the results. A study was carried out by the government in 2006 to establish parental attitudes towards the routine measurement of children's height and weight. This was a relatively small qualitative study, but the results highlighted that a family with an overweight child would be more likely to opt the child out of measurement. The parent interviewed in the study that had opted their child out was also overweight.

Activity box

What factors do you think influence the decision to opt out of such measurements?

Discussion points

Three factors which were highlighted in the government study were; trust in the school, perceived benefits of the exercise and views on the impact of the measurement exercise on the child. Parents trusted the school to carry out the exercise in a sensitive manner and those parents who viewed the measurement as positive step felt that it would improve children's health in general. Parents who perceived their child to have a healthy weight did not believe there was potential for a

negative impact on their child, however parents of overweight children felt that there could be negative impacts such as teasing. An overweight child could also put pressure on their parents to allow them to opt out of the process. A more recent study has shown that there were minimal adverse effects of feedback of weight information to parents and children, even when the children were overweight (Grimmett *et al.*, 2008).

Government data demonstrate that obesity prevalence for the period 1995 to 2004 increased from 14% to 24% for boys and from 15% to 26% for girls. Obesity prevalence in boys aged 2 to 10 increased from 10% in 1995 to 16% in 2004 and for girls from 10% in 1995 to 11% in 2004 (The information Centre, 2004). The NCMP will add to this data and assist local PCTs target their obesity strategies more strategically.

In 2004, the government produced **Choosing Health: Making healthy choices easier**, a white paper which proposed a number of actions aimed at increasing physical activity, improving diet and reducing obesity (DH, 2004). The **Choosing Health** paper was published along with a delivery plan and two action plans; **Choosing a Better Diet: a food and health action plan** (DH, 2005a) and **Choosing activity: a physical activity action plan** (DH, 2005b). In 2008 the government published **Healthy Weight, Healthy Lives: A cross-government Strategy for England** (Cross-Government Obesity Unit, 2008) which has a highly ambitious opening statement:

> Our ambition is to be the first major nation to reverse the rising tide of obesity and overweight in the population by ensuring that everyone is able to achieve and maintain a healthy weight. Our initial focus will be on children: by 2020, we aim to reduce the proportion of overweight and obese children to 2000 levels.

In the next sections we will look at the causes and consequences of obesity and some of the local and national strategies which have been developed to try and meet the targets of the **Choosing Health paper.**

Causes of obesity

The balancing act of body weight

Obesity is an emotive issue and the causes of obesity are especially so. The most common forms of obesity are multifactorial resulting from environmental, behavioural and genetic factors. However, in 99 out of 100 people there will be no medical reason for obesity and an imbalance of energy intake and energy output will be responsible for the weight gain — usually over many years. Let's think of body weight as a balancing act — a bit like a see-saw (Fig. 15.3). When the amount of energy taken in (food and drinks) equals the energy used by the body, **thermogenesis** (heat production), organ function, exercise etc) then we have weight maintenance. If either side

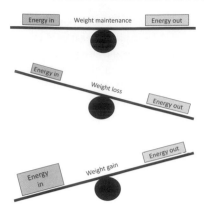

Fig. 15.3 The balancing act of weight maintenance.

of the see-saw is unbalanced, then weight gain or weight loss will occur. Obesity occurs when there is an increase in energy input and/or (usually and) a decrease in energy expenditure. This can be considered as 'environmental' factors — eating too much or an unhealthy diet and not using up enough energy.

There are some medical reasons for obesity such as **hypothyroidism** and **adrenal disorders**. A number of medications can also increase body weight by increasing appetite, such as some antidepressants (amitriptyline), **atypical antipsychotic drugs** (clozapine) and some drugs which are used in diabetes (insulin, rosiglitazone).

This 'see-saw' analogy assumes equal energy output for each situation. In real life, this is not usually the case as weight gain is often associated with increased energy intake and decreased energy output.

What about the genetic factors? Often, we attribute our physical (and intellectual) qualities! to our familial inheritance; 'I get my big hips from my Mum's side of the family' or 'everyone in our family is big' are phrases that are often used. There is some truth is these assumptions, our genes do have a role in determining our propensity for weight gain. There are some rare genetic disorders which lead to obesity, such as **Prader-Willi Syndrome** or deficiency of the hormone **leptin**, in both cases the brain signals which normally control appetite do not function normally. Syndromes like these are incredibly rare, in fact only a handful of individuals with leptin deficiency have been identified in the UK (Farooqi and O'Rahilly, 2005).

There is also good scientific evidence to suggest that there is hereditability of 40–70% in our BMI (Maes *et al.*, 1997). These studies have been carried out using **mono and dizygotic twins** (identical and non-identical respectively), biological parent-offspring and adoptive relative pairs — studies such as these can investigate the influence of nature versus nurture. However, the role of genetic factors in common obesity (that is in the absence of a known disorder such as Prader-Willi syndrome) is extremely complex as many genes are likely to be interacting (polygenic) and each of these may have a very small effect and only increase susceptibility to obesity when

working in combination with other environmental and behavioural factors such as physical activity and nutrient intake (Froguel, 2003).

The energy that we spend — our 'energy out' (Fig. 15.3) is influenced by our daily lifestyles. There have been enormous changes in the last thirty years in the way we work, travel and carry out day to day activities. Television viewing and computer work have increased, car ownership is relatively common, buildings have lifts and escalators and the introduction and availability of labour saving devices such as dishwashers have reduced our energy spent on household tasks. The media has been quick to highlight the sale of school playing fields in low income areas and link the reduction in these sports facilities with the increase in childhood obesity. A move to more sedentary lifestyles is an important causal factor in obesity.

Activity box

Can you think how you might encourage an individual to increase their physical activity? Remember, small changes can have an impact! How might an individual or professional measure changes in levels of physical activity?

Discussion points

Many PCTs have access to 'passport to leisure' (which can be accessed via GP prescription in some areas) programmes, or healthy heart activity sessions. These are leisure and activity programmes specially designed for groups of individuals who, for exampl e, have recently suffered from a heart attack or had a baby; 'pushy mums' is a popular walking group for women with young children. Encouragement to use the stairs rather than the lift or walk children/the dog more regularly can provide extra activity which costs little or nothing financially.

Measuring a change in physical activity is more difficult, pedometers can give an indication of steps per day (10,000 is recommended for an adult) but these are easily manipulated — especially in children. Assessment by a fitness trainer is the most accurate measurement; physical activity performance indicators, such as metres rowed in a minute, can be measured at intervals. This may be a useful tool in PCT weight loss programmes which are required to provide evidence of changes in individual's behaviour.

How can you encourage healthy diets?

National web sites describe strategies to support children and adults. Use these web sites and decide the best material for answering Case studies 15.3, 15.5 and 15.7.

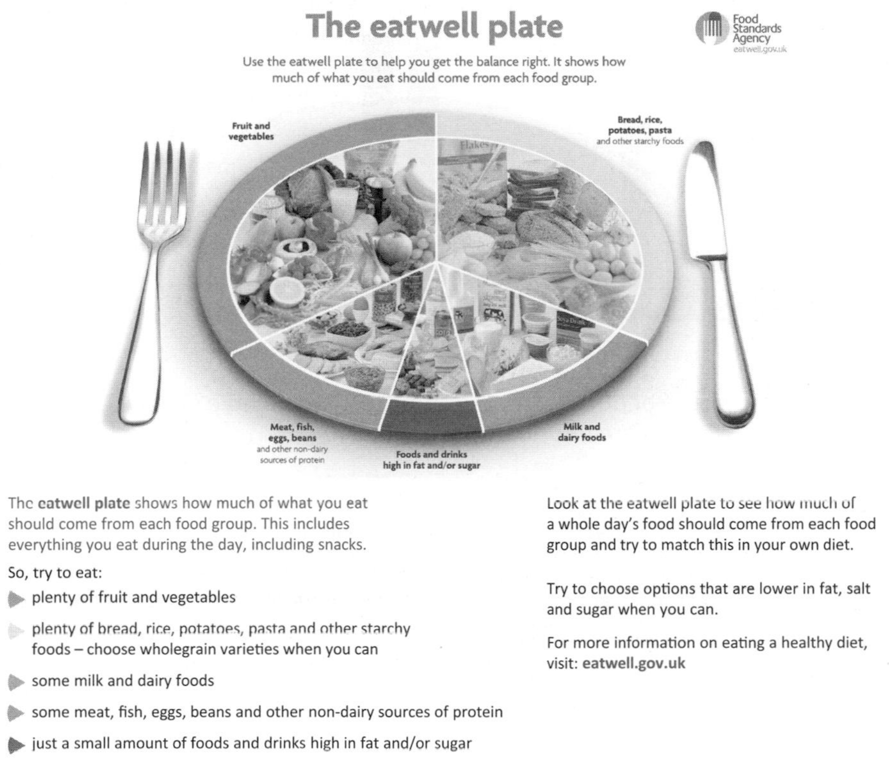

The eatwell plate
Food Standards Agency
eatwell.gov.uk
Use the eatwell plate to help you get the balance right. It shows how much of what you eat should come from each food group.
Fruit and vegetables
Bread, rice, potatoes, pasta and other starchy foods
Meat, fish, eggs, beans and other non-dairy sources of protein
Foods and drinks high in fat and/or sugar
Milk and dairy foods
The eatwell plate shows how much of what you eat should come from each food group. This includes everything you eat during the day, including snacks.
So, try to eat:
plenty of fruit and vegetables
plenty of bread, rice, potatoes, pasta and other starchy foods – choose wholegrain varieties when you can
some milk and dairy foods
some meat, fish, eggs, beans and other non-dairy sources of protein
just a small amount of foods and drinks high in fat and/or sugar
Look at the eatwell plate to see how much of a whole day's food should come from each food group and try to match this in your own diet.
Try to choose options that are lower in fat, salt and sugar when you can.
For more information on eating a healthy diet, visit: eatwell.gov.uk

Fig. 15.4 Eat well plate. Reproduced with permission from © Crown copyright.

Healthy cooking aimed at parents/adults:

a. UK-wide **http://www.eatwell.gov.uk/**

b. Wales **http://www.wales.nhs.uk/sites3/page.cfm?orgId=568&pid=14737**

c. Australia **http://raisingchildren.net.au/articles/childhood_obesity.html?highlight=obesity**

Aimed at professionals:

d. **http://www.physicalactivityandnutritionwales.org.uk/page.cfm?orgid=740&pid=34282**

Dietary changes have to be implemented with increased activity as the human body is designed to 'slow down' its metabolic rate if you diet. Increasing activity with a healthy diet aims to control weight gain.

Consider the **size** of food portions too. Many may mistakenly choose healthy diets but consume too much. The 'eat well' plate in Fig. 15.4 is designed to offer illustrations of appropriate portion sizes.

Psychological support

Psychological support is imperative to maintain the changes around diet. The 3 'S' strategy has been suggested, especially for children

- Slowly,
- Socially,
- Sitting.

This method describes how you can ONLY eat if **sitting down** (ie not walking as in a rush), and only in a 'social' setting. Hence family meals are encouraged and to avoid eating in front of the TV, back of car etc. Both aim to reduce snacking which occur unconsciously during our busy lives and often involve high calorie food (crisps, chocolate, sugary drinks). Eating **slowly** is advocated as many consume food so quickly that the unconsciously 'overeat', not allowing their body's natural regulatory mechanism to recognize when they are 'full' as this process takes time. Suggest talking between mouthfuls, use cutlery (as most people have to take time cutting food, as opposed to finger food which can be consumed rapidly). Successful weight control strategies even suggest using 'child size' cutlery as it takes even longer to use though this has to considered in the light of cultural sensitivities. Teenagers and adults may object to eating using child cutlery in public.

Remember anyone dieting will feel 'ravenous' and not merely hungry and will be tempted to avoid the 3 'S' principle, hence support will be important from peers or parents. Warn them that they may be more irritable on a diet as they will 'feel hungry', for different periods of the day, and avoiding

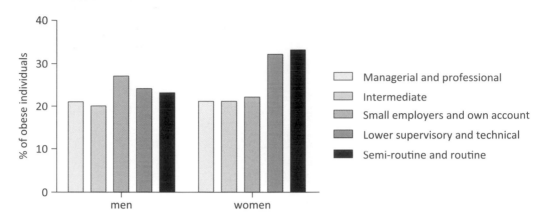

Fig. 15.5 Percentage of obesity by household income quintile in England, 2003. The Health and Social Care Information Centre, 2008

snacks is difficult. Consider the list of questions that you can ask (below). Solution focussed strategies built on similar questions will help develop strategies that empower people.

- **When** are the worst times of the day when they feel most hungry?
- **How** can they survive those times?
- **Who** helps them the most in 'surviving those times?

At risk groups

Are some groups or individuals more likely to become obese than other groups? The answer to this question is complicated, given the many factors which can impact on our risk of developing obesity. However, there is evidence to suggest that individuals from certain ethnic and socio-economic groups may be at increased risk of developing obesity.

Obesity rates vary considerably by household income in women in England (Fig. 15.5), with 12% more women in the lowest household income quintile being obese compared to the highest quintile. There was much less variation observed in men in England.

Research demonstrates preschool risk factors that are predictive of later adolescent obesity (Baird *et al.*, 2005). Similarly, risk factors in children up to 3 years of age demonstrated a degree of predictability for later obesity at 7 years of age (Reilly *et al.*, 2005).

Activity box

Can you think of reasons why lower socio-economic groups might have increased rates of obesity?

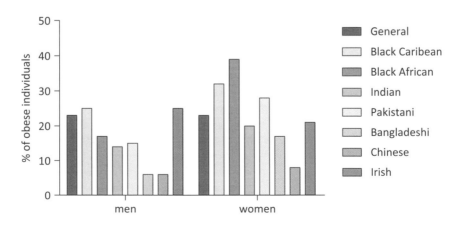

Fig. 15.6a Percentage of obesity by reported ethnicity, 2004. The Health and Social Care Information Centre (2008)

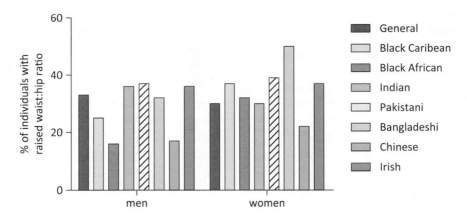

Fig. 15.6b Prevalence of raised waist:hip ratio (%) by reported ethnicity, 2004. The Health and Soial Care Information Centre, 2008

Discussion points

When we discuss obesity intervention strategies, we will have to consider the influence of factors such as educational level and socio-economic status as these will strongly influence the success of such strategies. There is evidence which recognizes that individuals in low income households are more likely to have patterns of food intake and a nutritional status which is likely to contribute to obesity. The reasons for this are complex, but involve factors such as knowledge of healthy food, access to shops and supermarkets and perceived financial cost of healthy food (Dobson *et al.*, 1996; Leather, 2003). An interesting factor highlighted in research by the Joseph Rowntree Foundation was that children in low income households were more likely to eat their preferred food (chips, burgers, fish fingers) compared to their more affluent friends. Parents attributed this to avoiding waste, as the children were more likely to eat their favourite foods (Dobson *et al.*, 1996). Households in the lowest income quintile in the UK have the lowest intake of vitamin C (Department of the Environment Food and Rural Affairs, 2008).

Worryingly, the effects of social inequalities appear to be influencing childhood obesity. A study in Plymouth, southern England, demonstrated a strong link between deprivation and obesity and this effect was particularly strong in girls, perhaps leading to the greater differences observed in women in lower income quintiles highlighted in Fig. 15.5 (Kinra *et al.*, 2000). You may not be surprised to learn that the same social inequalities which are associated with obesity, are also linked to under nutrition in childhood (Armstrong *et al.*, 2003). The government has set some initiatives, such as '5 A Day' and Food in Schools Programme to address some of these issues.

In England, there are some significant differences in the prevalence of obesity between different ethnic minority groups and gender. Compared with the general population, levels of obesity are much lower in Black African, Indian,

Pakistani, and, most markedly, Bangladeshi and Chinese men (Fig. 15.6a) (The Information Centre, 2008). Despite low levels of general obesity, Pakistani, Indian and Bangladeshi men, have similar levels of raised waist to hip ratio compared to the general population (Fig. 15.6b).

Obesity prevalence in women is higher for Black Caribbean, Black African and Pakistani women and low for Chinese women compared to the general population. Again the pattern is different for levels of central obesity (as measured by waist:hip ratio). Black Caribbean, Pakistani and Irish women all have levels of central obesity above that of the general female population, while Bangladeshi women are nearly twice as likely to have a raised waist to hip ratio as women in the general population (The Information Centre, 2008). The differences observed between obesity and **central adiposity** (measured as a raised waist:hip ratio) highlights the importance of assessing obesity by means other than BMI in certain ethnic minority groups. Studies from North America have demonstrated similar increases in the risk of obesity in certain ethnic minority groups (Ogden *et al.*, 2006; Turconi and Cena, 2007). Waist circumference of greater than 100cm in male and female adults increases the risk of insulin insensitivity and hence the metabolic syndrome.

Increased obesity in certain ethnic minority groups can be related to a number of factors including increasing consumption of less healthy food, genetic predisposition, lack of exercise, stress related to migration and settlement, changed meal patterns and altered working environment, including, longer hours and low pay (Gilbert and Khokhar, 2008). The transition from a traditional diet to a more 'westernized' diet containing high fat, salt and sugar has been observed in ethnic populations, particularly in younger generations. Many ethnic groups in the UK and indeed Europe belong to lower socioeconomic communities which can restrict food choice and lead to consumption of poor quality food.

197

Activity box

Do you think local and national initiatives to improve obesity rates in the UK consider ethnic minority groups? Can you think what provision might need to be made in an obesity intervention programme which was to be accessible by ethnic minority groups?

Discussion points

NICE has highlighted that person-centred care is of most importance when delivering a weight loss programme. In order to achieve this, provision for ethnic minority groups might include a translator for any taught sessions or a community food worker who has experience of foods and cooking styles from that particular culture. Cultural beliefs may need to be challenged, for example, the belief that obesity represents wealth and prosperity. Access to local programmes should be tailored for the local community, for example if the local population has a Muslim majority, avoiding holding the sessions on Fridays would be beneficial as this is the day that many Muslims attend the mosque.

We've been considering the incidence of obesity in ethnic minority groups residing in a host country, perhaps the UK, what about the countries of origin of these individuals? Is obesity just a consequence of moving to the UK or is the prevalence of obesity increasing throughout the world? It is difficult to compare between different countries worldwide as the classifications used to define obesity vary. Despite these difficulties, obesity appears to be increasing in the adult population of many countries, both westernized and developing. Within Europe there is a trend for an increase in the prevalence of obesity in both adults and children. When considering obesity alone (i.e. BMI >30), at least nine European countries have currently have male obesity rates above 20% including Greece and Cyprus reaching 27% (Lobstein *et al.*, 2005); this is surprising, given the promotion of the healthy 'Mediterranean' style diet.

The Center for Disease Control have data from 1985–2007 demonstrating a dramatic rise in obesity in the USA. In 2007, thirty states had a prevalence equal to or greater than 25per cent; three of these states (Alabama, Mississippi and Tennessee) had a prevalence of obesity equal to or greater than 30% (CDC, 2007). Have a look at the CDC website to see the progression of obesity in the USA in a mapped format. When ethnic minorities are considered, 58% of non-Hispanic black women aged 40 to 59 years were obese in 2003–2004 compared with about 38% of non-Hispanic white women of the same age (Ogden *et al.*, 2006).

What about the rest of the world? In certain Polynesian and Micronesian societies in the pacific the rates of obesity are almost 60% in adults, this is related to changing diets and impact of social status and prosperity. In rural Japan, China and Africa obesity is relatively rare (<5%).

Activity box

What factors do you think influence the low prevalence of obesity in these areas?

Discussion points

The low prevalence of obesity in rural Japan, China and Africa has been attributed to a diet which is low in saturated fats. Rural areas have less access to fast food restaurants and convenience stores and often the employment in these areas is more physically demanding than that of individuals living in urban Japan, China or Africa.

Physical, social and psychological impact of obesity

Obesity impacts on health, social and psychological well-being in a number of different ways. The influence of obesity on health and well-being affect not just the obese individual, but their family and also the general population.

Impact on physical health

Ultimately, obesity leads to morbidity and mortality. The consequences of obesity on health are well documented and include cardiovascular disease, insulin resistant (or type 2) diabetes, liver disease, reproductive problems and an increased risk of certain cancers (endometrial, breast, prostate, and colon) these are summarized in Table 15.2.

Table 15.2 Consequences of obesity on physical health

Hypertension	Coronary heart disease
Dyslipidaemia	Stroke
Congestive heart failure	Osteoarthritis
Gallstones	Cancer
Sleep apnoea	Diabetes
Women's reproductive health problems	

In obesity, the **relative risk** of hypertension increases to 2.1 and 1.9 in men and women respectively (National Institutes of Health, 1998). This in turn increases the risk of coronary heart disease and stoke in obese individuals. Obesity is associated with increased total cholesterol with a strong association with abdominal obesity (how would you measure abdominal obesity?), increased **plasma triglycerides**, decreased **low density lipoprotein** and increased **high density lipoprotein**. All of these changes increase the risk of cardiovascular disease.

There is an increased risk of developing non-insulin dependent (or type 2) diabetes in obesity — in particular with central adiposity. A BMI of 35 increases the risk of diabetes 40 fold. Losing weight can help to reduce the risk of developing diabetes — indeed; by altering their diet with the support of professionals, including diabetes specialist nurses and dieticians many individuals can manage (and perhaps prevent the development) non-insulin dependent diabetes.

Osteoarthritis is increased in obese individuals, not just in weight-bearing, but also, non-weight-bearing joints. The "cost" of osteoarthritis in obese individuals is considerable. Joint pain while moving will reduce ability to exercise and increase energy output, this will also limit the individuals ability to carry out employment.

One consequence of obesity which has been somewhat overlooked until recently is the effect on female reproduction. Obese women are more likely to have irregular or **anovulatory** (i.e. no ovulation) menstrual cycles and are more likely to require medical intervention during childbirth. A recent audit at a large hospital in Nottingham noted that over 18 months, 32 pregnant women were classified as extremely obese (BMI >50). This puts both mother and baby at risk during pregnancy and, in particular, during and post delivery. Overweight and obese girls are also more likely to enter puberty and commence menstruation earlier than girls of healthy weight. Increased **adiposity** alters **oestrogen signalling**, this is thought to be responsible for some of the effects on reproduction.

The consequences of obesity in childhood are similar to those in adults, but include an increased risk of developing or exacerbating asthma, foot abnormalities and increased risk of type-1 diabetes. There is also evidence to suggest that overweight or obese children will go on to become obese adults.

Case Study 15.2: Janice

James' mum, Janice, aged 30 discloses she and her husband have also been concerned about being 'big boned' but both have 'stressful' jobs. She weighs 100kg and is 5'5"tall. She also smokes. Her father died of a stroke aged 50 and was obese.

Exercise: Make a list of the main complications of adult obesity. List some reasons why being diagnosed with obesity may make Janice more likely to control her weight.

Discussion points

- Please refer to Chapter13 in this book for a more developed discussion about supporting people who want to stop smoking.
- Please refer to Table 15.2 in this chapter on adult complications of obesity.
- Discuss Janice's fears/aspirations around future health. A change in lifestyle is paramount but difficult given competing pressures in her life.
- Explain how Janice's efforts to control her weight will have a positive impact on James. Can she do it for 'James's sake'?
- Has she had her blood pressure and serum cholesterol/triglyceride profile measured?

The social cost of obesity

Obesity has a social 'cost; for the individual as well as society as a whole. Obesity is related to mobility limitations, which affect quality of life particularly with aging, this can limit certain daily activities and potentially employability (Visscher and Seidell, 2001). The House of Commons Health Select Committee (HSC) estimated that the health care cost of obesity and its consequences in England in 2002 was around £3340–3724 million. The cost of health and social care for obese individuals is great as there are higher levels of sickness and absence from work among obese individuals which reduces productivity and imposes costs on businesses. Premature mortality as a consequence of obesity reduces the national output relative to the level it would be in the absence of obesity (McCormick and Stone, 2007).

Lost earnings directly attributable to obesity were estimated to be £2350–2600 million. Obesity has a negative impact on employment, possibly because obesity is a debilitating health condition that reduces productivity and therefore employment or obese individuals may face discrimination in the work place (McCormick and Stone, 2007). Think about moving and handling — in order to move obese patients safely, some hospitals are buying and renting expensive equipment, other services such as police, fire brigades and ambulance services must also ensure that their equipment is capable of safely carrying obese individuals.

An American study has linked obesity during adolescence to negative social and economic consequences in adulthood, for example women who had been obese when aged 16–24 had completed fewer years of school, were less likely to be married, had lower household incomes and had higher rates of household poverty when assessed 7 years later (Gortmaker et al.., 1993). In the UK, obesity which does not persist beyond childhood has little impact on socioeconomic factors in adulthood, but persistent obesity in women has similar effects to the American study (Viner and Cole, 2005).

Activity box

If this is the case, which age group do you think should be a focus for prevention?

Discussion points

Childhood is the age group that the government is targeting with many strategies. In order to target obesity in childhood, programmes must involved parents, carers and families as children do not usually make the key dietary, budgeting and shopping decisions within a family.

Impact on psychological well-being

Despite the increase in prevalence of obesity it is still a stigmatized condition. Individuals may face discrimination in education, employment and health care (Wardle and Cooke, 2005). Historically, obesity was a consequence of wealth and obese individuals were perceived to be rich and able to afford expensive quantities of food. However, modern society associates success and attractiveness with slimness and therefore obese individuals are often stereotyped as being lazy or stupid, this can cause a substantial psychological burden. There have been many studies attempting to link obesity and depression; some have found a positive association, some negative and some believe the effect is gender specific. A link between obesity and depression has been demonstrated in extremely obese individuals (BMI >40) independent of gender and racial group (Dong et al., 2004).

The model proposed by Dong et al. proposes that candidate genes and environmental factors predispose individuals to both obesity and depression (Fig. 15.7). Low self esteem can feed into a cycle of over-eating and weight gain.

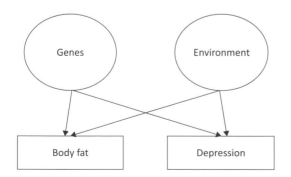

Fig. 15.7 Model linking common genes with obesity and depression. Dong et al., 2004.

Some drugs which are used to manage depression may themselves cause weight gain, for example the tricyclic antidepressants (e.g. amytriptyline) and this should be explained to clients who are initiated on such medications. Depression is covered in more detail in Chapter 17.

Activity box

Can you think of ways in which poor psychological well-being affect a clients ability to make changes to their lifestyle in relation to obesity?

Discussion points

Depression affects ability to make behavioural changes. Poor self-esteem and negative self-image perpetuate the cycle of emotional/comfort eating. Lack of social support, poor coping mechanisms, poor motivation. Trans-theoretical model—target interventions depending on where they are in cycle of change. Look at goal-setting and motivational interviewing.

The psychological impact of obesity in children is significant; children can develop a negative self-image, lowered self-esteem and a higher risk of depression. Almost all obese children will have experiences of teasing, social exclusion, discrimination and prejudice (Swanton and Frost, 2007).

There is a growing movement in the USA to promote acceptance of obesity, groups such as The National Association to Advance Fat Acceptance (NAAFA) work to eliminate discrimination based on body size and improve quality of life for obese individuals (NAAFA, 2008). NAAFA strongly discourages participation in weight-reduction diets (NAAFA, 2008). There is some opposition towards this movement, given the health risks of obesity and the benefits of even a small reduction in body weight. Take some time to consider what you think about this.

Case Study 15.3: Family and friends

Janice explained she always had 'puppy fat' but was never regarded as overweight. She remembered being bullied in secondary school for being 'fat' and regretted never managing to keep up with fashions as clothes never fit. She is worried about her future as her father died of what appeared to be obesity related problems, and recent media reports. She wants to 'get fit' especially as a group of work colleagues are keen to 'get together'. She is a secretary in a large law firm. Her husband, a taxi driver does not get time to exercise with the family.

Exercise : List the ways in which family and friends influence a persons weight control. What do you think is the role of the health care professional in involving family members and friends in helping weight control? Remember that most obese people should be managed through self help strategies, with a smaller proportion having attempted them and hence seek professional guidance. Most who approach professionals should have a degree of success with the minority requiring cognitive behaviour therapy, medication or surgery (consider a pyramid).

Discussion points

- Is there a work based scheme to support exercise/subsidized gym membership, employer related sessions on smoking cessation etc.

- Why do her colleagues want to control their weight/get fit? Identify motivating factors. Please see Chapter 13 on smoking.

- You are often limited to encouraging attendance at self-help groups. Please see NICE guidance http://www.nice.org.uk/CG43.

Prevention and intervention

The government has made clear national strategies for the reduction of obesity in the UK (DH, 2005b; DH, 2005a). A modest loss of 10% of body weight can have clinically significant benefits to an obese client, including reduction in blood pressure, reduction in cholesterol and even a reduction in overall mortality.

There are many small, local interventions which have not published their findings in the research arena, but are providing at a grass roots level, an appropriate service targeted at the local community. We will consider some of these strategies and how they fit with national government policy. Nationwide commercial weight loss programmes are available, many you will have heard of such as Weightwatchers and Slimming World. The weight loss industry in the UK is worth billions of pounds and is a lucrative business in many other countries. A quick search on the internet or in the local library will retrieve hundreds of diet books. Some are based on well known diet trends such as The Cabbage Soup Diet and The Atkins Diet and some are linked to media campaigns and television programmes. The evidence for the success of many of these books and programmes is questionable, but many desperate dieters will readily part with money to try out the latest celebrity supported 'miracle diet'.

Obesity should be managed as a chronic, relapsing disorder, with regular support and follow up from professionals as weight regain is an extremely common phenomena (Weiss et al., 2007). Losing weight which has previously been lost, then regained , is challenging for the client.

So what characteristics make a successful weight-loss intervention? The intervention must be **evidence-based** and also

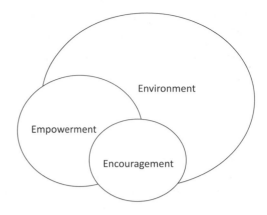

Fig. 15.8 The 3E's model proposed. Maryon-Davis, A. (2007)

cost effective, but most importantly and critical for success, an individual must be ready, able and motivated to make the necessary lifestyle changes (NICE, 2006). The care offered should be person-centred and will involve multi-agency teams.

NICE guidance on obesity intervention strategies state three key factors to consider when developing an intervention programme; is the client ready to begin such a programme, what barriers might prevent lifestyle change and tailoring the programme for individual groups. Many models for considering methods for making lifestyle changes are available and have been presented in other chapters. An appropriate model for obesity has been proposed by Maryon-Davis; the three 'Es' model (Fig. 15.8) has been proposed for lifestyle change which includes:

- encouragement,

- empowerment,

- and environment (Maryon-Davis, 2007).

Encouragement could include persuasion to make simple positive changes such as modifying diet and taking more exercise; the encouragement could be given by nurses and other professionals such as food workers. Many media campaigns can also successfully provide encouragement. I'm sure you can think of several. The British Heart Foundation recently campaigned for thirty minutes activity a day for older adults and the '5 A Day' campaign. Knowledge of healthy eating and the skills required to make lifestyle changes will empower individuals; again, nurses are in an ideal position to deliver this information following some specialist training.

Finally environment refers to the cultural, social, physical and economic environments which are required for an individual to make lifestyle changes. This is the area in which nurses may have the least input, but by working as part of a multi-disciplinary team with other professionals and agencies such as community food workers and dieticians, sports and leisure services and local religious leaders, environmental challenges can be overcome. Family culture and social life can be addressed by encouraging whole families to adopt healthy lifestyles, thus facilitating a favourable environment for change. Ultimately, the 3 E's must be delivered together to produce successful modifications (Maryon-Davis, 2007).

Local interventions

The benefit of small local interventions is that they can appropriately target key groups in the community for support. One potential drawback of such interventions is that the outcomes are often unpublished and the success rates unknown outside the PCT or management group. A toolkit has been developed by the National Heart Forum in conjunction with the NICE guidelines to help develop local strategies to tackle overweight and obesity in children and adults (Swanton and Frost, 2007). Behavioural and cognitive behavioural strategies combined with exercise and weight loss strategies are particularly successful in helping obese individuals lose weight (Shaw *et al.*, 2005).

A recent publication has described the success of a community-based family intervention for obesity in children. Twenty seven overweight or obese children and their families took part in the programme which was facilitated by a number of professionals including a health visitor and school nurse. This programme had an emphasis on parenting and relationship skills. Evaluation at nine months after the start of the twelve week programme demonstrated a significant reduction in BMI z score.

National and commercial interventions

National government strategies to help reduce obesity include **Sure Start**, **Healthy Start**, the **Food in Schools Programme** and work to improve the promotion of food to children through the media.

There are some published reports of the success of some nationally available commercial weight loss programmes which provide evidence of successful weight loss in motivated adults. Highly motivated individuals who were randomized to four well known commercial weight loss programmes (Slim-Fast plan, Weight Watchers pure points programme, Dr Atkins' new diet revolution, Rosemary Conley's eat yourself slim diet and fitness plan) demonstrated similar levels of weight loss over six months (~8kg) (Truby *et al.*, 2006). At twelve months, more participants on 'unsupported' diets (Atkins and Slimfast) had changed programmes, suggesting that group support has some advantages. Many PCTs cannot support all obese individuals who wish to make lifestyle changes and referral to supported weight-loss programmes may be a suitable alternative.

Activity box

Can you think what sort of benefits (social and psychological) there are of being part of a supported weight-loss group?

Medical and surgical interventions

As well as a behavioural approach to weight loss, there are medical and surgical treatments available such as drugs and gastric bypass surgery. The area of medicine dealing with obesity is called **bariatrics**, this word is derived from the Greek *baros* weight/heavy (think of barometer). According to the British National Formulary, anti-obesity drugs should only be considered for obese individuals who have attempted three months of unsuccessful managed care (supervised diet, exercise, and behavioural modification). Drugs should not be used as mono-therapy and clients should be fully supported and regularly monitored for weight change (BNF, 2008).

Anti-obesity drugs fall into two categories, those which affect the absorption of fat across the gastro-intestinal (GI) tract and those which act centrally. Sibutramine (Reductil) acts centrally by inhibiting the re-uptake of noradrenaline and serotonin and acts as an appetite suppressant. This drug has now been withdrawn from European markets due to safety concerns with an increased risk of cardiovascular problems. It may be purchased on the internet, so please be aware of concerns. A drug you may have heard of is Orlistat (trade names Xenical and Alli) which inhibits the absorption of dietary fat; Orlistat is used in conjunction with a low-calorie diet. Fats which are not absorbed across the GI tract are excreted via the bowels, leading to some rather nasty side effects including flatulence, faecal urgency and oily leakage from the rectum. Many clients lose weight while taking Orlistat as they reduce their fat intake to attenuate some of the side effects.

The most drastic treatment for obesity is surgery — often classified as bariatric surgery. **The Cochrane Collaboration** state that surgery for **morbid obesity** does lead to weight loss, but it is unclear which surgical procedure is safest and most effective operation (Cochrane Database, 2009). Surgery must also be associated with behavioural changes. The most common types of bariatric surgery options are **laparoscopic gastric bypass, laparoscopic adjustable gastric banding, sleeve gastrectomy, duodenal switch** and **open gastric bypass**. Surgery is a drastic option and comes with its own risks to the clients' health. Although risk of morbidity and mortality during and after surgery are increased in obese individuals surgery is currently considered to be only effective long-term treatment for obesity.

Case Study 15.4: Medication

Janice has heard about 'medication' that can help her lose weight. What do you advise?

Exercise: List medication that can be used. What are the indications for use? What are the side effects?

Discussion points

See NICE guidance http://www.nice.org.uk/CG43. You and she will need to discuss this with her GP for further guidance if she remains keen to proceed

Role of the nurse

Hopefully in the previous sections you've developed a sense of where a nurse can support obese individuals to make positive lifestyle changes, we will now consider some more specific aspects of the role and values of nurses. Nurses, particularly in the primary care setting, are often required to take measurements such as height and weight for general assessments such as for new patients in a GP surgery or as part of a routine check-up. This, theoretically, presents the nurse with an opportunity to discuss weight management issues with the patient; but do nurses necessarily take these opportunities to discuss obesity issues? The primary care setting provides an ideal setting for nurses to promote healthy eating and exercise, obesity prevention and management is in fact a priority for primary care nursing development. However, a study from Sheffield has demonstrated that very few of the nurses studied had received any training or support for obesity management.

This training should also address beliefs and attitudes about obesity and obese clients (Brown *et al.*, 2007). Smoking cessation clinics are often successfully run by nurses (see Chapter 13) and offer an additional opportunity for promotion of other aspects of a healthy lifestyle. Although giving up smoking is associated with an increase in body weight, the benefits of stopping smoking should be considered a priority and weight management, if appropriate, could be initiated by the same nurse as part of the programme.

Studies of nurses' attitudes towards obesity included self-assessment of the nurses BMI. The BMI of the nurses in this study had an impact on their beliefs and behaviours around obesity management, suggesting that there is a relationship between a health professionals own personal health status and their professional health promotion practices (Hoppé and Ogden, 1997). A criterion for entry into a number of nursing courses is to have an appropriate weight for their height; can you remember what a healthy weight is according to the WHO BMI categories?

Case Study 15.5: The role of the nurse

You are a school nurse and have been contacted by a practice nurse regarding James aged 11 years. He is reportedly being bullied in school as he is obese. He is the 3rd child in that school reported to have obesity related problems.

Exercise:

A) What initiatives can you introduce to **prevent** obesity.

B) What initiatives can you introduce to **tackle** obesity (these can overlap).

Discussion points

Please see NICE guidance http://www.nice.org.uk/CG43

Case Study 15.6: The role of the health visitor

You are a health visitor and have been contacted by a keen school nurse. That school nurse wants to collaborate in devising a local weight control programme. She has recently started a school based programme following an episode of bullying. She suggested that obesity was a **preschool** issue too and needed to ensure any programme she devised conformed to initiatives you devise.

Exercise: What principles should you use to define a preschool obesity prevention programme? When would you need to refer a child under 2 to a doctor for obesity related concerns?

Discussion points

Please see NICE guidance http://www.nice.org.uk/CG43

Case Study 15.7: The role of the midwife

You are a midwife and have been tasked with developing an education programme as part of your antenatal classes around preventing obesity in infancy. You realize many of the mothers are also obese.

Exercise: What are the principles you will adopt?

Discussion points

Please see NICE guidance http://www.nice.org.uk/CG43

PSA targets

The Public Service Agreement (PSA) on obesity (2004) aimed to halt the year-on-year rise in obesity among children under 11 by 2010 in the context of a broader strategy to tackle obesity in the population as a whole. This target is jointly owned by the Department of Health, Department for Education and Skills and the Department for Culture, Media and Sport. The obesity PSA strategy included universal and targeted interventions:

- Universal interventions are preventative interventions aimed at all children with the ambition of halting the rise in childhood obesity. The universal interventions are supported with programmes such as promotion of breastfeeding, healthy school food and the Physical Education, School Sport and Club Links strategy.
- Targeted interventions are aimed at treating obese children and their families, the guidance from NICE (NICE, 2006) should be followed when initiating a programme.

The progress of the PSA targets will be tracked by the Health Survey for England as well as through the The National Child Measurement Programme; as yet it is too early to tell whether the PSA targets are being achieved.

Summary

This chapter has explored definitions of obesity and examined the epidemiological evidence on the prevalence of obesity in the UK and how to measure obesity in adults and children. It has examined some of the causes of obesity and its impact, both at individual and societal level. Local and national strategies designed to prevent obesity as well as the role of the nurse in their delivery have also been examined.

Obesity is defined as a BMI greater than 30; there are increasing rates of obesity among adults and children in the UK with specific socioeconomic and ethnic minority groups more likely to develop obesity than others. The government has set ambitious targets to tackle obesity, particularly in childhood and many local initiatives have been developed to address these targets. Person-centred care is at the centre of any weight loss programme, which should be adapted to meet the cultural, religious and social requirements of the local or target population. Other therapeutic tools are available, such as weight loss drugs and bariatric surgery, the NICE guidelines outline the

selection criteria for these treatments (NICE, 2006). As the population of the UK becomes more obese, the role of the nurse in supporting weight loss in individuals as well as group programmes is likely to become more complex.

Online Resource Centre

For more information on tackling obesity visit the Online Resource Centre —
http://www.oxfordtextbooks.co.uk/orc/linsley/

Further reading

http://www.nhsdirect.nhs.uk/magazine/interactive/bmi/index.aspx
http://www.who.int/bmi/index.jsp
http://www.iaso.org/popout.asp?linkto=http%3A//www.iotf.org/media/euobesity2.pdf
http://iotf.org/index.asp
http://www.cdc.gov/nccdphp/dnpa/obesity/trend/maps/index.htm
http://www.dh.gov.uk/en/publichealth/healthimprovement/obesity/index.htm
http://www.eatwell.gov.uk/healthissues/obesity/
http://www.nice.org.uk/CG43
http://www.nationalobesityforum.org.uk/
http://www.nhlbi.nih.gov/health/dci/pods/podcasts.html (obesity podast)
http://www.healthyfuture.org.uk/obesity.html
http://www.cochrane.org/reviews/en/ab003817.html
http://www.cochrane.org/reviews/en/ab001871.html
http://cochrane.org/podcasts/review_summaries/2008issue3/Issue3_2008_exercise.html (PODCAST)
http://www.naafaonline.com/dev2//index.html
www.heartforum.org.uk
http://www.bhf.org.uk/news_and_campaigning/our_campaigns/30_a_day_campaign.aspx
http://www.eatwell.gov.uk/foodlabels/trafficlights/
http://www.5aday.nhs.uk/topTips/default.html
Armstrong, J., Dorosty, A. R., Reilly, J. J., Child Health Information, T. & Emmett, P. M. (2003). Coexistence of social inequalities in undernutrition and obesity in preschool children: population based cross sectional study. Arch Dis Child, 88: 671–675.
Baird, J., Fisher, D., Lucas, P., Kleijnen, J., Roberts, H. & Law, C. (2005). Being big or growing fast: systematic review of size and growth in infancy and later obesity. BMJ, 331: 929.
British National Formulary (2008). British National Formulary, London: BMJ Group.
Brown, I., Stride, C., Psarou, A., Brewins, L. & Thompson, J. (2007). Management of obesity in primary care: nurses' practices, beliefs and attitudes. Journal of Advanced Nursing, 59, 329–341.
CDC (2007). Overweight and obesity: Obesity trends — U.S. obesity trends 1985–2007. Washington DC: Centers for Disease Control.

Cochrane Database Syst Rev. (2009) Apr 15(2):CD003641.

Cole, T. J., Bellizzi, M. C., Flegal, K. M. & Dietz, W. H. (2000). Establishing a standard definition for child overweight and obesity worldwide: international survey. *BMJ*, 320: 1240.

Cross-Government Obesity Unit (2008). Healthy Weight, Healthy Lives: a Cross-Government Strategy for England. London: Department of Health and Department of Children Schools and Families (Ed.). HMSO.

Department of Health (2004). *Choosing Health: Making healthy choices easier*. London: HMSO.

Department of Health (2005a). Choosing a better diet: A food and health action plan. London: HMSO.

Department of Health (2005b). Choosing activity: a physical activity action plan. London: HMSO.

Department of Health (2008). The National Child Measurement Programme.London: The Stationery Office.

Department of the Environment Food and Rural Affairs (2008). Family Food Report 2006. Department of the Environment Food and Rural Affairs (ed.). London: HMSO.

Dobson, B., Beardsworth, A., Keil, T. & Walker, R. (1996). Diet, choice and poverty: Social cultural and nutritional aspects of food consumption among low-income families. The Family Policy Studies Centre with the Joseph Rowntree Foundation.

Dong, C., Sanchez, L. & Price, R. (2004). Relationship of Obesity to Depression: a Family-based Study. *International Journal of Obesity*, 28: 790–795.

Farooqi, I. S. & O'rahilly, S. (2005). Monogenic obesity in humans. *Annual Review of Medicine*, 56: 443–458.

Froguel, P. (2003). Do our genes make us fat? IN: Voss, L. & Wilkin, T. (Eds.) *Adult obesity: a paediatric challenge*. New York, USA: Taylor and Francis.

Gilbert, P. A. & Khokhar, S. (2008). Changing dietary habits of ethnic groups in Europe and implications for health. *Nutrition Reviews*, 66: 203–215.

Gortmaker, S. L., Must, A., Perrin, J. M., Sobol, A. M. & Dietz, W. H. (1993). Social and Economic Consequences of Overweight in Adolescence and Young Adulthood. *N Engl J Med*, 329: 1008–1012.

Grimmett, C., Croker, H., Carnell, S. & Wardle, J. (2008). Telling Parents Their Child's Weight Status: Psychological Impact of a Weight-Screening Program. *Pediatrics*, 122: e682–688.

Hoppé, R. & Ogden, J. (1997). Practice nurses' beliefs about obesity and weight related interventions in primary care. *International Journal of Obesity*, 21: 141–146.

Kinra, S., Nelder, R. P. & Lewendon, G. J. (2000). Deprivation and childhood obesity: a cross sectional study of 20 973 children in Plymouth, United Kingdom. *J Epidemiol Community Health*, 54: 456–460.

Leather, S. (2003). Social inequalities, nutrition and obesity. In: Voss, L. & Wilkin, T. (Eds.) *Adult obesity: a paediatric challenge*. New York: Taylor and Francis.

Lobstein, T., Rigby, N. & Leach, R. (2005). EU Platform on diet, physical activity and health: IOTF EU Platform Briefing Paper. Brussels: European Association for the Study of Obesity.

Maes, H. H. M., Neale, M. C. & Eaves, L. J. (1997). Genetic and Environmental Factors in Relative Body Weight and Human Adiposity. *Behavior Genetics*, 27: 325–351.

Maryon-Davis, A. (2007). Weight management in primary care: how can it be made more effective? *Proceedings of the Nutrition Society*, 64: 97–103.

Mccormick, B. & Stone, I. (2007). Economic costs of obesity and the case for government intervention. *Obesity Reviews*, 8: 161–164.

National Association to Advance Fat Acceptance (2008).

National Institute for Health and Clinical Excellence (2006). *Obesity: the prevention, identification, assessment and management of overweight and obesity in adults and children*. London: NICE.

Ogden, C. L., Carroll, M. D., Curtin, L. R., Mcdowell, M. A., Tabak, C. J. & Flegal, K. M. (2006). Prevalence of Overweight and Obesity in the United States, 1999–2004. *JAMA*, 295: 1549–1555.

Reilly, J. J., Armstrong, J., Dorosty, A. R., Emmett, P. M., Ness, A., Rogers, I., Steer, C., Sherriff, A., Parents, F. T. A. L. S. O. & Children Study Team (2005). Early life risk factors for obesity in childhood: cohort study. *BMJ*, 330: 1357.

Shaw, K., O'rourke, P., Del Mar, C. & Kenardy, J. (2005). Psychological interventions for overweight or obesity. *Cochrane Database of Systematic Reviews*, Issue 2.

Stevens, J. (1998). Studies of the impact of age on optimal body weight. *The Journal of Nutritional Biochemistry*, 9: 501–510.

Swanton, K. & Frost, M. (2007). *Lightening the load: Tackling overweight and obesity*. In: National Heart Forum in Association with the Faculty of Public Health and the Department of Health (Ed.). Department of Health.

The Information Centre (2004). *Health Survey for England 2004. Updating of trend tables to include childhood obesity data*. London: The Information Centre.

The Information Centre (2008). *Statistics on Obesity, Physical Activity and Diet: England*. London: The Information Centre.

Truby, H., Baic, S., Delooy, A., Fox, K. R., Livingstone, M. B. E., Logan, C. M., Macdonald, I. A., Morgan, L. M., Taylor, M. A. & Millward, D. J. (2006). Randomized controlled trial of four commercial weight loss programmes in the UK: initial findings from the BBC "diet trials". *BMJ*, 332: 1309–1314.

Turconi, G. & Cena, H. (2007). Epidemiology of obesity. In Bagchi, D. & Preuss, H. G. (Eds.) *Obesity: Epidemiology, Pathophysiology and Prevention*. Boca Raton: CRC Press, Taylor and Francis Group.

Viner, R. M. & Cole, T. J. (2005). Adult socioeconomic, educational, social, and psychological outcomes of childhood obesity: a national birth cohort study. *BMJ*, 330: 1354.

Visscher, T. L. & Seidell, J. C. (2001). The public health impact of obesity. *Annual Review of Public Health*, 22: 355–375.

Wardle, J. & Cooke, L. (2005). The impact of obesity on psychological well being. *Best Practice & Research Clinical Endocrinology & Metabolism*, 19: 421–440.

Weiss, E. C., Galuska, D. A., Kettel Khan, L., Gillespie, C. & Serdula, M. K. (2007). Weight Regain in U.S. Adults Who Experienced Substantial Weight Loss, 1999–2002. *American Journal of Preventive Medicine*, 33: 34–40.

Who Expert Consultation (2004). Appropriate body-mass index for Asian populations and its implications for policy and intervention strategies. *The Lancet*, 363: 157–163.

Chapter 16
Improving sexual health

Sheena MacRae and Jill Ladlow

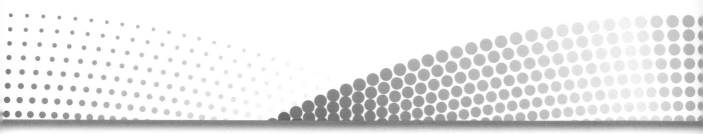

Introduction

What is sexual health?

Sexual health can feel like a difficult subject. As an issue it poses a lot of questions when we first consider how to approach it in our practice.

- What is **sexual** health?
- What can be done to improve sexual health?
- How does sexual health affect my practice?

In truth much of our practice regarding sexual health will relate to our own attitudes, values and confidence with the topic therefore it is important to realize and reflect on this. Some practitioners can feel uncomfortable dealing with issues of sexuality and sexual health with their patients. Others feel that sexual health does not fit into their role. These thoughts and feelings are natural about any topic as intimate as sexual health but in reality the skills required to meet these needs are as easily practised and honed as any other part of practice.

This chapter aims to enable practitioners to begin to develop an understanding of the components that contribute to sexual health in order to maximize the health of all patients regardless of the setting in which they work. Why? Because an individual's sexuality is an intrinsic part their overall well-being.

What does it mean to experience good sexual health? Defining sexual health, like health in general, is more complex than you would perhaps think. Good sexual health goes beyond avoiding illness and enters the realms of equity, entitlement and enjoyment.

There are a number of elements which contribute to an individual's sexuality and their experience of a fulfilling sexual life. Unfortunately, it is all too easy to think about sexual health in terms of the absence of disease or the access to appropriate health care, contraception and treatments. This view does not take into account identity, pleasure and social welfare, for example. Human sexual behaviour is complex and diverse and as such requires a wide range of responses from professionals. If nurses are to work towards supporting the population to achieve optimum sexual health, then a progressive holistic approach to this area is needed.

In the UK, Jo Adams and Carol Painter developed the following to aid practitioners understanding of the complexities of human sexuality.

This model highlights the need to be mindful of the huge range of factors that will contribute to an individual's sexuality and therefore their sexual health. We can begin to see that actions relating to wider health will lead to consequences for sexual health. We will return to this later.

Activity box

What might be the consequences of poor sexual health?

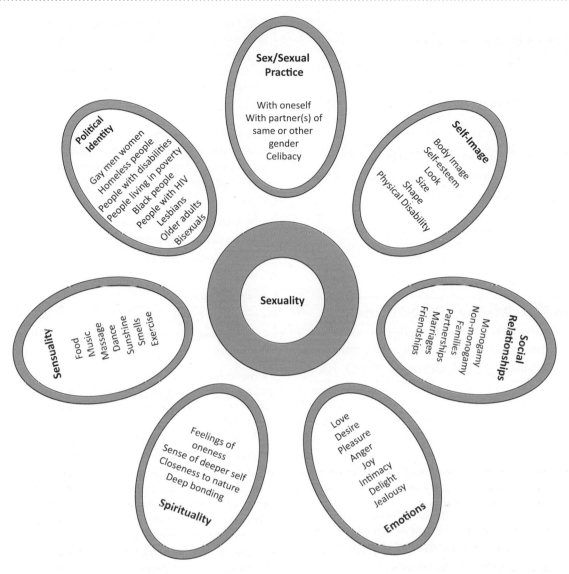

Sex/Sexual Practice

With oneself
With partner(s) of same or other gender
Celibacy

Political Identity

Gay men women
Homeless people
People with disabilities
People living in poverty
Black people
People with HIV
Lesbians
Older adults
Bisexuals

Self-Image

Body Image
Self-esteem
Look
Size
Shape
Physical Disability

Sexuality

Sensuality

Food
Music
Massage
Dance
Sunshine
Smells
Exercise

Social Relationships

Monogamy
Non-monogamy
Families
Partnerships
Marriages
Friendships

Spirituality

Feelings of oneness
Sense of deeper self
Closeness to nature
Deep bonding

Emotions

Love
Desire
Pleasure
Anger
Joy
Intimacy
Delight
Jealousy

Fig. 16.1 The Sexual Health Flower. The petals add up to how we define ourselves as sexual beings. Sexuality involves our relationships with ourselves, those around us and the society in which we live — whether we identify as gay, heterosexual, lesbian, bisexual or celibate. Adams, J. and Painter, C. (2001).

Discussion points

There are many consequences of poor sexual health including:

- Social impacts:
  - including exploitation, violence, unwanted pregnancies, poor academic attainment, impact on employment prospects.

- Physical impacts:
  - ill health e.g. pelvic inflammatory disease, HIV, various cancers, forms of hepatitis, herpes.

- Psychological consequences:
  - poor mental health e.g. depression, low self-worth, poor self image.

Although the issues related here could happen to anyone, like other health issues, they are not evenly distributed in the population. The people most burdened by sexual ill health are:

- women,

- gay men,

- teenagers,

- young adults,
- black and minority ethic groups.

National Strategy for Sexual Health and HIV (DH, 2001a)

In 2002, the World Health Organization (WHO) convened a technical consultation with sexual health professionals from across the world to try to do the following:

- define sexual health and related issues,
- identify barriers to sexual health promotion,
- suggest strategies to address these barriers.

This group provided a set of working definitions which aimed to support public health professionals in addressing sexual health concerns in their populations.

> **Box 16.1** Working definitions, from 'Defining Sexual Health — Report of a technical consultation on sexual health, 28-31 January 2002, Geneva,' (WHO, 2002)
>
> **Sex**
>
> Sex refers to the biological characteristics that define humans as female or male. While these sets of biological characteristics are not mutually exclusive, as there are individuals who possess both, they tend to differentiate humans as males and females.
>
> **In general use in many languages, the term sex is often used to mean 'sexual activity', but for technical purposes in the context of sexuality and sexual health discussions, the above definition is preferred.**
>
> **Sexuality**
>
> Sexuality is a central aspect of being human throughout life and encompasses sex, gender identities and roles, sexual orientation, eroticism, pleasure, intimacy and reproduction. Sexuality is experienced and expressed in thoughts, fantasies, desires, beliefs, attitudes, values, behaviours, practices, roles and relationships. While sexuality can include all of these dimensions, not all of them are always experienced or expressed. Sexuality is influenced by the interaction of biological, psychological, social, economic, political, cultural, ethical, legal, historical, religious and spiritual factors.
>
> **Sexual health**
>
> Sexual health is a state of physical, emotional, mental and social well-being in relation to sexuality; it is not merely the absence of disease, dysfunction or infirmity. Sexual health requires a positive and respectful approach to sexuality and sexual relationships, as well as the possibility of having pleasurable and safe sexual experiences, free of coercion, discrimination and violence. For sexual health to be attained and maintained, the sexual rights of all persons must be respected, protected and fulfilled.
>
> **Sexual rights**
>
> Sexual rights embrace human rights that are already recognized in national laws, international human rights documents and other consensus statements. They include the right of all persons, free of coercion, discrimination and violence, to:
>
> - the highest attainable standard of sexual health, including access to sexual and reproductive health care services;
> - seek, receive and impart information related to sexuality;
> - sexuality education;
> - respect for bodily integrity;
> - choose their partner;
> - decide to be sexually active or not;
> - consensual sexual relations;
> - consensual marriage;
> - decide whether or not, and when, to have children; and
> - pursue a satisfying, safe and pleasurable sexual life.
>
> The responsible exercise of human rights requires that all persons respect the rights of others.

As you can see, the professionals convened by WHO gave a very broad account of all the elements contributing to sexual health, reflecting the complexity and diversity of human sexuality. It is important therefore to be mindful of this when approaching sexual health in practice.

Public health responses to sexual health in the UK

The profile of sexual health as a public health issue has risen dramatically over the last thirty years. The impact of HIV and the rise of other sexually transmitted infections (STIs) coupled with consistently high rates of both unintended and teenage conceptions have triggered the launch of a number of strategies and programmes designed to reduce these statistics and their consequent impact on public health.

The emergence of HIV in the 1980s set in motion a range of public health responses designed to reduce the spread of the virus. In an unprecedented step, a national campaign was launched with leaflets sent to every household in the UK with accompanying television adverts highlighting what people must do to avoid HIV (see following weblink). Condom advertising started appearing on mainstream British television and the concept of safer sex began to be widely promoted.

Initially, much of the press focus on HIV centred on groups of people who at this time were deemed to be more at risk of contracting the virus, particularly gay men and injecting drug users. In response to the fear and discrimination bred by misunderstandings in the popular media HIV prevention work began to focus on high risk behaviours rather than high risk groups. Much of this work was driven by grass roots HIV organizations, such as Terence Higgins Trust, supporting people in communities across Britain.

> **Box 16.2** HIV Web sources
>
> For further information about the history of HIV in the UK go to http://www.avert.org/uk-aids-history.htm
>
> To view the original 'Tombstone' public health film go to http://www.nationalarchives.gov.uk/films/1979to2006/filmpage_aids.htm
>
> To view current Department of Health guidance in England on HIV go to http://www.dh.gov.uk/en/Publichealth/Healthimprovement/Sexualhealth/HIV/HIVgeneralinformation/index.htm

Key strategic responses to sexual health in the UK

By the late 1990s, pressure was building within sexual health services. Sexually transmitted infections were on the increase, and although within Western Europe our rates of HIV were comparatively low, diagnoses were rising steadily. It appeared that either the messages of the previous decade were losing their power or that messages were not getting through at all. In 2001, the Department of Health (DH) published its first response to this developing sexual health crisis. The National Strategy for Sexual Health and HIV (DH, 2001a) aimed to set out clear goals to address sexual health in the population.

The Medical Foundation for AIDS and Sexual Health

(MedFASH, 2005) recommended standards for NHS HIV services alongside the 'NHS Operating Framework 2006/7' 48 hour GUM access target. The national strategy was designed to drive the modernization of sexual health services and reverse the negative trends which were being tracked in the United Kingdom (UK).

These strategies were not alone in addressing sexual health concerns in the population. In England, in June 1999,

> **Box 16.3** The National Strategy for Sexual Health and HIV (DH, 2001a)
>
> Aims:
> - reduce the transmission of HIV and STIs,
> - reduce the prevalence of undiagnosed HIV and STIs,
> - reduce unintended pregnancy rates,
> - improve health and social care for people living with HIV,
> - reduce the stigma associated with HIV and STIs.

the Government's Social Exclusion Unit produced a national teenage pregnancy strategy with two goals:

1. To halve the rate of conceptions among those under 18 years old in England by 2010 and set a firmly established downward trend in the conception rates for under 16s by 2010.

2. To achieve a reduction in the risk of long-term social exclusion for teenage parents and their children.

From a public health perspective **Choosing Health: Making Healthy Choices Easier** (DH, 2004a) outlined the Government's intention to launch a major new sexual health campaign and to accelerate progress for a national programme of screening for Chlamydia. Box 16.4 collates the key targets for sexual health improvement in the UK in the last decade from all the strategic documents outlined here.

> **Box 16.4** Summary of sexual health Strategy targets*, from *Progress and Priorities — working together for high quality sexual health. Review of National Strategy for Sexual Health and HIV.* (MedFASH, 2008)
>
> - Reduce by 25% the number of newly acquired HIV and gonorrhoea infections by the end of 2007.
> - By the end of 2004, all Genitourinary Medicine (GUM) clinic attendees to be offered an HIV test on their first screening for sexually transmitted infections (and subsequently according to risk):
>   - Increase uptake of the HIV test by those offered it in GUM clinics to 60% by the end of 2007;
>   - Reduce by 50% the number of previously undiagnosed HIV infected people attending GUM clinics who remain unaware of their infection after their visit by the end 2007.

- Increase the uptake of hepatitis B immunization in homosexual and bisexual men attending GUM clinics as follows:
  - Uptake of the first dose of hepatitis B vaccine, in those not previously immunized, to be 90% by the end of 2006.
  - Uptake of the three doses of hepatitis B vaccine (i.e. the full course), in those not previously immunized, to be 70% by the end of 2006.
- For women who meet the legal requirements, access to an abortion within three weeks of the first appointment with the referring doctor.

* In line with the move to minimize the number of centrally determined targets following Shifting the balance of power, the 'targets' in the 2001 Strategy were amended to 'standards' and 'goals' in the implementation action plan published in 2002.

Scotland' first national response to emerging sexual health issues *Respect and Responsibility: Strategy and Action Plan for Improving Sexual Health* was launched in January 2005. Its funding was extended by the Scottish Government until 2011 and it set out to achieve.

- reduced levels of regret and coercion;
- reduced levels of unintended pregnancy, particularly in those under 16 but also to see a reduced number of repeat abortions in all ages;
- reduced levels of sexually transmitted infections, recognizing that there will first of all have to be an increase due to increased testing;
- increased access to sexual health information and uptake of services;
- reduced levels of HIV transmission, particularly amongst men who have sex with men;
- reduced levels of undiagnosed HIV transmission, particularly men who have sex with men and African populations (Scottish Executive 2005).

It is hoped the action plan will deliver 'a balance between what government should do to help people avoid contracting or spreading sexually transmitted disease or an unintended pregnancy and the individual's responsibility for their own health and the safety of others'.

The Welsh Government responded to its populations sexual health needs setting up the All Wales Sexual Health Network in 2000. Its role was to implement the Welsh Sexual Health Strategy and this work was managed by Public Health Wales. The Strategy sought to address the high rates of teenage pregnancy and increasing rates of sexually transmitted infections (STIs) in Wales. The aims of the strategy are:

- To improve the sexual health of the population of Wales;
- To narrow inequalities in sexual health;
- To enhance the general health and emotional well-being of the population by enabling and supporting fulfilling sexual relationships.

'The Sexual Health Strategy proposed an action plan with a number of objectives including one to: 'promote a more supportive environment, which encourages openness, knowledge and an understanding about sexual issues and fosters good sexual health'. The All Wales Sexual Health network was established in response to this objective.
See: http://www.shnwales.org.uk/

Northern Ireland launched its Sexual Health Promotion Strategy and Action Plan 2008–2013 on 1 December 2008. The strategy aimed to improve, protect and promote the sexual health and well-being of the whole population in Northern Ireland. Its objectives were as follows:

- Enable all people to develop and maintain the knowledge, skills and values necessary for improving sexual health and well-being.
- Promote opportunities to enable young people to make informed choices before engaging in sexual activity and, especially, empowering them to delay first intercourse until an appropriate time of their choosing.
- Reduce the number of unplanned births to teenage mothers by seeing that all people have access to sexual health services.
- Reduce the incidence of sexually transmitted infections, including HIV. DHSSPSNI (2008).

The strategy calls for the establishment of a Sexual Health Promotion Network to consider and advise on the approach to encouraging better sexual health in Northern Ireland.
See: http://www.dhsspsni.gov.uk/dhssps_sexual_health_plan_front_cvr.pdf

The epidemiology of Sexually Transmitted Infections (STIs)

The graphs below illustrate the trends in diagnoses for a variety of different sexually transmitted infections.

Fig. 16.2 shows the trend in the number of estimated and observed HIV and AIDS diagnoses, HIV-infected people accessing care and deaths among people infected with HIV in the UK from 1997 to 2006. The number of new HIV diagnoses increased quite significantly from under 3,000 in 1997 to almost 8 in 2005 but has since started to plateau. This has been paralleled with an increase in the number of HIV infected persons accessing care, from around 15,000 in 1997 to over 50,000 in 2006. AIDS diagnoses and death among people

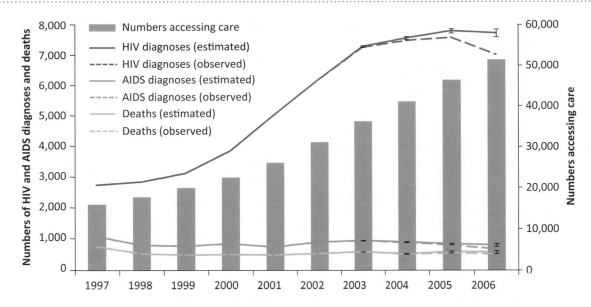

Fig. 16.2 HIV/AIDS diagnoses and death reports, and annual survey of HIV-infected persons accessing HIV care. Testing Times (HPA, 2007)

infected with HIV have remained relatively stable at well under 1,000 per year over this ten-year period.

In Fig. 16.3, the number of new HIV and AIDS diagnoses are broken down by different population groups. In 1997 the majority of new diagnoses were among men who have sex with men (MSM) followed by heterosexual people and to a much lesser extent intravenous drug users (IDU) children, through vertical transmission (ie mother-to-child transmission immediately before or after birth or during the perinatal period) and blood product recipients. Infection among

these latter three groups has remained low throughout the ten year period.

The number of new infections amongst MSM has increased quite steadily reaching around 2,500 in 2006 whilst infections to the heterosexual population have increased much more dramatically particularly between 1999 and 2003, when they started to level off.

Fig. 16.4, shows the rates (number per 100, 000 population) of gonorrhoea diagnoses in the UK by sex and age group from 2002 to 2006.

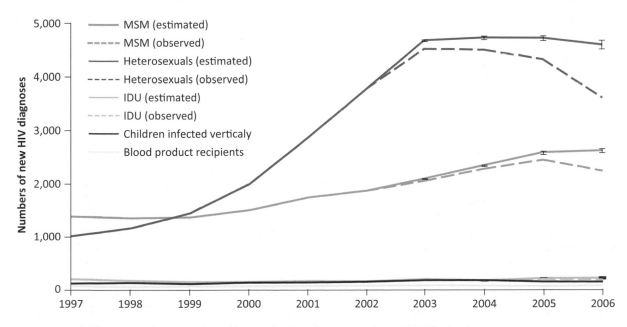

Fig. 16.3 HIV/AIDS diagnoses and death reports. Testing Times (HPA, 2007)

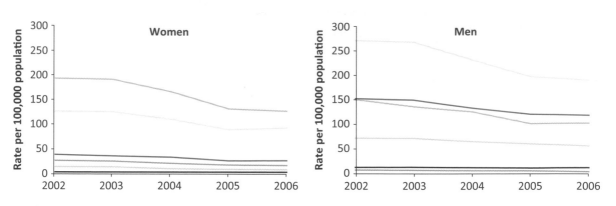

Fig. 16.4 Rates of gonorrhoea diagnoses by sex and age group, UK. Testing Times (HPA, 2007)

In both sex groups, rates fell steadily between 2002 and 2006. Rates are higher amongst men particularly in the 20–24 age group. In women, the highest rates are seen in the 16–19 age group followed by the 20–24 year old group; rates are much less significant in women under 16 or 25 and above.

Fig. 16.5 shows rates of genital chlamydia in the UK, by sex and age group from 1997 to 2006.

Rates of chlamydia diagnoses increased steadily in both sexes between 1997 and 2006. In women the incidence is highest in the 16–19 year old group followed by women aged 20–24 years old. In men, infection rates are much more significant in the 20–24 year old group.

Fig. 16.6 shows the number of diagnosed cases of syphilis in England and Wales and Scotland, by sex, between 1997 and 2006. In 1997, numbers of diagnoses were much higher in

men in England and Wales than in any of the other sub-groups shown. Numbers then fell, quite dramatically until 1989, when they levelled off. Interestingly, again amongst men in England and Wales, numbers infected with syphilis have increased very significantly to almost 3,000 in 2006.

Fig. 16.7, shows the number of diagnoses of genital warts (first attack) in GUM clinics by sex and sexual orientation in the UK from 1997 to 2006.

Numbers have increased fairly steadily from around 35,000 in 1997 to around 40,000 in women and slightly higher in heterosexual men in 2006. The number of diagnoses amongst MSM is much lower.

Fig. 16.8 shown the number of diagnoses of genital herpes (first and recurrent episodes) in GUM clinics by sex, in England and Wales from 1977 to 2005. Between 1997 and 1990 the

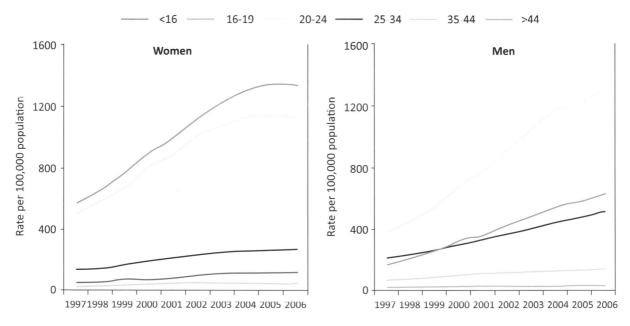

Fig. 16.5 Rates of genital chlamydia diagnoses by sex and age group. Testing Times (HPA, 2007)

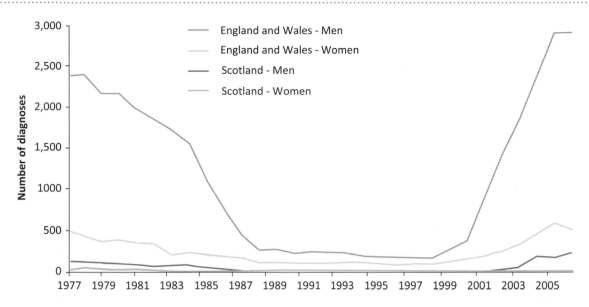

Fig. 16.6 Diagnoses of syphilis in GUM clinics by sex, England, Wales, and Scotland. Testing Times (HPA, 2007)

trend in men and women followed a similar pattern increasingly significantly in both groups but being higher amongst men. Since 1990 the numbers of genital herpes diagnoses have continued to increase but this has been much more marked amongst the female population.

Fig. 16.9 shows diagnosis rates of chlamydia, gonorrhoea, syphilis, genital warts, genital herpes and HIV in young adults (16–24) in the UK, from 1997 to 2006. (Note the different scales used for each of the infections.)

Chlamydia diagnoses have increased the most steadily and are currently the most significant in the younger population: in 2006 around 1,100 per 100, 000 young people aged 16–24 received a positive diagnosis. Although rates of gonorrhoea increased between 1997 and 2002, they have since started to fall.

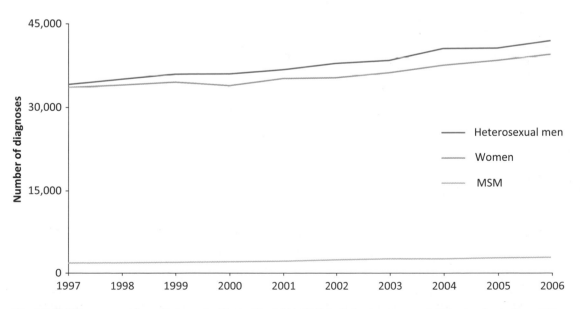

Fig. 16.7 Diagnoses of genital warts (first attack) in GUM clinics by sex and sexual orientation, UK. Testing Times (HPA, 2007)

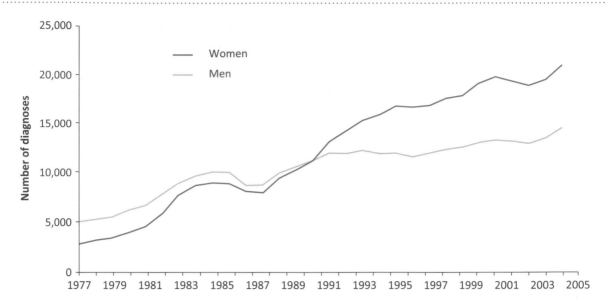

Fig. 16.8 Number of diagnoses of genital herpes (first and recurrent episodes) in GUM clinics by sex, England and Wales. Testing Times (HPA, 2007)

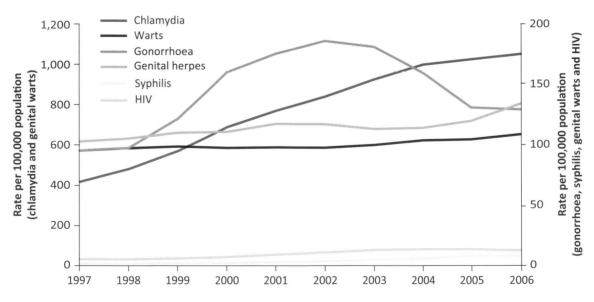

Fig. 16.9 Diagnosis rates of chlamydia, gonorrhoea, syphilis, genital warts, genital herpes and HIV in young adults (16-24), UK. STI data from genitourinary medicine clinics, and HIV/AIDS diagnoses and death reports

Testing Times (HPA, 2007)

Activity box

What group of people in the population accounts for more than 50% of STI diagnoses?

What might be the reason this group is more predisposed to infection?

Rates of STIs are increasing in the over 45s. What reasons are there for this rise?

Discussion points

Young people account for more than 50% if STI diagnoses (despite making up only 12% of the population) (HPA, 2008)

It is thought this can be attributed higher levels of sexual activity in young people and possible increased susceptibility to infection (HPA, 2008). According to the second **National Survey of Sexual Attitudes and Lifestyles** (Wellings *et al.*, 2001), young people generally have higher numbers of partners and a higher frequency of partner change than older people. They are considered vulnerable as they may not have the skills and confidence to understand and negotiate safer sex. They may also be at risk to coercion by a manipulative partner.

Risk taking in sexual behaviour is not confined to young people this and the fact that increasing numbers of older people are single are thought to be driving the trend of STIs are increasing in the over 45s. In addition, condoms are often not used by this older age group due to lack of concern relating to pregnancy due to menopause or surgical forms of contraception (HPA, 2008).

Mussen *et al.* (1998) shows that an individual's behaviour may directly affect their sexual partner, through transmission of an infection or unintended pregnancy. Specific sexual health promotion Government targets have been set, but concentrate on 'high risk' groups. Therefore, other population groups, such as the older age group are ignored. Sexual health messages should be aimed at all the sexually active populations to truly achieve a reduction in STI rates.

International perspectives on sexual health

Sexual health matters are of concern internationally not least with the global impact of HIV weighing heavily on medical resources world wide. The World Health Organization embeds sexual health improvement work internationally through its Millennium Development Goals (2000) particularly:

Target 5.A: Reduce the maternal mortality ratio by three quarters between 1990 and 2015 and

Target 5.B: Achieve, by 2015, universal access to reproductive health.

This work is the responsibility of the Department of Reproductive Health and Research including the UNDP/UNFPA/WHO/World Bank Special Programme of Research, Development and Research Training in Human Reproduction (HRP). The following are the main areas of concern to address:

- adolescent sexual and reproductive health,
- aging and sexual health,
- cancers related sexual and reproductive health,
- family planning,
- female genital mutilation and other harmful practices,
- infertility,
- maternal and perinatal health,
- reproductive tract infections, STIs, HIV/AIDS,
- unsafe abortion.

This work intersects with programmes supporting work with emergency situations, ethical issues, gender equality and human rights.

http://www.who.int/reproductivehealth/en/

Determinants and distribution of sexual ill health

As with general health, sexual health is acknowledged to be influenced by a range of social, economic and cultural factors. Poorer sexual health outcomes can be closely mapped to deprivation and inequality which is reflected in a range of statistics from STI prevalence to teenage pregnancy (HPA, 2005). Why is this the case? The social determinants of health are discussed in more detail in chapter? However, where there is poverty and lack of opportunity health outcomes suffer. It can be argued that this happens due to lack of available service provision but as seen in the petal diagram earlier in the chapter an individual's self esteem is also a strong contributing factor to their sexual well-being. These elements are only part of a complex picture however and do not account for the overall level of sexual ill health and unplanned pregnancy in the UK.

The UK has higher rates of teenage pregnancy than the rest of Europe but we also top the polls in terms of use of drugs and alcohol as well as poor mental health outcomes in young people. Why would these issues be considered alongside sexual health? Well clearly all of these issues would impact on an individual's ability to make well considered choices. The next question that should follow however is why do we as a nation have such poor health relating to mental health and drug alcohol? Chapters 17 and 18 consider this in more detail but we can see from these enquiries that a range of public health issues interrelate closely and do not stand alone. Mental well being and risky behaviours relating to substances and sex are closely linked and therefore holistic practice should be utilized to encourage better health overall.

If we were to consider the sexual health of Britain as a whole the range of factors influencing it would overwhelm us. It is for this reason that our approach to sexual health is targeted at different diverse groups within the population, to best meet their needs. This approach is not without difficulty as the initial HIV work proved in the UK. Messages regarding sexual health particularly around prevention need to be tailored to meet the demography of the population and their specific concerns.

It is important that sexual health services are easily accessible to those most at need but how do we identify those most in need. According to the Health Protection Agency national data and documents *Mapping the Issues* (HPA, 2005); *A Complex Picture* (HPA, 2006) and *Testing Times* (HPA 2007a) groups requiring targeted prevention are listed as:

• women;

• men who have sex with men (MSM);

• black and minority ethnic populations;

• pregnant women;

• young people;

• injecting drug users.

These groups were identified as being disproportionally affected by sexual ill health. Other people who could be considered to be 'at risk' of poor sexual health outcomes include HIV-positive patients; victims of sexual assault; those with needle-stick injuries and sexual partners of individuals who are high risk or positive to blood borne viruses.

As with a range of other health issues we know the population can reduce the risks of unplanned pregnancy and STIs by practising 'safer sex' so what is the problem and why are the rates so high? Similar to the concerns regarding smoking, often the public are well informed of sexual health risks however knowledge does not necessarily lead to changes in individual behaviour.

Poor sexual health is costly on the National Health Service (NHS). Health economics examine how best to use resources and the need to do this is based on the undeniable fact that resources in the NHS are overstretched and can not meet all needs. Therefore, choices have to be made on what services are provided (FPA, 2005). Hence, preventing poor sexual health has significant potential not just to improve health, but also to better manage scarce resources.

Approaches to health promotion activity and relevant models to assist this work, has already been discussed within this book. Sexual health promotion focuses on two main areas: the individual and societal change. In order to bring about change, the health professional and the patient firstly need to acknowledge the impact of risk taking behaviour on sexual health. The

nurse should consider an individual plan of care aimed at improving the client's knowledge and understanding of sexual health issues, promoting 'safer sex,' and for those who continue to take risks, plan strategies to help reduce that risk. For example, offering Hepatitis B immunization to clients who undergo high risk activities, such as sex workers and men who have sex with men (MSM). Or as a school nurse ensuring young people are aware of where to access emergency contraception, in the case of unprotected sexual intercourse (UPSI).

Although 'at risk' groups are identified as being higher risk of poor sexual health, it must be acknowledged that all sexually active people are at risk of ill health, especially if they participate in unprotected sex. People with multiple partners who fail to access health services put themselves at increased risk of infections, whether or not they are symptomatic. This highlights the importance of raising sexual health and STI awareness and providing safer sex messages and increasing the access of sexual health services at both a local and national level. Table 16.1 provides an overview of the main bacterial and viral STIs that exist, as well as minor illness linked to the genital tract, for example candidal infections.

Key interventions to improve sexual health

The National Chlamydia Screening Programme

Health Protection Agency (HPA) statistics reveal that Chlamydia is the most common bacterial sexually transmitted infection and is most prevalent in the 16 to 24 age group, where it has been diagnosed in one in ten people (HPA, 2008; National Chlamydia Screening Programme, 2006). Between 1999 and 2008, Infection rates have risen by over 149% in men and 84% in women (HPA, 2008). In order to stem this rise, the National Chlamydia Screening Programme was established in 2003, and is central to the implementation of National Strategy for Sexual Health and HIV. The programme aims to:

• Prevent and control chlamydia through early detection and treatment of asymptomatic infection;

• Reduce onward transmission to sexual partners;

• Prevent the consequences of untreated infection. See **http://www.chlamydiascreening.nhs.uk/ps/about/aims. html**

The programme was instigated as a result of the sharp rise in chlamydia diagnoses recorded in GUM settings throughout the latter half of the 1990s. Chlamydia is a bacterial infection

Table 16.1 Sexually Transmitted Infection - Symptoms + Treatment

STI	Symptoms		Treatment
	Male	**Female**	
Bacterial Infections			
Chlamydia	*Acute* • Urethral discharge • Dysuria • Testicular pain *Chronic* • Epididymitis • Orchitis • < Fertility • Reactive Arthritis • Reiter's Syndrome	*Acute* • Bleeding between periods • Heavier periods • Dyspareunia (painful sex) • Post-coital bleeding • Lower abdominal (pelvic) pain • Dysuria • Abnormal vaginal discharge *Chronic* • Pelvic Inflammatory Disease (PID) • Blocked fallopian tubes/risk of ectopic pregnancy • Bacterial Hepatitis • < Fertility • Reactive Arthritis • Reiter's Syndrome (less common in females)	*First-line Antibiotics/ antibacterials* • Azithromycin • Erythromycin • Doxycycline
Non-Specific Urethritis *(males only)*	*Acute* • <50% caused by Chlamydia • Urethral discharge • Dysuria/Frequency • Testicular pain *Chronic* If caused by Chlamydia, same chronic symptoms as above		*First-line Antibiotics/ antibacterials* • Azithromycin • Erythromycin • Doxycycline
Gonorrhoea	*Acute* ~10% have no symptoms Yellow/green urethral discharge Dysuria Testicular pain Balanitis *Chronic* Orchitis Prostatitis < Fertility Reactive Arthritis Reiter's Syndrome Meningitis	*Acute* ~50% have no symptoms Yellow/green vaginal discharge Lower abdominal pain Bleeding between periods/heavier periods *Chronic* Pelvic Inflammatory Disease (PID) Blocked fallopian tubes/ectopic pregnancy Infertility Reactive Arthritis Reiter's Syndrome Meningitis	*First-line Antibiotics/ antibacterials* Cefixime and Azithromycin Ceftriaxone
Bacterial Vaginosis *(females only)*		*Acute* Thin, white or grey discharge with fishy odour and high (alkaline) pH Vaginal soreness	*First-line treatments:* Metronidazole Clindamycin

(Contd.)

217

		Chronic Pelvic Inflammatory Disease (PID) Blocked fallopian tubes/ectopic pregnancy Infertility Pregnancy problems	Partner also requires treatment with Metronidazole
Viral Infections			
Genital Herpes	*Acute* Flu-like symptoms Soreness, stinging, tingling or itching in the genital/anal area Small fluid-filled blisters bursting after 1-2 days to small red painful sores Dysuria *Recurrent Episodes* Usually milder and less painful	*Acute* Flu-like symptoms Soreness, stinging, tingling or itching in the genital/anal area Small fluid-filled blisters bursting after 1-2 days to small red painful sores Dysuria *Recurrent Episodes* Usually milder and less painful	*Treatment – Anti-virals:* First-line: Aciclovir Valaciclovir
Genital Warts	Fleshy growths of variable sizes Approximately 30 types of genital warts - caused by the human papilloma virus (HPV)	Fleshy growths of variable sizes Approximately 30 types of genital warts - caused by the human papilloma virus (HPV)	*First-line treatments:* Cryotherapy Warticon Cream Aldara cream
Fungal Infections			
Thrush	Erythema, soreness under prepuce White curdy secretion under prepuce	Thick white curdy discharge Vulval itching and soreness Vaginal soreness	First-line treatments: Clotrimazole Fluconazole
Balanitis **(males only)**	Erythema, soreness under prepuce Eczema/dermatitis-like symptoms		Treatment depends upon cause: Clotrimazole Aqueous Cream
Parasitic Infections			
Pubic Lice	Tiny parasitic insects living in pubic hair. Yellow-grey colour 2mm long. Symptomatic Itching, irritation and inflammation to affected areas Black powdery lice droppings Brown eggs on pubic/body hair Sky-blue spots and specks of blood on skin	Tiny parasitic insects living in pubic hair. Yellow-grey colour 2mm long. Symptomatic Itching, irritation and inflammation to affected areas Black powdery lice droppings Brown eggs on pubic/body hair Sky-blue spots and specks of blood on skin	Treatment is by cream, lotion and shampoo
Scabies	Scabies caused by tiny parasites 0.4mm long that burrow into the skin and lay eggs. Intense itching in affected areas Itchy rash or tiny spots	Scabies caused by tiny parasites 0.4mm long that burrow into the skin and lay eggs. Intense itching in affected areas	Treatment by cream and lotions

(Contd.)

Table 16.1 Sexually Transmitted Infection - Symptoms + Treatment *(Contd.)*

STI	Symptoms		Treatment
	Male	**Female**	
Parasitic Infections			
	Inflammation or raw broken skin caused by scratching Fine silvery lines where mites have burrowed	Itchy rash or tiny spots Inflammation or raw broken skin caused by scratching Fine silvery lines where mites have burrowed	
Trichomonas Vaginalis (TV)	TV is a tiny parasite found in the urethra. Thin and white discharge from penis Dysuria Inflammation of foreskin (uncommon)	TV is a tiny parasite found in vagina and urethra. Vaginal soreness, inflammation and itching Thick or thin frothy yellow discharge with strong smell Dysuria	Metronidazole
Blood Borne Infections			
Human Immuno-deficiency Virus (HIV)	HIV weakens and damages the immune system <50% report flu-like symptoms after recent exposure (sero-conversion) Often no signs or symptoms Usually initially diagnosed when non-resolving infections are being investigated. Earlier diagnosis advantageous in achieving early monitoring, management and treatment	HIV weakens and damages the immune system <50% report flu-like symptoms after recent exposure (sero-conversion) Often no signs or symptoms Usually initially diagnosed when non-resolving infections are being investigated. Earlier diagnosis advantageous in achieving early monitoring, management and treatment	Untreated – can lead to mild to serious illness due to immuno-suppression, which can eventually lead to death. If patient complies with combination therapies (anti-retrovirals) the prognosis is favourable. These patients are advised to lead a 'healthy lifestyle' to avoid immuno-suppression.
Syphilis	*Acute: First Stage Syphilis* Very infectious Usually 2-3 weeks after exposure 'Chancre' appear (painless sores) – mainly on genitalia Less commonly sores to mouth, lips, tonsils, fingers or buttocks *Second Stage Syphilis* Painless rash can spread all over body or in patches (commonly palms of hands/soles of feet).	*Acute* Very infectious Usually 2-3 weeks after exposure 'Chancre' appear (painless sores) – mainly on genitalia Less commonly sores to mouth, lips, tonsils, fingers or buttocks *Second Stage Syphilis* Painless rash can spread all over body or in patches (commonly palms of hands/soles of feet).	*Strong antibacterial/ antibiotic therapy:* Benzylpenicillin Treatment very effective for first and second stage syphilis.

(Contd.)

	Flat warty-looking growths on anus Flu-like symptoms and swollen glands (weeks/months) White patches on tongue Patchy hair loss *Third Stage/Latent Syphilis* Serious damage to heart, brain, eyes, internal organs, bones and nervous system Death	Flat warty-looking growths on vulva Flu-like symptoms and swollen glands (weeks/months) White patches on tongue Patchy hair loss *Third Stage/Latent Syphilis* Serious damage to heart, brain, eyes, internal organs, bones and nervous system Death	Latent syphilis can be treated, but any damage already done to body will be permanent
Hepatitis B	*Acute* Short mild flu-like illness Nausea and vomiting Diarrhoea Loss of appetite Weight loss Yellow jaundice skin and itching In severe cases hospitalisation *Chronic* Chronic hepatitis Liver cirrhosis Liver cancer	*Acute* Short mild flu-like illness Nausea and vomiting Diarrhoea Loss of appetite Weight loss Yellow jaundice skin and itching In severe cases hospitalisation *Chronic* Chronic hepatitis Liver cirrhosis Liver cancer	Most adults infected with Hepatitis B virus fully recover and develop lifelong immunity. 2-10% of adults will become chronic carriers. Antiretroviral therapy to treat.
Hepatitis C	Asymptomatic for many years, although liver damage can be developing. Chronic condition leading to cirrhosis of the liver. 1 in 4 people naturally resolve condition.	Asymptomatic for many years, although liver damage can be developing. Chronic condition leading to cirrhosis of the liver. 1 in 4 people naturally resolve condition.	Anti-viral drug therapy, that is effective on ≥ 50% of people treated. Antiretroviral therapy to treat.

which is relatively easy to treat, but left untreated can lead to a range of complications including:

- pelvic inflammatory disease (PID),
- ectopic pregnancy,
- tubal factor infertility (in women),
- epididymitis (in men),
- Reiter's syndrome (reactive arthritis).

A key factor in the concerns over the rise in diagnoses of Chlamydia was the fact that it was often asymptomatic. This could mean that for every case identified there would be many unaware of their infection with potentially complex and costly needs in the future. The programme began to role out in ten pilot sites in 2003, with another twenty six areas in 2004 before going nationwide 2006/7, (NCSP 2006; NCSP 2007).

Due to the hidden nature of Chlamydia, it was imperative that a model of practice was developed which would maximize the numbers of people tested. The programme has achieved this through promoting opportunistic screening in non-traditional settings as well as in established health care settings linking with a range of partners in other settings who come into contact with young people, for example youth services, schools and colleges.

As well as non-traditional settings for screening, the programme has used novel methods to engage with their intended client group. Examples include self-testing designed to increase access for those in rural areas or maximizing engagement with patients fearful of intrusive examination.

In 2007, the National Chlamydia Screening Programme and the Health Protection Agency highlighted the specific need to engage young men into the screening programme. In 2006/7, only 21.1% of all screens were from young men and whilst this was a clear improvement on the 7% in 2003/4, it was clear

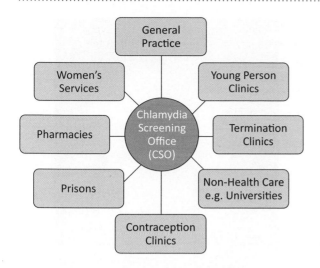

Fig. 16.10 The range of venues at which chlamydia screening is available. Adapted from © National Chlamydia Screening Programme

work needed to be done to address this. 'Men too' (NCSP, 2007), was subsequently launched. This strategy aimed to:

- raise awareness of the importance of screening men, both for their own sexual and reproductive health and to contribute to preventing reproductive morbidity in women;

- engage with the local NHS to ensure men can access screening;

- develop best practice in providing chlamydia screening for men.

In order to facilitate the achievement of these aims, a toolkit is being developed to enable practitioners to best meet the needs of young men.

Overall, the National Screening programme is now expected to screen 17% of the 15–25 population. In so doing, it is hoped that chlamydia screening will eventually become a routine facet of health care for all young people in this age group.

Sexual health prevention campaigns

To engage young people into service, the Department of Health has had to compete with a myriad of marketers, advertisers and entertainment providers all vying for the attention of this audience. As outlined in the 2001 National Strategy for Sexual Health and HIV, a major campaign was established to raise awareness in young people of the need to protect their sexual health. The overall campaign split young people into three distinct demographics with specifically targeted sub-campaigns designed to communicate appropriate key messages according to their perceived needs.

RUThinking

Target audience: 13–17 year old sexually inexperienced young people.

Aims: To provide consistent accurate information about sex and relationships in order to dispel myths and to correct false beliefs.

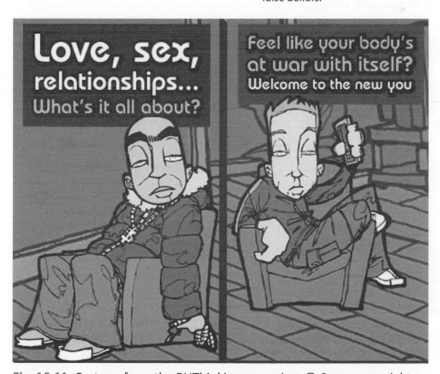

Fig. 16.11 Cartoon from the RUThinking campaign. © Crown copyright

Key messages:

- supports delaying the onset of sexual activity;
- highlights need for contraception in all sexual activity;
- outlines the range of contraception available to young people;
- promotes condom use to prevent STIs.

Website: http://www.ruthinking.co.uk/

Want respect?

Target audience: 16–18 year old sexually active young people.

Aims: To promote condom use by association with social success and consequently link lack of use with negative peer response.

Key messages:

- Want respect? Use a condom;
- Lose respect if you don't.

Website: None at present but utilizes TV, cinema and other media.

Condom Essential Wear

Target audience: 18–24 year olds engaging in sexually risky behaviour.

Aims: To normalize condom possession and use.

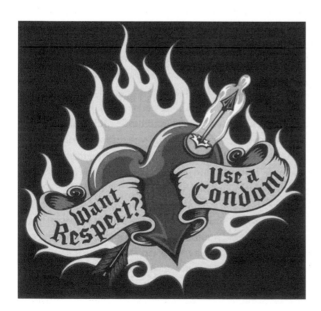

Fig. 16.12 Cartoon from the Want respect? campaign. © Crown copyright.

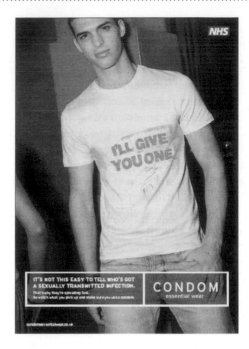

Fig. 16.13 Poster from the Condom Essential Wear campaign. © Crown copyright

Key messages:

- Sex is great but if not protected can lead to harm;
- Outlines the real risks of unprotected sex.

Website: http://www.condomessentialwear.co.uk/

The campaigns have been running now for a number of years and have explored a range of platforms in order to communicate effectively with young people. The effectiveness of these campaigns is being monitored on an ongoing basis by the Department of Health in consultation with young people themselves and sexual health professionals from the individual Strategic Health Authorities across England.

The targetting of the three campaigns to three discreet demographic groups is a key aspect of an approach known as social marketing.

> **Box 16.5** Social marketing
>
> Definitions and examples of social marketing in practice can be found at
>
> **http://www.nsms.org.uk/public/default.aspx**

HPV vaccination programme

The human papilloma virus (HPV) is extremely common and at least 100 genotypes of the virus have been identified to date, including forty which are linked to sexual acquisition and two key strains (16 and 18) which are thought to be responsible for 70% of cervical cancers in women.

In 2007 the Department of Health announced the launch of an immunization programme designed to reduce morbidity and mortality associated with cervical cancer in the UK. The programme would target young women aged 12–13 and immunize against the two key strains of HPV linked to cervical cancer (DH, 2008a).

Box 16.6 Immunization controversy

Despite clear intentions to reduce serious health problems in the population this programme was not met with universal approval. Parents, practitioners and some religious groups opposed the programme fiercely on the grounds that it would promote sexual promiscuity and early onset of sexual activity. What do you think of these concerns?

Some clinical professionals have criticized the choice of vaccine used in the programme. In the UK, a bivalent vaccine Cervarix has been chosen which protects against strains 16 and 18, instead of Gardasil, a quadravalent product which protects additionally against strains 6 and 11 which are also linked with genital warts. What do you think of this decision?

Are there any other aspects of this programme which you feel would need to be addressed in future? Do you feel immunizing only young women is equitable?

The role of the nurse

Today nurses need to develop a holistic approach to nursing care, were sexual health issues should be addressed alongside all other health concerns. The role of the nurse is crucial in creating a safe environment were patients feel comfortable to speak freely and in confidence regarding all health matters including their sexual health and sexuality. Nurses with limited knowledge should therefore make appropriate referral, with patient consent, to a sexual health service or health professional who can offer further advise, support and care to meet specific patient needs.

Nurses from any field with a special interest in sexual health can develop their skills by attending specific courses, which may include family planning and contraception, child protection, HIV/AIDS and genito-urinary medicine (GUM).

According to the best practice document *Effective Commissioning of Sexual Health and HIV Services* (DH, 2003) nurses are pivotal to the successful delivery of the *Strategy for Sexual Health and HIV* (DH, 2001a). They have a key role in educating, managing and supporting service users and patients across both clinical and non-clinical settings. Nurses involved in sexual health provision therefore need a sound knowledge base to successfully engage confidently with patients and their families in the promotion of sexual health. This requires many skills including obtaining thorough sexual histories, examining, screening/investigations, undertaking microscopy, treating, information sharing and dealing sensitively with very personal and confidential issues. Effective communication is paramount to ensure individual sexual health needs of the patient are recognized and managed appropriately.

Discussion box

How would you feel discussing sexual health matters with a patient?

What qualities would you need to address sexual health issues with a patient?

What are the benefits of addressing sexual health issues with patients?

Appropriately trained nurses who may provide sexual health care as part of their role include specialist Sexual Health Nurses, Family Planning Nurses, Practice Nurses, School Nurses, Gynaecology Nurses, Prison Nurses, Health Visitors and Midwives. Some trained nurses may also perform genital examinations and screening as part of their role. Within the Sexual Health Service, nurses, as key health professionals, are vital to the achievement of sexual health targets, set by policies at both national and local level.

There are several key documents, which have attributed to the advancement of nurses working in the field of sexual health. The documents are *Making a Difference* (DH 1999a), *The NHS Plan* (DH, 2000a), *The National Strategy for Sexual Health and HIV* (DH, 2001a), *Choosing Health: Making Healthy Choices Easier* (DH, 2004a), which are all drivers for change and the development of increased nurse-led sexual health services. Finally, the Medfash *Recommended Standards for Sexual Health Services* (2005), BASHH *Standards for Sexual Health Services* (BASHH, 2005) and *The 10 High Impact Changes for Genitourinary Medicine (*DH, 2006; DH, 2008b*),* placed nursing and sexual health on the national agenda. The National Strategy set out three levels of service provision (refer to Box 16.7). Level One services should be available in all GP Practices, Level Two at GP practices who maintain a special interest and Level Three at Centres for Sexual Health. The nurses working within the difference practices will therefore reflect different levels of competence, depending on their training and job description.

> **Box 16.7** Levels of sexual health service provision
>
> **Level One**
>
> • Sexual history taking and risk assessment,
> • STI testing for women,
> • HIV testing and counselling,
> • Pregnancy testing and referral,
> • Contraceptive information and services,
> • Assessment and referral of men with STI symptoms,
> • Cervical cytology screening and referral,
> • Hepatitis B immunization.
>
> **Level Two**
>
> All level one plus:
>
> • Intrauterine insertion (IUD/Coil),
> • Testing and treating STIs,
> • Vasectomy,
> • Contraceptive implant insertion,
> • Partner notification,
> • Invasive STI testing for men
>
> **Level Three**
>
> All of level one and two plus:
>
> • Outreach of STI infection prevention,
> • Outreach contraception services,
> • Specialized infections management, including coordination of partner notification,
> • Highly specialized contraception,
> • Specialized HIV treatment and care.

Nurses who provide sexual health support and promotion

Nurses play a vital role in sexual health promotion and HIV prevention (RCN, 2001). They build awareness of sexual health and help patients access the information and services they need.

• **Sexual Health Nurses** — These are nurses who work in the field of genito-urinary medicine caring and managing clients with suspected and diagnosed STIs and HIV. There are several levels of nursing ranging from the Staff Nurse, Senior Nurse and Health Advisor to Specialist Nurse, Nurse Practitioner and Consultant Nurse. All have vital roles offering sexual health advice, screening, treatments, contraception and contact tracing to address the Social Exclusion Unit (1999) report on *Teenage Pregnancy* and *The National Strategy for Sexual Health and HIV* (DH, 2001a).

• **Family Planning Nurses** — Many nurses/midwives choose to study and obtain a family planning qualification to enhance their roles. For example, a family planning trained practice nurse or school nurse may supply contraception and sexual health promotion and education to patients as part of their role or may work in a specific family planning clinic.

• **School Nurses** — *Saving Lives* (DH, 2000b) and *Making a Difference* (DH, 2001b) supports the public health role of school nurses. The role promotes healthy living of children and young adults and includes health screening and surveillance and therapeutic interventions for individuals, including meeting sexual health needs.

• **Midwives** — Midwives are essential providers of sexual health education. They provide preconception, antenatal, parentcraft, healthy living and post-natal care, and play a crucial role in antenatal STIs and HIV screening.

• **Prison Nurses** — Nurses working in prisons provide sexual health promotion and treatments. Prisoners receive screening for STIs and blood-borne viruses and are offered Hepatitis B immunization. Some prisons offer nurses a lead role in sexual health.

• **Health Visitors** — In *Saving Lives* (DH, 2000b), these public health professionals are identified as having a key role in the delivery of health improvement, providing information, advice and support on issues such as parenting, personal relationships, healthy lifestyles and sexual health.

> ## Nursing Practice box
>
> *The Code* set by the Nursing and Midwifery Council (2008) reiterates the requirement to be non-judgemental in practice. Nurses need to be sensitive in their approach to recognizing client's individual needs and avoid being judgemental.

Evidence-based practice

As a nurse, it is essential that you remain updated with policies and guidance in relation to client care and management, to ensure that best care is provided. Often, the choice of treatment is based not only upon the effectiveness of the therapy, but also the cost and availability of the medication, considering the current climate where monetary constraints exist within the National Health Service (NHS). Implementing evidence based practice is a complex but valued process that requires support for nurses to make it a reality in care delivery. This requires effective and updated local and national guidance on service delivery. To assist Sexual Health Services and individuals with the identification of 'best practice', the British Association for Sexual Health and HIV (BASHH) have developed and regularly update comprehensive guidelines for the treatment and suppression of STIs and HIV.

Details can be found at http://www.bashh.org

Understanding confidentiality

According to the Nursing and Midwifery Council *The Code* (NMC, 2008) a duty of confidence arises when one person discloses information to another in circumstances where it is reasonable to expect that the information will be held in confidence. This duty is derived from both common law and statute law.

All clients seeking sexual health services should be certain that their right to confidentiality would be respected and maintained in line with *The Code* (NMC, 2008). *The National Health Service Venereal Disease Regulations (SI 1974 No.29)* is key legislation now part of the *NHS Trusts and Primary Care Trusts (Sexually Transmitted Diseases) Directions 2000*, to ensure health authorities take necessary steps to protect the individual client's identity from disclosure when accessing sexual health services, (DH, 2000c).

> ## Box 16.8 Respect people's confidentiality
>
> NMC (2008)
>
> - You must respect people's right to confidentiality.
> - You must ensure people are informed how and why information is shared by those who will be providing their care.
> - You must disclose information if you believe someone may be at risk of harm, in line with the law of the country in which you are practising.

As a nurse you therefore have a duty of confidentiality. This means that you must not disclose anything learned from a client, whom you have consulted, examined or treated, without that person's consent (RCGP, 2000).

Within the sexual health service, GPs are not routinely informed of any attendance/diagnosis/treatment provided,

unless shared care is agreed, for example, to link in with follow-up treatment.

Considerations for sexual health work with young people

Fraser guidelines

As a nurse, you can provide advice and treatment to under 16s, as long as you are satisfied that the young person is competent and fully aware and consenting to all care provided. These guidelines were initially compiled to enable health professionals to provide contraception to under 16s and were issued in 1985, as part of Lord Fraser's judgement. As a result, the Fraser Guidelines continue to support practitioners in their decisions to treat young people under 16 respecting their individual rights to confidentiality (DH, 2004b).

> ## Box 16.9 The Fraser guidelines
>
> It is considered good practice for workers to follow the *Fraser Guidelines* when discussing personal or sexual matters with a young person under 16. The framework provides guidance to doctors, social care and health professionals in England and Wales on providing advice and treatment to young people under 16 years of age. These hold that sexual health services can be offered without parental consent providing that:
>
> - The young person understands the advice that is being given.
> - The young person cannot be persuaded to inform or seek support from their parents and will not allow the worker to inform the parents that contraceptive advice is being given.
> - The young person is likely to begin or continue to have sexual intercourse without contraception.
> - The young person's physical or mental health is likely to suffer unless they receive contraceptive advice or treatment.
> - It is in the young person's best interest to receive contraceptive advice and treatment without parental consent.
>
> See: http://ww.brook@org.uk/content/M6_4_undersixteens.asp

However, where a health professional believes that there is a risk to the health, safety or welfare of a young person, locally agreed child protection protocols exist and should be followed. Ideally disclosure should take place after consulting the young person, unless in exceptional circumstances, were informing the young person may lead to further harm occurring until support mechanisms are put in place.

The law and sex

The legal age for young people to have sex is still sixteen, whether they are heterosexual, gay or bi-sexual. According to *The Sexual Offences Act 2003* (OPSI, 2003), the aim of the law is to protect the rights and interests of young people, and make it easier to prosecute people who pressure, entice or force others into having unwanted sexual relationships. The Law is not intended to prosecute mutually agreed teenage sexual activity between two young people of similar age. Importantly, those professionals providing sexual health advice and care to young people should be reassured that they are acting lawfully if they act for the purposes of:

- Protecting the child from sexually transmitted infections, or
- Protecting the physical safety of the child, or
- Preventing the child from becoming pregnant, or
- Promoting the child's emotional well-being by the giving of advice.

Sexual Offences Act 2003, Section14 (2) and(3)

Informing clients of the legal situation

Young people should be aware of the legislation concerning their sexual activity to help them make informed choices about their behaviour. However, as young people may be deterred from accessing help for fear that their partner could face prosecution, information about the law should not undermine the essential message that the service remains confidential unless the professional undertaking the assessment believes that the young person is at risk of harm.

For further guidance on practice with young people see Open University website.

Remember clients should have the assurance of confidentiality with regard to their consultations, regardless of age, gender, sexual orientation, religion or ethnicity, unless the clinician has concerns about client well-being and/or safety (FFPRHC, 2006).

Box 16.10 Confidentiality — key points

- Know 'The Code' — your professional body's standards of conduct, performance and ethics (Nursing and Midwifery Council, 2008).
- Familiarize yourself with the confidentiality policy of the workplace. In sexual health clinics and family planning clinics it is recommended to display the confidentiality statement in the premises.
- You should be provided with sexual health training if you work within the sexual health service.
- You should be provided with specific training to work with young people and vulnerable adults and be aware of local and national policies (General Medical Council, 2004).
- Prior to working with the under 16s, you should be familiar with the *Fraser Guidelines* and the Legal Issues (DH, 2004b; OPSI, 2003).
- *The Sexual Offences Act 2003* does not affect the ability of health professionals working with young people to provide confidential advice or treatment within the field of sexual and reproductive health.
- Child Protection training days are held within hospitals and also accredited courses are held at colleges and universities to equip staff with the appropriate skills to deal with the recognition and management of children in need. A local 'safeguarding children nursing team' should be accessible to all nurses, where concerns can be discussed and advice sought. Don't panic! If worried, discuss concerns with your mentor/colleagues/nurse in charge.
- Never discuss information with anyone outside the service unless specific permission/consent has been sought from the client. Practice within safe professional boundaries.

Case Study 16.1: A 15 year old young man

A 15 year old young man asks the Practice Nurse for condoms. What advice and support do you think he should be offered?

Discussion points

Guidance for practice answers

- Establish confidentiality and any potential limitations i.e. services are confidential to under 16s, except where the individual is being harmed or suspected of harming some-one else.

- Reiterate law on sex, discussing consensual sex.
- Establish age of partner in order to rule out coercion.
- Demonstrate condom use and check client's understanding.
- Determine competence using Fraser guidance.
- If unprotected sex disclosed discuss access to local sexual health services.
- Discuss 'safer sex', love, relationships and risky behaviours.
- Dispense condoms and invite client to return for further supplies.

Sexual health in other nursing roles

Although there are specific nursing roles pertaining to sexual health promotion and care, all nurses should remain mindful of sexual health in their practice in order to provide holistic care for their patients. Nurses need to recognize that sexuality and sexual health is an important area of nursing care and that we all have a professional and clinical responsibility to address it. For example, nurses working in a residential care home for the elderly, must not assume that the patient's need for sexual expression has ceased. Such ignorance could lead staff not to recognize signs of sexual abuse, as they believe older people to be a 'no risk' group. Similarly, the nurses should consider the needs of all patient groups, including those with physical disabilities or with mental health issues.

'Providing sexuality and sexual health care can be an inti-mate process and nurse typecasting can lead to misunder-standing from patients and colleagues. It is therefore important for nurses to maintain a professional and non-judgemental attitude in their work'
RCN, 2000:1

Nurses should remain observant and familiar with the signs and symptoms of sexual abuse and exploitation, including the recognition of vulnerable young people and adults. This may include disaffected young people, sex workers, older people, patients with disabilities (whether learning or physical) or those with mental health problems. An understanding of these factors further enhances the importance of sexual health promotion and education geared towards the individ-ual and wider population.

When dealing with sexual health issues, the nurse needs to work within safe professional boundaries and must abide by his/her job description and policies within the workplace. For example, if two people are having sex and one or both has

learning difficulties or physical difficulties, the nurse has a duty of care to ensure it is consensual sex between both parties and not just make assumptions. Also, if both parties are consenting to sex and of the legal age, privacy and dignity must be consid-ered. In such cases, a team approach may be adopted and the sexual health needs included in the care plans. This will also provide peer support to individual key workers involved in the provision of care.

The Family Planning Association (FPAa) provide a very informative website on sexual health, pregnancy choices (including abortion), planning a pregnancy, contraception methods and sexually transmitted infections (STIs). **http://www.fpa.org.uk**

Contraceptive methods

The prevention of an unwanted pregnancy is a prime concern of many couples and individuals worldwide. Contraception plays an important role in modern society. John Guillebaud (2007) a highly respected professor of family planning and reproductive health and author of several reputable books on contraception reiterates that sex education must promote (as recognized in the Netherlands) the societal norm that sex is a feature of a good relationship only with the existence of ade-quate contraception.

Nurses, Midwives and Health Visitors are in key positions to either signpost patients to appropriate contraceptive services or provide advice and contraception within their role. Many obstacles preventing people accessing contraceptive services is that they are unaware, or do not understand the choices available too them. During patient consultation the clinician should discuss the full range of contraceptive options available from condoms to long-acting reversible contraceptives (LARC) and tailor to meet individual needs. Taking a thorough medical and sexual history, considering lifestyle, age, sexuality, career choice and past and present contraceptive use are all factors to be considered. For example a young woman commencing a three year university course may benefit from a LARC method of contraception such as the implant, whilst a mother breast-feeding her baby might consider a progestogen-only pill or an intrauterine devise.

Methods of contraception

Box 6.11 Method of contraception

Barrier
- male and female condoms.
- diaphragms/caps with spermicide.

Combined hormonal contraceptives

- containing two female sex hormones, oestrogen and progestogen,
- combined oral contraceptive pill— commonly called 'the pill',
- contraceptive patch,
- vaginal ring.

Progestogen-only methods

- Progestogen-only pill, commonly called 'the mini-pill'.
- emergency contraception.

Long-acting Reversible Contraceptives (LARC)

- contraceptive injection Depo-Provera (progestogen-only) lasts for 12 weeks.
- implant (progestogen-only) lasts for three years.
- intrauterine system (IUS) — known as the 'hormonal coil' (progestogen-only). Works for five years.
- intrauterine device (IUD) traditional coil with no hormone. Can stay 3-10 years depending on type.

Natural family planning — using fertility indicators shows when you can have sex without risking pregnancy.

Female and male sterilization — the fallopian tubes in women or the vas deferens tube in men are cut (vasectomy).

With increasing numbers of unplanned pregnancies leading to abortion reported by the Office for National Statistics and Department of Health (2008) there is a government push to increase use of Long Acting Reversible Contraception (LARC). This is supported by the National Institute for Health and Clinical Excellence (NICE, 2005).

Medicines management

The *NHS Plan* (DH, 2000a) emphasizes the necessity to organize and deliver services around the needs of the patients. One area in which an increase in nurse-led activity can be identified as improving the quality and continuity of patient care, is in medicines management (DH, 2005).

Since *The Crown Report* (DH, 1998 and1999b), specific nurses can now be trained to either prescribe or supply and administer medication under strict guidance. A combination of independent prescribing, supplementary prescribing and Patient Group Directions (PGDs) can be used to enable patients to receive STI treatment and contraception from nurses. Further information on medicines management for nurses can be found on the National Prescribing Centre (NPC) website: **http://ww.npc.co.uk/non_medical.htm**

Managing unplanned pregnancies

The National Strategy for Sexual Health and HIV (DH, 2001a) acknowledged a strong link between social deprivation and STIs, abortions and teenage conceptions. It also identified how unintended pregnancies increase the risk of poor social, economic and health outcomes for both mother and child.

The determinants of teenage unplanned pregnancies are complex and multifaceted . However, there are strong socio-economic links to high rates in the population. Preventing teenage unplanned pregnancies is therefore more complex than simply providing accessible contraceptive services and sex education. Nevertheless, the provision of accessible sexual and reproductive health services for young people is an important part of any programme aiming to reduce teenage pregnancy rates.

One of the key aims of *The Sexual Health and HIV Strategy* (DH, 2001a) is to reduce the number of unintended pregnancies, through better access to contraception. The Department of Health (2004b) includes the national target, set out in the Government service agreement "to reduce the under 18 year old's conception rate by 50% by 2010, as part of a broader strategy to improve sexual health." Also, for those women seeking an abortion and who meet the legal requirement, accessing an early abortion requires prompt onward referral. Improvements to access to abortions are therefore necessary. The Commissioning document (DH, 2003) recommends that services offer arrangements which minimize delay, such as telephone referral systems and direct access from referral sources other than GPs, including self-referral. As a nurse, it is beneficial to familiarize yourself with abortion referral services in the local area. This will enable you to signpost the patient to the appropriate service. Printed information on abortion services should also be available in GP Practices, Health Centres, Family Planning and Sexual Health Services. Abortions are usually provided by an NHS hospital or specialist provider such as the British Pregnancy Advisory Service (BPAS) or Marie Stopes (non profit-making organizations).

Nurses have an important role to play in the provision of abortion services. As a family planning nurse, midwife, practice nurse, sexual health nurse or gynaecology nurse you may be the person who performs the pregnancy test confirming the pregnancy and then discusses pregnancy options and referral to pregnancy advisory or maternity services, as necessary. Although the requirements of the Abortion Act 1967, as amended, is that a pregnancy may only be terminated by a registered medical practitioner, generally it is a nurse, who will provide physical and psychological support to the patient. Nurses who do not wish to be involved in the abortions are able to make a conscientious objection. However, as a nurse, there is a moral and professional responsibility to direct a woman to a nurse/doctor who can give unbiased information and support for abortion if requested.

> **Box 16.12** Medical abortion versus surgical abortion
>
> • Early medical abortion is a preferable option to surgery, as it carries significantly reduced risk of complications and can be less distressing.
>
> • Medical abortion is a more cost-effective use of NHS resources.
>
> • Some patients prefer the idea of not being awake during the procedure, which a surgical termination would offer.
>
> • Waiting for a surgical procedure may lead to a late abortion.

Summary

The chapter has identified how nurses play a vital role in the provision of sexual health services. Sexual health promotion and HIV prevention support the Government's *NHS Plan* (DH, 2000a) and *HIV and Sexual Health* Strategy (DH, 2001a). These documents provide opportunities for nurses to work in new ways to deliver holistic care to clients. Nurses, midwives and health visitors need to have a basic understanding of sexual health so that they can identify a patient's individual sexual health needs. Employers have a duty to provide training to enable the nurse to identify and provide care or refer to appropriate professionals as necessary. Nurses can successfully address teenage and unwanted pregnancy rates and rising STI rates in their local area by raising awareness of sexual health issues and helping individuals to access the information and services they need.

Online Resource Centre

For more information on sexual health visit the Online Resource Centre —
http://www.oxfordtextbooks.co.uk/orc/linsley/

References

Adams, J. (2001). *Doing it! Toolkit: Practical Strategies for Sexual Health Promotion* Sheffield: Sheffield Centre for Sexual Health.

British Association for Sexual Health and HIV (2005). *Consultation for the Standards for Sexual Health Services.* London: BASHH.

Department of Health (1998). *A Report on the Supply and Administration of Medicines under Group Protocol (Crown Report, Part 1).* London: DH.

Department of Health (1999a). *Making a Difference: Strengthening the Nursing Midwifery and Health Visiting Contribution to Health and Healthcare.* London: DH.

Department of Health (1999b). *Review of Prescribing, Supply and Administration of Medicines (Crown II) Final Report.* London: DH.

Department of Health (2000a). *The NHS Plan: A Plan for investment, A Plan for Reform.* London: DH.

Department of Health (2000b). *Saving Lives: Our Healthier Nation.* London: DH.

Department of Health (2000c). *NHS Trusts and Primary Care Trusts (Sexually Transmitted Diseases) Directions 2000.* London: DH.

Department of Health (2001a). *The National Strategy for HIV and Sexual Health: Better Prevention, Better Services, Better Sexual Health.* London: DH.

Department of Health (2001b). *Making a Difference in Primary Care.* London: DH.

Department of Health (2003). *Effective Commissioning for Sexual Health Services.* London: DH.

Department of Health (2004a). *Choosing Health: Making Healthy Choices Easier.* London: DH.

Department of Health (2004b). *Best Practice Guidance for Doctors and Other Health Professionals on the Provision of Advice and Treatment to Young People under 16 on Contraception, Sexual and Reproductive Health.* July. London: DH.

Department of Health (2005). *Evaluation of Extended Formulary Independent Nurse Prescribing: Executive Summary.* Southampton: University of Southampton School of Nursing and Midwifery.

Department of Health (2006) *10 Impact Changes for Genitourinary Medicine 48 hour Access.* London: DH.

Department of Health (2008a). *HPV in Immunization Against Infectious Disease 'the Green Book'.* London :Health Protection Agency.

Department of Health (2008b). *Genitourinary Medicine 48 hour access: Getting to Target and Staying There.* London: COI

Department of Health, Social Services and Public Safety Northern Ireland (2008). Sexual *Health Promotion Strategy and Action Plan 2008–2013.* Belfast: DHSSPS.

Faculty of Family Planning and Reproductive Health Care (2006). Service Standards for Sexual Health Services. January 2006. www.ffprhc.org.uk

Family Planning Association (2005). *The Economics of Sexual Health: Findings.* London: FPA. www.fpa.org.uk

General Medical Council (2004). *Guidance on Good Practice — Confidentiality: Protecting and Providing Information.* London: GMC. www.gmc-uk.org

Guillebaud J. (2007). *Contraception Today.* Sixth Edition. London: Martin Dunitz.

Health Protection Agency (2005). *Mapping the Issus: HIV and other Sexually Transmitted Infections in the United Kingdom.* London: HPA. www.hpa.org.uk

Health Protection Agency (2006). *A Complex Picture.* London: HPA.

Health Protection Agency (2007a). *Testing Times: HIV and other Sexually Transmitted Infections in the United Kingdom.* London: HPA.

Health Protection Agency (2007b). *Health Protection Report* 1:35. London: HPA.

Health Protection Agency (2008). *Sexually Transmitted Infections and Young People in the UK*. London: HPA

Medical Foundation for Sexual Health and HIV (2005). *Recommended Standards for Sexual Health Services*. London: Medfash.

Medical Foundation for AIDS and Sexual Health. (2008). *Progress and Priorities — Working Together for High Quality Sexual Health. Review of the National Strategy for Sexual Health and HIV*. London: Med FASH

Mussen J., Naidoo J., Wills J. (1998). *Sexual Health Promotion in Practising Health Promotion*. London: Bailliere Tindall.

National Assembly for Wales (2000). *A Strategic Framework for Promoting Sexual Health in Wales*. London: Health Promotion Division.

National Chlamydia Screening Programme (2006). *New Frontiers: Annual Report of the National Chlamydia Screening Programme in England 2005/06*. London: Health Protection Agency.

National Chlamydia Screening Programme (2007). *Men Too*. London: NCSP.

National Institute for Health and Clinical Excellence (2005) *Clinical Guideline No.30: Long-acting Reversible Contraception*. London: NICE.

Nursing & Midwifery Council (2008). *The Code: Standards for Conduct, Performance and Ethics*. London: NMC. **www.nmc-uk.org**

Office for National Statistics & Department of Health (2008). Statistical Bulletin, Abortion Statistics: England and Wales 2007. London: ONS.

Office of Public Sector Information (2003) The Sexual Offences Act. London: OPSI (Home Office).

Royal College of General Practitioners and Brook (2000). The Confidentiality and Young People Toolkit. Londn: RCGP.

Royal College of Nursing (2000). Sexuality and Sexual Health in Nursing Practice: An RCN Ddiscussion and Guidance Document for Nurses who want to Develop their Nursing Practice in the Field of Sexuality and Sexual Health. London: RCN.

Royal College of Nursing (2001) RCN Sexual Health Strategy: Guidance for Nursing Staff. London: RCN.

Scottish Executive (2005). Respect and Responsibility: Strategy and Action Plan for Improving Sexual Health. Edinburgh: SE.

Social Exclusion Unit (1999). The Teenage Pregnancy Strategy. London: Social Exclusion Unit.

Wellings, K. et al., Johnson, A.M., Mercer, C.H., Erens, B., Copas, A.J., & McManus, S., (2001). Sexual Behaviour in Britain: Partnerships, Practices and HIV Risk Behaviours. Lancet 2001; 358(9296):1835–1842.

World Health Organization (2002). Defining Sexual Health: Report of a Technical Consultation on Sexual Health, Geneva: WHO Press.

Chapter 17
Mental health

Paul Linsley and John Hurley

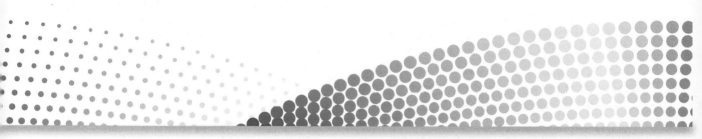

Introduction

Many of us will know of someone who has suffered a mental health problem, although we may not have recognized it as such. It is likely that some of us will have felt uncomfortable or even frightened by these people — wondering what to them and whether it is safe to ask them how they feel? These feelings can often arise from not understanding why people experience such problems and how to support and respond to those who have a mental illness.

The following chapter provides you with an introduction to mental health and in particular mental health promotion. It looks at the complexities of providing care to people with a mental health problem and the challenge this presents for nurses as part of their everyday practice. Major policy initiatives pertaining to mental health are discussed as are a series of measures to promote positive mental health. The chapter also looks at the role of the nurse in supporting those people with a mental health problem and the contribution that people can make to maintain their own mental well being.

Defining mental ill health

Mental illness is a term that describes a broad range of mental and emotional conditions that significantly interfere with a person's ability to conduct the tasks needed for day-to-day living (Corey, 2002). It is a collective term that refers to all the different types of mental conditions, including those that affect mood, thinking and behaviour. Mental disorders are of different types and different degrees of severity. To be classified as a mental illness a condition must cause functional impairment in people, in one or more areas of their life, such as in work, in relationships or in social situations.

Box 17.1 Classes of mental ill health

Mental ill health is based on the symptoms a person experiences and the clinical features of the illness (WHO, 2007; American Psychiatric Association, 1994). The main classes of mental ill health are:

Psychotic disorders
These disorders impair a person's sense of reality, the most notable example of a psychotic disorder being schizophrenia, although other classes of disorder can be associated with psychosis at times.

Mood disorders
These include disorders that affect how the person feels, such as persistent sadness or feelings of elation. Mood disorders include clinical depression and bipolar disorder.

Anxiety disorders
Anxiety is an emotion characterized by the anticipation of future danger or an extreme feeling of being ill at ease. Examples include panic disorder, obsessive-compulsive disorder, specific phobias and generalized anxiety disorder.

Cognitive disorders

These disorders affect the person's ability to think and reason. They include delirium, dementia and memory problems. The most well known cognitive disorder is Alzheimer's disease.

Developmental disorders

Developmental disorders cover a wide range of problems that usually first begin to make themselves known in early childhood or adolescence. They include autism, attention deficit disorder and learning disabilities. Although they come under the same group, there is not necessarily a relationship between these disorders.

Personality disorders

A personality disorder is an enduring pattern of behaviour that is dysfunctional and leads to distress or impairment, such as anti-social personality disorder.

Dissociative disorders

This is a type of disorder in which a person's sense of self is disrupted, such as when there are physical symptoms in the absence of a clear physical cause, such as hypochondriasis.

The term 'serious mental illness' is sometimes used to refer to a more severe, long-lasting disorder, such as schizophrenia, whilst the phrase 'mental health problem' is used to refer to milder, more transient problems such as anxiety or mild depression (WHO, 2008).

Someone can experience a mental illness over many years. The type, intensity and duration of symptoms vary from person to person. They come and go and do not always follow a regular pattern, making it difficult to predict when symptoms

---

Box 17.2 Older people and mental health problems

Mental health problems are among the most common forms of ill health. They place a heavy burden on individuals, their families and friends and the community at large. They also impose substantial economic costs on the Health Service. The National Institute for Mental Health in England (NIMHE, 2005) estimates that 40% of older people seeing their general practitioner, 50% of older people staying in general hospitals, and 60% of care home residents may have a mental health problem. Other age groups are affected by mental health issues. It is estimated that as many as 1 in 6 people at any point in time suffer from a diagnosed condition such as depression or anxiety (NICE, 2006; WHO, 2008).

---

and functioning will flare-up, even if treatment recommendations are followed.

Causes of mental ill health

We do not know for sure what causes mental ill health but most studies suggest that a combination of factors contribute to the onset, recovery, and severity of most mental health problems. The factors that influence well-being are interrelated (NICE, 2005). For example, a job provides not just money but purpose, goals, friendships and a sense of belonging. Some factors also make up for the lack of others; for example, a good marriage can compensate for a lack of friendships, while religious beliefs may help a person come to terms with physical illness. Many of these factors lie outside the control of the health and social services, and indeed of government. The natural capacity of people to make decisions about what is or is not good for them can be compromised by either internal or external factors, or both. Factors which may compromise mental or emotional well-being include:

Genetic factors

Some mental health problems may occur more often in families where there is a history of mental illness. For example, schizophrenia is said to be 'familiar' within generations of some families (Drake and Lewis, 2005; Barnes and Pant, 2002). Suicide rates are higher in males than females, across all age groups (WHO, 2008).

Biological factors

Age and gender are believed to affect the rates and prevalence of mental illness especially when combined with other environmental factors (NIMHE, 2007). For example, some studies suggest that young gay or lesbian people may have an increased risk of suicidal behaviour, possibly through being more likely to experience prejudice, homelessness, depression and substance use.

Psychological factors

Low self-esteem and self-worth, an inability to cope with stress and organize thoughts and make sense of feelings can all contribute to mental illness. For example, substance use — alcohol and other drugs—can exacerbate other mental illnesses and may decrease inhibitions and increase impulsive and risky behaviour (WHO, 2005a).

Environmental factors

Stresses due to finances, relationships, family background, and access to health care and social supports are all believed to affect mental health (WHO, 2008). Some examples might include recent loss of a significant person, relationship break-down, or disciplinary or legal crisis.

Divorce or separation may leave family members feeling isolated and vulnerable and increase the risk of depression (Arroll, Khin and and Kerse, 2004). Marital discord, family conflict, and domestic violence can all have serious repercussions, as does child abuse.

Social disadvantage and economic disadvantage may increase the risks of mental health problems and suicidal behaviour.

Mental health problems and the risk of self-harming behaviours may be higher among young people who are disengaged from school, which may result in non-participation, early school-leaving, truancy and suspension (Selekman, 2006).

Social Isolation, due to unemployment, or homelessness, or living in a remote place can all impact on the mental health of a person.

Physical factors

Symptoms of mental illness can be found to occur in people with a physical illness (Kendal, 2006). For example, people who experience a chronic physical illness may also experience depression. In turn, a person's experience of a physical illness may be affected by their mental health.

Having a risk factor for mental illness increases the chances of getting a condition but does not always lead to mental illness. Some factors such as poverty and community conflict affect people than others to a greater extent. Some factors affect us irrespective of age, such as family breakdown, sexual or emotional abuse, social exclusion or discrimination, domestic violence or bullying. Others have particular affects at different stages of our lives — during childhood, young adulthood and when we are older.

Discussion points

Sally is a student nurse in the second year of her studies. Her standard of work has deteriorated over the last couple of weeks; she seems to lack any energy and is finding it difficult to apply herself. It is known amongst her peers, that Sally has recently split up with her husband and is finding it difficult to cope with their two children who are missing their father. There are early indications that Sally might be suffering from a **reactive depression** owing to her change in circumstances.

Questions:

- How do you think you would feel towards Sally?
- How do you think that you would respond to Sally's deteriorating situation?
- Should you 'get involved'?

Mental health approaches generally assume that problems are multi-causal, that everyone is vulnerable to stressful life events, and that any disability or problem may arise as a consequence (Soundy, Faulkner and Taylor, 2007). For example, four vulnerable people can face a stressful life event, such as the collapse of a marriage, as Sally did, but all experience very different consequences. One person may become severely depressed, the second may be involved in a car accident, the third may resort to increasing their consumption of alcohol, and the fourth suffer no ill effects at all, but find the whole event liberating.

Nursing Practice box

If you become concerned about an individual's mental health and well-being think about why this is.

According to the Centre of Excellence in Inter-Disciplinary Mental Health (CEIMH), typical signs that someone may be in difficulty include:

- **The individual telling you or someone else that he/she has a problem.**
- **Changes in the pattern or standard of work.**
- **Significant changes in appearance such as loss or gain of weight, deterioration of personal hygiene or signs of sleeplessness.**
- **A noticeable change of smell, which may result from increased use of alcohol or non-prescription drugs.**
- **Change in the way he or she sounds (for example flat tone, very quiet, loud, and agitated).**
- **Change of mood from previous experience of him or her (for example very up and down, miserable, tired).**
- **Other people, such as friends, housemates, relatives or other colleagues, expressing concern to you.**
- **Talk or evidence of self-harming behaviour such as arm cutting.**

(CEIMH 2009)

People develop different ways of coping during the course of their life. They learn to manage the demands made of them and exercise control over their choice and decision-making Lifestyles are built around patterns of response that have been established to cope with stressful situations and threats. These lifestyles are highly individual and necessary to protect and maintain a person's sense of well-being.

When challenged, people will often revert to coping strategies that have proved successful over time and from which they have found reward. Coping activities take a wide variety of forms including all diverse behaviours that people engage in to meet actual or anticipated challenges (Barker, 2009). Available coping mechanisms are those that people usually use when they have a problem. They may sit down and try to think the problem through or talk it over with a friend. Some might cry out their frustrations or try to get rid of their feelings of anger and hostility by swearing, kicking a chair, or slamming a door. Others may get into verbal battles with family and friends. Some may react by temporarily withdrawing from the situation in order to reassess the problem, while others will throw themselves into some form of activity in an effort not to think about their problem or difficulty.

These are just a few of the many coping methods people use to relieve tension and anxiety when faced with a problem. Each has been used at some time in the developmental past of the individual, has been found effective in maintaining emotional control and has become part of his or her lifestyle in meeting and dealing with the stresses of daily living.

Activity box

Watch the video on the Online Resource Centre of Mandy.

Mandy has a number of current anxieties that are impacting on her general well-being. Can you identify any of these from the video?

Stigma

There is no universally agreed cut-off point between normal behaviour and behaviour associated with mental illness. What is considered abnormal behaviour or an abnormal reaction to circumstances differs between cultures, social groups within the same culture, and even different social situations (NIMHE, 2004). Often, the only way to know whether someone has been diagnosed with a mental illness is if they tell you. The majority of the public are likely to be unaware of how many mentally ill people they know and encounter every day.

Stigma refers to the negative qualities and perceptions that are attributed to people with mental health problems. Stigma is often associated with discrimination, prejudice, and stereotypes (Barker, 2009). The label mental illness is highly stigmatizing. People often avoid or delay medical care and treatment for their mental health problems because of stigma and the fear others will see them as 'weak' or 'different' (WHO, 2005b). It encourages people to think of 'the mentally ill' as different, rather than seeing them as ordinary people who have more severe emotional difficulties to cope with. Popular misconceptions, fuelled by the media, see mentally ill people as violent and dangerous (WHO, 2005b). These stereotypes are contradicted by ordinary people's experiences of mental health problems affecting themselves, their friends, family and colleagues.

Looking at mental illness — a public health approach

Increasing recognition of mental illnesses, notably depression, as a major public health issue has led national and international public policies to place greater emphasis on improving the population's mental and emotional health status (Hope, 2004). Mental and physical health are deeply intertwined and interdependent While the need for evidence-based actions to tackle mental health problems is acknowledged, there is growing recognition of the need to better understand and conceptualize how to actively engage in mental health promotion as an integral part of public health (WHO, 2001). The actions taken increasingly rely on a public health approach that emphasizes the importance of the quality of societal and community life. These policies adopt a health improvement approach, which takes a broader view than the traditional psychiatric model of mental health. This approach aims to support people to achieve and maintain good mental health, as well as improve the well-being of communities.

Donovan et al. (2006) state that 'mental health promotion is attracting attention as health authorities become increasingly concerned with the rise in mental illnesses'. Accordingly, the National Institute for Health and, Clinical Excellence (2007) stated that mental health promotion was either the subject or a key feature of numerous recent policy and guidance documents, including:

- The **Disability Discrimination Act** 2005;
- **From Here to Equality: A Strategic Plan to Tackle Stigma and Discrimination on Mental Health Grounds, 2004–2009** (NIMHE, 2004);
- **Celebrating Our Cultures for Mental Health Promotion with Black and Minority Ethnic Communities** (DH 2004).

The Department of Health's National Service Framework for Mental Health, launched in 1999, is a long-term strategy to improve specific areas of mental health care. The framework is divided into seven standards which span five related areas:

1. Health promotion and stigma,
2. Primary care and access to specialist services,
3. The needs of people with severe and enduring mental illness,
4. Carers' needs,
5. Suicide reduction.

DH, 1999

Standard 1 in the National Service Framework for Mental Health (DH 1999) states that health and social care services should:

- Promote mental health for all, working with individuals and communities;
- Combat discrimination against individuals and groups with mental health problems, and promote their social inclusion.

If nurses and other health care professionals are serious about promoting mental health, they also need to consider and combat the discrimination and exclusion encountered by people who experience mental distress. In this way they can also start to address unseen mental health problems and promote well-being. Promoting well-being is a significant aspect of mental health promotion in which the focus is on wellness and enabling individuals to take control of their lives.

The Scottish Executive and the Welsh Assembly also emphasize the importance of mental health promotion. The Scottish Executive's **National Programme for Improving Mental Health and Well being 2003–2006** (Scottish Executive 2003) has four key aims:

1. Raising awareness and prompting mental health and well being;
2. Eliminating stigma and discrimination;
3. Preventing suicide;
4. Promoting and supporting recovery.

On the same theme, the Welsh Assembly's **Mental Health Promotion Action Plan for Wales** consultation document states that:

'Mental health promotion targets the whole population. It goes beyond treating mental ill health to proactively promoting well being and good mental health. The mental health status of an individual or population is constantly changing. It will respond to the circumstances confronting an individual or community such as employment status, quality of housing, access to leisure and a sense of security. It will also vary in accordance with an individual's ability to deal with these factors. This is often terms 'resilience'.
Welsh Assembly Government, 2006: 5–6

Similarly in Northern Ireland, the document **Promoting Mental Health: Strategy and Action Plan 20032008** (DHSSPS, 2003) outlines an integrated approach that addresses wider social, economic and cultural contexts of mental health. In particular it focuses on tackling inequalities under the headings:

- policy development,
- raising awareness and reducing stigma,
- improving knowledge and skills,
- preventing suicide.

These reports are built on the broad notions of health that recognize the range of social, economic and environmental factors that contribute to health. Mental health is understood not in terms of illness and disease but in terms of people's capacity to define, assess and analyze the determinants that influence their health (DH, 2001), and to access the resources they need to act on those determinants (see Chapter 3). When these conditions are met, people are enabled to adapt, respond to or control the challenges and changes in the environments that surround them (Keleher and Murphy, 2004).

If a determinants approach is taken to defining mental health promotion, then it is necessary to recognize the importance to mental health of ensuring people can develop the capacity to adapt to, respond to and/or control life's challenges and changes, and have the necessary resources to act on the circumstances that determine their mental health and well-being.

Consistent with health promotion generally, mental health promotion actions need to be multi-level and inter-sectoral, and concerned with systems change, policy and the development of evidence about what population-based programmes work. A key message for practitioners is that the inclusion in general health promotion programmes, of mental health promotion outcomes, will enhance their ability to achieve equity and tackle inequities (Mittelmark, 2003; Tilford, Delaney and Vogels, 1997). It involves looking beyond prevention, to the relationship between mental health and mental well-being as well as the mental health impact of public policies, programmes and plans.

Taken together the above reports aim to:

- Improve people's mental and emotional well-being, in particular that of people at risk or vulnerable, and people with identified mental health problems, their carers and families.
- Prevent, or reduce the incidence and impact of, mental and emotional distress, anxiety, mental illness and suicide.
- Raise awareness of the determinants of mental and emotional health at public, professional and policy making levels and reduce discrimination against people with mental health problems.
- Ensure that all those with a contribution to make are knowledgeable, skilled and aware of effective practice in mental and emotional health promotion.

Key aims of mental health promotion

Mental health promotion is concerned with achieving positive mental health and quality of life. The focus is on promoting positive mental health in the whole population and on strengthening protective factors and enhancing well-being. Mental health is often narrowly defined as the absence of mental illness, but it is more than that. It includes emotional

235

health, **mental functioning, self-determination,** positive personal relationships and **resilience.**

Mental health is a state of well being in which the individual realizes his or her own abilities, can cope with the normal stresses of life, can work productively and fruitfully, and is able to make a contribution to his or her community
WHO, 2001

It is:

'the emotional and spiritual resilience which enables us to enjoy life and to survive pain, disappointment and sadness. It is a positive sense of well being and an underlying belief in our own and others' dignity and worth'
Stuart and Laraia, 2006

As such, mental and emotional health is a resource which we need for everyday life, and which enables us to mange our lives successfully. Factors which support or influence our mental health and emotional well-being include: a stable and secure environment; the ability to engage in lasting meaningful relationships and maintain self-esteem; the emotional skills to manage change and survive difficulties in our lives; coping and life skills to enable us to control our lives and deal with stressful circumstances effectively. Mental health promotion is underpinned by understandings of what constitutes mental health, and is frequently located in broad health and social development work, and distinguishes population-wide mental health promotion from the early intervention and prevention strategies of the mental illness movement.

Mental health promotion is essentially concerned with:

- How individuals, families, organizations and communities think and feel;
- The factors which influence how we think and feel, individually and collectively;
- The impact that this has on overall health and well-being.

Naidoo and Wills, 2005

Effective mental health promotion involves not only attending to the needs of those with mental health difficulties, but also promoting the general mental well-being of all. This can range from self-help, community and voluntary groups to specific locally inspired activity on health related issues, such as a lobby group for responding to a drugs problem on a housing estate.

Mental health promotion works at three levels: and at each level, is relevant to the whole population, to individuals at risk, vulnerable groups and people with mental health problems (Whitehead, 2006).

Strengthening individuals

This includes 'person-based strategies', increasing emotional resilience through interventions to promote self-esteem,

life and coping skills, e.g. communicating, negotiating, relationship and parenting skills. This is the area that most nurses will focus their efforts on.

Strengthening communities

This includes collective responses to external hazards, such as increasing social inclusion and participation, improving neighbourhood environments, developing health and social services which support mental health, anti-bullying strategies at school, workplace health, community safety, childcare and self-help networks. This is achieved by maximizing the important role of family, friends, voluntary agencies and the community as a whole. The need for social cohesion and the need to create conditions for communities to work cooperatively are important here. This is an area that practitioners are expected to support and encourage.

Improving access to essential facilities and services

Policies are needed to establish the foundations for health including housing, clean water, health care, education and employment and training. One example might be health advocacy through alliances to improve services and access to them. Practitioners here may be involved in a health alliance or through their professional or union bodies lobbying for policy changes.

Encouraging macro-economic and cultural change

This refers to a whole population approach to reducing inequality rather than individual, group or locality based approaches. One example might be, labour marker policies such as the European minimum wage. This is an area that the practitioner is least likely to influence directly.

Mental health promotion also includes application of the nursing process, with a focus on the primary prevention of maladaptive coping responses associated with an identified stressor. As such, it incorporates the following aspects:

- **Assessment:** identification of a stressor that precipitates maladaptive responses and a target population group that is vulnerable or at risk for it.
- **Planning:** elaboration of specific strategies of prevention and relevant social institutions and situations through which the strategies may be applied.
- **Implementation:** application of selected interventions aimed at decreasing maladaptive responses to the identified stressor and enhancing adaption.
- **Evaluation:** determining the effectiveness of the nursing interventions with regard to short-term and long-term outcomes, use of resources and comparison with other prevention strategies.

Levels of prevention

'The concepts of primary, secondary, and tertiary prevention provide a framework for discussing contemporary mental health nursing practice and mental health promotion.'
Naidoo and Wills, 2005

Primary prevention

Primary prevention involves lowering the incidence of illness in a community by changing causative factors before they can do harm. It is a concept that precedes disease and is applied to a generally healthy population. It includes health promotion, illness prevention and protection against disease. Within this area lie many of nursings' independent functions, which are intended to decrease individual's vulnerability to illness and strengthen their capacity to withstand stressors. Direct nursing care activities in this area include the following:

- Teaching about the principles of mental health;
- Effecting changes in living conditions, poverty levels and education;
- Educating consumers in such areas as normal growth and development and sex education;
- Making appropriate referrals before mental disorder occurs based on assessment of potential stressors and life changes and events;
- Helping patients in a general hospital setting to avoid future psychiatric problems;
- Working with families to support family members and group functioning;
- Becoming active in community and political activities related to mental health.

Secondary prevention

Secondary prevention involves reducing illness by early detection and treatment of a problem. Direct nursing care activities in this area include the following:

- Screening and evaluation services;
- Home visits for preadmission or treatment services;
- Emergency treatment and psychiatric services in a general hospital;
- Creation of a therapeutic milieu;
- Supervision of patients receiving medication;
- Suicide prevention services;
- Counselling on a time limited basis;
- Crisis intervention;
- Family support;
- Intervention with communities and organizations based on an identified problem.

Tertiary prevention

Tertiary prevention involves reducing the residual impairment or disability resulting from an illness. Direct nursing care activities in this area include the following:

- Promoting vocational training and rehabilitation;
- Organizing aftercare programmes for a patients' discharge from psychiatric facility to ease transition from hospital to the community;
- Providing partial hospitalization options for patients, for example, attending a college educational programme whilst still a patient of a ward.

In addition to direct nursing care functions, nurses engage in indirect care that affects all three levels of prevention. These activities include teaching nursing personnel in various educational programmes; consulting with colleagues, other professionals, consumer groups, community care-givers, and local and national agencies and researching clinical problems in the field.

Mental health promotion is most effective when Departments and Agencies work together to provide information and support. The messages can be reinforced in a wide range of settings including the media, the workplace, primary care, schools, libraries, and places of worship, leisure centres and other community settings.

As a primary prevention strategy, supporting social systems does not attempt to remove or minimize the stressor or risk factor within someone's life but rather an attempt to strengthen social supports as a way of buffering or cushioning the effects of a potentially stressful event (Donovan et al., 2006). It is an important concept for all levels of intervention — primary, secondary and tertiary — and it has implications for:

- Tertiary prevention — helping one to deal with chronic mental and physical illness;
- Secondary prevention — reducing the occurrence of potentially stressful events;
- Primary prevention — encouraging health promotion behaviour helping people seek assistance earlier.

Social support systems can be helpful in emphasizing the strengths of individuals and families and focusing on health rather than illness (Barry and Jenkins, 2006). Given the goal that social support should be maximized, how can this be achieved? First, how much social support a high risk group needs must be determined and compared with the amount of social support available. Although the question is straightforward, it is complicated by the fact that there are multiple determinants of each element. The need for social support is influenced by the nature of the stressors, and the availability of other coping resources such as economic assets, individual abilities and skills, and defensive techniques. The availability of social supports is similarly influenced by age, gender, socioeconomic status, the nature of the stressor, and the characteristics of the environment. Changes or stressors viewed in a positive way by the individual's social network, such as a birth of a baby or a promotion, may elicit a great deal of support, whereas a negative event, such as a sudden death, may generate little support. In addition, the quality of type of social support that meets one need may not meet another.

Furthermore, social support patterns can be used to assess communities and neighborhoods to identify problem areas and high risk groups. Not only will information about the quality of life be gained, but the social isolation of a particular group might become apparent, as well as central to individuals who may be enlisted to help develop community-based programmes.

A second preventative intervention would be to improve links in community support systems and formal mental health services. Often health professionals are not aware or comfortable with the existence of functioning or community support systems. They should be taught how to use and mobilize community resources and social support systems. All health care providers need to recognize where patients need social support to provide them with access to appropriate community support systems.

Another type of intervention is to strengthen natural, existing care giving networks (Laverack, 2007). Health professionals and nurses can provide information and support to informal caregivers in the community, who serve a very important and somewhat different function than more formalized and organized support systems. Informal support systems can provide the following:

- A natural training ground for the development of problem-solving skills;
- A medium in which people grow and develop by learning to direct the process of change for themselves;
- A supportive milieu that capitalizes on the strength of existing ties among people in communities, rather than fragmenting intact social units on the basis of diagnosed needs or specialized services.

Additionally, health promotion may serve to help the person or group develop, maintain and use a network.

Effective interventions will also take account of the specific needs of minority ethnic groups and people with disabilities (NIMHE, 2004). For example, the mental health needs of people with a learning disability can often be overlooked or attributed to their other identified difficulties; deaf children who

have limited access to the kinds of incidental hearing that support the development of social understanding may need particular support and help to build confidence and develop problem solving skills.

Since childhood mental distress is strongly predictive of poor mental health and social outcomes in adult life, preventive interventions for children have clear potential to bring long-term psychological, social and economic benefits (Scriven, 2005).

Effective interventions for children from disadvantaged communities and high risk families/children include:

- High quality preschool and nursery education;
- Support visits for new parents; supporting bereaved families and
- Home based programmes to strengthen the relationship between the child, parent or care giver.

Approaches which have proved to be effective include:

Young people

A number of effective school-based programmes have been developed and evaluated (McDowall, Bonnel and Davis, 2006; Scriven, 2005). These are characterized by:

- Focusing on improving social skills;
- Reducing substance misuse and aggressive behaviour;
- Developing coping skills to deal with life situations, for example, problem solving and parenting;
- Promoting good social relationships, for example, through training for social skills, assertiveness, communication and relationships;

Participation in creative arts has also proved to benefit young people experiencing personal, social and behavioural problems.

Research has shown that both being a bully or a victim of bullying is a good predictor for later problems (Rivers et al., 2009; Bonner, 2006). Effective anti-bullying schemes involving the whole school have been shown to be effective and have significant long-term impacts on criminal behaviour, alcohol misuse, depression and suicidal behaviour.

Adults

There is a range of effective interventions to promote the mental well-being of adults. These include:

- General health promotion programmes involving the whole community in a participatory manner on healthy living;
- Community based support groups for the mildly depressed, divorced or separated people, unemployed, carers and recently bereaved people;
- Home visiting programmes focusing on parenting skills and specific interventions to reduce post-natal depression;

- Positive working conditions, including increased control at work, greater social support and pre-retirement interventions.

Brief interventions, such as simple advice, have proved to be effective in reducing excessive alcohol consumption (O'Conner and Whaley, 2007; Anton *et al.*, 2006). More severe alcohol related problems can be reduced by approaches which focus on skilled or specialist help, for example, in primary care services, addiction services or self-help groups.

Physical activity, either alone or as part of organized programmes, can improve emotional well-being for all age groups. It can also prevent the onset of mental health problems and improve the quality of life for people with such problems.

Recovery

Since the mid-1980s, a great deal has been written about mental health recovery from the perspective of the consumer (client), family member and mental health professional. The amount of research of various aspects of recovery continues to grow. Early research by Courtney Harding (1987) and others challenged the belief that severe mental illness is chronic and that stability is the best one could hope for. They discovered there are multiple outcomes associated with severe mental illness and that many people did progress beyond a state of mere stability. As such, the concept of recovery began to obtain legitimacy (Sullivan, 1997). Anthony (1993) identifies recovery as:

'a deeply personal, unique process of changing one's attitudes, values, feelings, goals, skills and/or roles. It is a way of living a satisfying, hopeful, and contributing life even with limitations caused by the illness. Recovery involves the development of new meaning and purpose in one's life as one grows beyond the catastrophic effects of mental illness'.

In this sense, recovery is a personal process for tackling the adverse impacts of experiencing mental health problems, despite their continuing presence. It involves personal development and change, including acceptance there are problems to face, a sense of involvement and control over one's life, the cultivation of hope and the support of others, and direct collaboration in joint problem solving between service users, workers and families. Recovery starts with the individual and works from the inside out.

Within the context of mental health the concept of recovery moves beyond the traditional boundaries of simply returning to a level of **pre-morbid functioning**. Rather recovery in this sense takes a wider and perhaps deeper view. While many do 'recover' from illness in the traditional sense recovery within mental health encompasses the communicated attitude that regardless of symptomology, those with mental illness can and should have a hopeful, meaningful and fulfilling life.

According to Judith Boxer cited in Barker (2003), core skills associated with current mental health promotion are based on an ability to be adaptable, in contrast to the more rigid traditional model in which practitioners tell other people what they should do to improve their health.

The ultimate goal of the recovery movement, and of psychiatric rehabilitation, is the re-establishment of normal roles in the community, the development of a personal support network, and an increased quality of life. The primary methods used to achieve this goal include:

- building on the existing strengths of each individual,
- facilitating reintegration into the community.

Mutual support and self-help enhance this goal by adding an emphasis on the individual's right to direct their own affairs, including the mental health services they receive. This treatment strategy is different from the traditional approach which focuses more on individual deficiencies instead of strengths; stabilization instead of recovery; connections to the treatment system instead of the community; and compliance with the regimes mandated by treatment authorities instead of individuals taking an active part in their treatment and in directing their own affairs (Campbell and Schraiber, 1989).

The Recovery Model is built upon principles articulated by Anthony of Boston University (Spaniol *et al.*, 1994):

- Recovery can occur without professional intervention;
- People who recover have people who stand by them and believe in them;
- Recovery can occur whether ones sees mental illness as biological or environmental;
- Recovery can occur even though symptoms may reoccur;
- Recovery often changes the frequency and duration of symptoms;
- Recovery is not a linear process;
- Recovery from the consequences of being ill is often more difficult that recovering from the illness itself;
- Recovery does not mean that one did not have a mental illness.

Ultimately, because recovery is a personal and unique process, everyone with a psychiatric illness develops his or her own definition of recovery. However, certain concepts or factors are common to recovery. Some of these are listed below.

Hope

Having a sense of hope is the foundation for ongoing recovery from mental illness. Even the smallest belief that we can get better, as others have, can fuel the recovery process — recognizing and accepting that there is a problem, committing to change, focusing on strengths rather than on weakness or the possibility of failure, looking forward rather than ruminating on the past, celebrating small shifts rather than expecting seismic change, reordering priorities and cultivating optimism.

Early in the recovery process, it is possible for a treatment provider, friend, and/or family member to carry hope for a consumer. At some point, however, the person must develop and internalize their own sense of hope.

While many people are frustrated by the process of finding the right medications and the side effects of medications, most persons with a psychiatric disorder indicate that medications are critical to their success (Sullivan, 1997). For many, the goal is not to be medication-free, but to take the least amount necessary.

Likewise, mental health consumers often report that mental health professionals and treatment programmes are valuable to their recovery; especially when the person feels they are engaged in a partnership with their treatment provider and are involved in their treatment planning.

Empowerment

Empowerment is the belief that the person has power and control in their life, including over their illness. Empowerment also involves taking responsibility for self and advocating for self and others. As the person grows in their recovery, they gain a greater sense of empowerment in their lives (Barker, 2009). People with mental health problems must be afforded and have **control and choice** in their own care.

Barker, Stevenson and Leamy (2000) describe, what they call, an empowering interactions framework. This, they state, is built on certain assumptions:

- People should be treated as equals and the relationship should be based on collaboration;
- The person is an expert on his or her life, its problems and potential resolutions;
- The person is able to make personally appropriate choices;
- The person retains a problem solving capacity;
- The person has responsibility for beginning, controlling and ending the therapeutic contact.

They go on to state that power is an inevitable component of human relationships and that sharing power is central to the cultivation of hope and the development of a sense of control and therefore empowerment.

Power, control, learning and defining a sense of self are about choice but also, as pointed out in the review, are about clients making mistakes and being allowed to fail in order to learn.

Support

Support from peers, family, friends and mental health professionals is essential to recovery from mental illness. It is especially beneficial to have multiple sources of support. This not only reduces a person's sense of isolation, but also increases their activity in the community, allowing them to obtain an integral role in society. Repper (2000) states that a common factor in recovery is the presence of people who believe in and stand by the individual. These people are described as those who try to listen, understand and encourage recovery without forcing it or becoming frustrated when nothing seems to change.

In addition to support from individuals, participation in support groups is an important tool for recovery. Numerous informal support groups exist. They may include church groups, civic organizations, clubs, women's groups or work and neighbourhood supports. Self-help groups are becoming more common as members organize themselves to solve their own problems. The members all share a common experience, work together toward a common goal and use their strengths to gain control over their lives. The processes involved in self-help groups are social affiliation, learning self-control , modelling methods to cope with stress, and acting to change the social environment (Yanos, Primavera and Knight, 2001).

Self-help groups such as Alcoholics Anonymous, Weight Watchers are family to the public. They have demonstrated their ability to help people experiencing mental health problems. Because self-help groups use a variety of methods and membership criteria, each group should be addressed individually for its general effectiveness and appropriateness for particular individuals and families.

Self-help

While most people recognize the value of professional treatment, self-help is often viewed as the conduit to growth in recovery (Ridgway, 2001). Self-help can take many forms including learning to identify symptoms and take actions to counteract them, reading and learning about an illness and its treatment, learning and applying coping skills, and attending support groups and developing a support system to rely on when necessary.

Employment/meaningful activity

Frequently, when we meet new people, they ask 'what do you do?' Whether it is fair or not, what we do shapes others' opinions of who we are. As a result, it is common for a person's identity to be significantly impacted by what they do. Likewise, what a person does influences his/her confidence, esteem, social role, values, etc. The experience of work, in and of itself, has proven to be a significant facilitator in the recovery process. Simply put employment/meaningful activity afford most people the opportunity to regain a positive identity, including a sense of purpose and value (Barker, 2009).

Social inclusion

Above all, there is a need to fight stigma and seek social inclusion for those suffering from a mental health problem. Anthony (1993) suggests that the barriers and discrimination that people experience as a consequence of their difficulties can limit life far more than a person's cognitive and emotional problems.

Repper (2000) agrees with this and cites a lack of access to a decent income, housing, work and friends as holding back the process of recovery. She further states that public attitudes are changed very little by public education and that it is personal acquaintance with people who have found ways of coping with their mental health problems that changes personal prejudices.

The physical health of mental health service users

Good mental health is a prerequisite for good physical health. The uptake of behaviours to improve physical health, including effective self-management of acute or chronic disease, is intimately connected to an individual's mental health and well being. **Not All in the Mind** is the title of a report by Mentality (2003) which examines the physical health of mental health service users. It points out that:

'There is a growing body of research that demonstrates the impact of mental health on physical health'
Marmot and Wilkinson, 1999, cited in Mentality 2003.

Service users with serious and enduring mental health problems frequently have poor physical health, yet their physical problems can remain largely undetected. Ohlsen *et al.*, (2005) suggest that physical health problems amongst the mentally ill population have become a pressing issue in recent years, but little is done to put systems in place to screen for them. Stronger links between primary and secondary care services need to be forged to ensure that 'mentally ill patients with physical health problems receive holistic care packages' (Olshen *et al.*, 2005)

The National Service Framework for Mental Health (DH 1999) recommends that the physical needs of people with serious and enduring mental illness should be monitored. One way of doing this is through screening by primary care

services. None-the-less there is limited evidence that health promotion is being systematically attempted in this group of service users. Therefore there is a clear need for attention to be paid to physical health (Panesar, 2006).

A helping relationship

It is through communication that **helping relationships** are formed, problems are identified and discussed, and information is conveyed. There are two aspects to communication, verbal and non-verbal. Verbal communication is principally achieved through the spoken word, including the underlying emotion, context and connotation of what is actually said. It can be used to convey information accurately and efficiently. However, it is a less effective means of communicating feelings or nuances of meaning, and it represents only a small segment of total human communication.

People will often assume that they are on the same 'wavelength' when talking to each other; however this is not always the case. Because words are only symbols, they seldom mean precisely the same thing to two people. If the word represents an abstract idea such as 'depressed' or 'hurt', the chance of misunderstanding or misinterpretation is increased. That is why it is important for nurses to listen carefully to what the person has to say by checking their interpretation and incorporating information from the non-verbal level as well.

The way in which we listen (or fail to listen) can be a major barrier to our interpersonal relationships. If we are to fully understand the person and their needs, we need to learn to listen effectively; that is we need to listen not only to words, but also to the hidden feelings and intentions that are expressed. The health care worker indicates active listening through their verbal and non-verbal communication and sensitivity to these is important.

The importance of communication as a nursing intervention is highlighted by the contemporary acceptance of nursing being a relationship or partnership with the client. This relationship can be the difference between a client losing the hope for wellness, or the client moving toward wellness. Health care givers must be aware that we bring our personal values, beliefs, experiences and characteristics to these professional relationships. Schinkel and Dorrer (2007) offer the following as important characteristics for engaging with people who experience mental illness.

- Listening that is active and interactive;
- Interpersonal qualities such as caring, patience and humility;
- Belief in and encouragement of change;
- Focus on the individual rather than being a collection symptoms;
- Understanding what the other person may be experiencing;

- Knowledge about illness, interventions and resources;
- Bringing out the other person's strengths;
- Good life skills and experience;
- Non-judgemental and open minded attitude;
- A sense of humour.

Two important issues dictate the effectiveness of employing these crucial aspects of ourselves. First, we must be aware of the characteristics we have, both helpful and non-helpful. Secondly we must be able to communicate our helpful characteristics to others. Consequently it is vital to be able to look at ourselves honestly, evaluate our helpful and unhelpful characteristics and then develop health communication skills. This use of self therefore means that we must be able to not only recognize our thoughts and feelings but exercise control over their use so that our thoughts and feelings are employed only for the betterment of those around us.

Recipients of nursing interventions will assess the behaviours of the nurse toward them. This assessment will predominantly be focused on problem solving ability, verbal ability and social competence. Social competence demonstrated through acceptance, sensitivity and the ability to admit errors would be at the forefront of client's experience.

Barker (2006) defines effective support as:

- The presence of a close confidant;
- Active ongoing emotional support from that confidant;

A further insight into effective forms of social support is given by Barbee (1990). She investigated the ways in which a helper provided support to a distressed friend, two of which helped, and two which did not. The behaviours that helped were:

- **Problem solving**: Asking about stressful events and circumstances and making suggestions about how to cope.
- **Emotional support**: Giving encouragement, affirming the person's ability, and accepting the person's feelings as valid.

Behaviours which did not help were:

- **Belittling the person's problem**: Telling the person that his or her problems are not important, or substituting the problem with one's own. Some health workers behave in this way, mistakenly believing they are empathizing ('I know how you feel, I've experienced that too').
- **Taking over the person's life**: Not allowing the person to make decisions for themselves; refusing requests and denying access to people, 'you're not up to seeing them just yet.'

Summary

Mental illness is more common than is frequently thought and there is a need for health care workers to safeguard against stigma and ensure a high level of care. Even small improvements in mental well-being can achieve emotional benefits through improvements in physical health, productivity and quality of life. There is a need for all nurses to be mindful of, and promote, the mental and emotional health needs of those that they care for and support.

 # Online Resource Centre

For more information on mental health visit the Online Resource Centre —
http://www.oxfordtextbooks.co.uk/orc/linsley/

References

American Psychiatric Association (2008). Diagnostic and Statistical Manual IV — Text Revision. NY: American Psychiatric Association (Pub).

Anton, R. F., O'Malley, S. S., & Ciraulo, D. A. *et al.* (2006). Combined pharmacotherapies and behavioral interventions for alcohol dependence: the COMBINE Study: a randomized controlled trial. *Journal of the American Medical Association*, 295, 17: 2003–2017.

Anthony, W. A. (1993). Recovery from mental illness: The guiding vision of the mental health service system in the 1990's. *Psychosocial Rehabilitation Journal,* 16, 4: 11–23.

Arroll, B., Khin, N., & Kerse, N. (2004). Screening for depression in primary care with two verbally asked questions: cross sectional study. *BMJ* 327:1144–6.

Barker, P. (2009). *Psychiatric and Mental Halth Nursing. The Craft of Caring* (2nd ed) London: Hodder Arnold.

Barnes, T. R. E. & Pant, A. (2002). Long-term course and outcome of schizophrenia. *Psychiatry* 1, 9: 34–36.

Barry, M. & Jenkins, R. (2006). *Implementing mental health promotion: a practical guide to planning, implementing and evaluating mental health promotion programmes*. London: Churchill Livingstone.

Beck, A. T. & Freeman, A. (1990). *Cognitive Therapy of Personality Disorders*. New York: Guilford.

Beck, A. T. Wright, F. D. & Newman, C. F. (1993). *Cognitive Therapy of Substance Misuse*. New York: Guilford.

Boxer, J. (2003). Mental Health Promotion. In P. Barker (ed.) *Psychiatric and Mental Health Nursing: The Craft of Caring*. London: Hodder Arnold.

Campbell, J. & Schraiber, R. (1989). *In Pursuit of Wellness: The Well being Project.* Sacramento, CA: California Department of Mental Health.

Centre of Excellence in Interdisciplinary Mental Health (CEIMH) (2009). *Guidance on Promoting Mental Health and Well being*. Birmingham: University of Birmingham.

Cochran, S. D. & Mays, V. M. (2000). Lifetime prevalence of suicidal symptoms and affective disorders among men reporting same-sex sexual partners: results from the NHANES III. *Am J Pub* Health, 90:573–578.

Corey, K. (2002). The mental health continuum: from languishing to flourishing in life. *Journal of Health and Social Behaviour* 43: 207–222.

Cox, J. L., Holden, J. M. & Sagovsky, R. (1987). Detection of post-natal depression: development of the Edinburgh Postnatal Depression Scale. *British Journal of Psychiatry*. ISO. 782–786.

Department of Health (1999). *National Service Framework for Mental Health: Modern Standards and Service Models*. London: DH.

Department of Health (2001). *A Guide to Delivering Mental Health Promotion*. London: DH.

Department of Health (2002). *Mental health policy implementation guide. Community mental health teams*. London: DH.

Department of Health (2004) *Celebrating Our Cultures for Mental Health Promotion with Black and Minority Ethnic Communities*. London: DH.

Department of Health, Social Services and Public Safety (2003). *Promoting Mental Health: Strategy and Action Plan 2003–2008*. Belfast: DHSSPS.

Donovan, R. J., James, R., Jalleh, G. & Sidebottom, C. (2006). Implementing Mental Health Promotion: The Act-Belong-Commit Mentally Healthy WA Campaign in Western Australia. *The International Journal of Mental Health Promotion*, 8, 1, 33–42.

Drake, R. J. & Lewis, S. W. (2005). Early detection of schizophrenia. *Current Opinion in Psychiatry* 18. 2, 147–150.

Harding, C. (1987). The Vermont Longitudinal Study of Persons with Severe Mental Illness. *American Journal of Psychiatry* 144: 727–734.

Harding, C. M., Brooks, G. W., Asolaga, T. S. & Breier, A. (1987). The Vermont longitudinal study of persons with severe mental illness. *American Journal of Psychiatry*, 144: 718–726.

Hawton, K., Sutton L., Haw, C. *et al.*, (2005). Schizophrenia and suicide: systematic review of risk factors. *British Journal of Psychiatry* 187(Jul), 9–20.

Her Majesty's Government (2005). *The Disability Discrimination Act 2005*. London: Her Majesty's Stationery Office.

Hope, R. (2004). *The Ten Essential Shared Capabilities: A Framework for the Whole of the Mental Health Work Force*. London: National Institute for Mental Health in England/The Sainsbury Centre for Mental Health Joint Workforce Support Unit.

Keleher, H. & Murphy, B. (eds.) (2004). *Understanding health: a determinants approach*. Oxford: Oxford University Press.

Kendal, W. S. (2006). Suicide and cancer: a gender comparative study. *Annuals of Oncology*, 18, 2: 381–387.

Laverack, G. (2007). *Health promotion practice: Building empowered communities*. London: Open University Press.

MacDowall, W., Bonnell, C. & Davies, M. (2006). *Health Promotion Practice*. London: Open University Press.

MacLaren, J. (2004). A kaleidoscope of understandings: spiritual nursing in a multi-faith society. *Journal of Advanced Nursing*, 45, 5: 457–462.

Mentality, (2003). *Not all in the Mind. The Physical Health of Mental Health Service Users*. London: Mentality.

Mittelmark, M. B. (2003). Five strategies for workforce development for mental health promotion. *IUHPE — Promotion and Education*, 1: 20–22.

Morgan, O. W. C., Griffiths, C. & Majeed, A. (2004). Association between mortality from suicide in England and antidepressant prescribing: an ecological study. *BMC Public Health* 4:63.

Naidoo, J. & Wills, J. (2005). *Public Health and Health Promotion*. London: Bailliere Tindall.

National Institute for Health and Clinical Excellence (2004). *Anxiety: management of anxiety (panic disorder with or without agoraphobia and generalized anxiety disorder in adults in primary, secondary and community care*. London: NICE.

National Institute for Health and Clinical Excellence (2005). *Depression: management of depression in primary and secondary care*. Clinical Guidance No. 23. London: NICE.

National Institute for Health and Clinical Excellence (2006). *Brief Interventions and referral for smoking cessation in primary and other care settings*. London: NICE.

National Institute for Mental Health in England (NIMHE) (2004). *From Here to Equality: A Strategic Plan to Tackle Stigma and Discrimination on Mental Health Grounds, 2004–2009*. Leeds: NIMHE.

National Institute for Mental Health in England (2007). *Mental disorders, suicide, and deliberate self-harm in lesbian, gay and bisexual people a systematic review*. Leeds: NIMHE.

O'Connor, M. J. & Whaley, S. E. (2007). Breif Intervention for Alcohol Use by Pregnant Women. *American Journal of Public Health*, 97, 2: 252–258.

Ohlsen, R. I., Peacock, G. & Smith, S. (2005). Developing a service to monitor and improve physical health in people with serious mental illness. *Journal of Psychiatric and mental Health Nursing*, 2, 5: 614 -619.

Panesar, N. P. (2006). A survey of the physical health screening of all in-patients in a residential rehabilitation population. *The Journal of the Royal Society for the Promotion of Health* 126: 38–40.

Repper, J. (2000). Adjusting the Focus of Mental Health Nursing: Incorporating Service Users' Experiences of Recovery. *Journal of Mental Health*, 9, 6: 575–587.

Ridgway, P. (2001). ReStorying Psychiatric Disability: Learning from First Person Recovery Narratives. *Psychiatric Rehabilitation Journal*, 24, 4: 335–343.

Rivers *et al.*, (2009). Observing bullying at school: The mental health implications of witness status. *School Psychology Quarterly*, 24, 4: 211.

Sainsbury Centre for Mental Health (2001). Cultural Sensitivity Audit tool for mental health service. London: SCMH.

Schinkel, M. & Dorrer, N. (2007). *Towards Recovery Competencies in Scotland: The Views of Key Stakeholder Groups*. Edinburgh: Edinburgh Scottish Executive.

Scriven, A. (2005). *Health Promoting Practice, The Contribution of Nurses and Allied Health Professionals*. London: Palgrave Macmillan.

Scottish Executive (2003). *National Programme for Improving Mental Health and Well being: Action Plan 2003–2006*, Edinburgh: Scottish Executive.

Selekman, M. W. (2006). *Working with Self-Harming Adolescents: A Collaborative Strengths-Based Therapy Approach*. New York: Norton.

Soundy, A., Faulkner, G. & Taylor, A. (2007). Exploring Variability and Perceptions of Lifestyle Physical Activity Among Individuals with Severe and Enduring Mental Health Problems: A Qualitative Study. *Journal of Mental Health*, 16: 493–503.

Spaniol, L., Koehler, M., & Hutchinson, D. (1994). *The Recovery Workbook; Practical Copying and Empowerment Strategies for People with Psychiatric Disability*. Boston: Center for Psychiatric Rehabilitation.

Stuart, G. W. & Laraia, M. T. (2009). *Principles and Practice of Psychiatric Nursing* (8th edn.). Philadelphia, Pa: Mosby.

Sullivan, W. P. (1997). A long and winding road: The process of recovery from severe mental illness. In L. Spaniol, C. Gagne & M. Koehler (eds.), *Psychological and social aspects of psychiatric disability* (pp. 14–24). Boston: Center for Psychiatric Rehabilitation.

Tilford, S., Delaney, F. & Vogels, M. (1997). *Effectiveness of mental health promotion interventions: a review*. London: Health Education Authority.

Tones, K. & Green, J. (2004). *Health Promotion: Planning and Strategies*. London: Sage Publications.

Welsh Assembly Government (2006) Mental Health Promotion Action Plan for Wales (Draft for consultation). Cardiff: WAG.

Whitehead, D. (2006). *Health Promotion in Health Service Settings, A Guide for Health Professionals*. London: Palgrave MacMillan.

World Health Organization (2005). *Promoting Mental Health: Concepts, Emerging evidence, Practice: A report of the World Health Organization, Department of Mental Health and Substance Abuse in collaboration with the Victorian Health Promotion Foundation and the University of Melbourne*. Geneva: WHO.

World Health Organization (2005). *WHO Resource Book on Mental Health: Human rights and legislation*. Geneva: WHO.

World Health Organization (2007) *The ICD-10 Classification of Mental and Behavioural Disorders. Clinical descriptions and diagnostic guidelines*. Geneva: WHO.

World Health Organization (2008). Depression: Facts and Figures. European Regional Office. Geneva: WHO.

Woodside, J. & Byrne, C. (2001), Meaning, Relationships and Control. *Journal of Psychosocial Nursing*, 39, 1: 46–53.

Yanos, T., Primavera, L. & Knight, E. (2001). Consumer-Run Service Participation, Recovery of Social Functioning and the Mediating Role of Psychological Factors. *Psychiatric Services*, 52, 4: 493–500.

Chapter 18

Alcohol: reducing harm

Damian Mitchell and Iain Armstrong

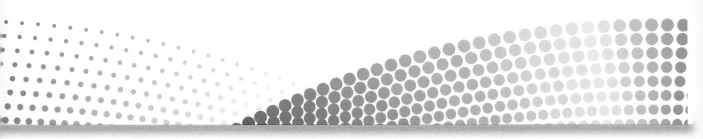

Introduction

This chapter will describe the extent and cost of alcohol-related harm in the UK and the approaches that government takes to address it. It will outline the health interventions that are in place to help people who drink too much and the role nurses can play in facilitating behaviour change. It will then go on to describe some specific skills and activities associated with 'Identification and Brief Advice' (IBA), which is known to be have a cost-effective impact on alcohol harm at a population level.

Alcohol misuse is a major cause of disease and injury. Worldwide it accounts for 9.2% of disability-adjusted life years (premature death) with only tobacco smoking and high blood pressure as higher risk factors. Health inequalities are clearly evident as a result of alcohol-related harm where analysis of Office for National Statistics (ONS) data indicates that alcohol-related death rates are about 45% higher in areas of high deprivation (DH, 2007). For the NHS in England alone, the estimated financial burden of alcohol misuse is around £2.7 billion in hospital admissions, attendance at A&E, primary care, treatment of hypertension, etc. (DH 2008). When taking into account crime and anti-social behaviour, loss of productivity in the workplace and social problems experienced by alcohol misusers and their families this cost increases around £20 billion a year in the UK (Cabinet Office, 2003):

- The Scottish Government has estimated the annual cost of alcohol misuse in Scotland to be around £2.25 billion every year (Scottish Government, 2009).

- In England, alcohol-related illness or injury accounts for nearly a million hospital admissions per year and this number is rising.

- In Wales:
  - 15% of all hospital admissions are due to alcoholic intoxication;
  - 30,000 hospital bed days are related to alcohol every year;
  - Liver disease (of which alcohol is a major cause) is responsible for around 1,600 admissions every year;
  - The estimated health service cost in Wales of alcohol related chronic disease and alcohol related acute incidents is between £70 million and £85 million each year. (Welsh Assembly Government, 2008)

The strategic approaches taken by the UK Governments to tackle alcohol-related harm are broadly similar in that they are based on mutually reinforcing components which are known to have an impact. In England for instance, the Government's approach is described in its refreshed alcohol strategy **Safe. Sensible. Social. The next steps in the National Alcohol Strategy** (DH, 2007). The strategy presents a cross-government approach to tackling the harms and cost of alcohol misuse using a number of linked components — including considerations of price and availability of alcohol, enforcement and planning measures, point of sale information, public education and health interventions.

A strain is being placed on hospital A&E departments where research has shown that up to 35% of all A&E attendance and ambulance costs may be alcohol-related and up to 70% of A&E attendances at peak times on the weekends (between midnight and 5am) (Cabinet Office, 2003). Common reasons for alcohol related attendance at A&E Departments include:

- a violent assault,
- incident involving weapons,
- road traffic accidents,
- psychiatric emergencies,
- deliberate self harm episodes.

Cabinet Office (2003)

However, although alcohol-related violence and its effects are significant issues and tend to command public attention, in health terms acute conditions only account for about 10% of alcohol-related hospital admissions. The majority of alcohol-related ill health is chronic. As well as a number of diseases which, by definition, are wholly attributable to alcohol consumption,

such as alcohol poisoning and alcoholic liver disease, there are a number of conditions to which alcohol is a significant contributory factor. Some are listed in Table 18.1.

The predominant cause of chronic alcohol-related ill health and therefore, of the majority of the health harms and costs, is regular and frequent alcohol misuse. The number of people in the UK who drink at levels likely to present risk to their health has risen steadily over recent decades and NHS Hospital Episodes Statistics (HES) data indicate that rates of chronic alcohol-related illness are rising steadily year on year. Due to the non-instantaneous impact of alcohol on such conditions the trend is set to continue to rise, which many see as a health time bomb. Unless defused, this threatens to exacerbate health inequalities, shorten healthy lives and place an intolerable burden on the NHS. Alcohol misuse is recognized therefore as a public health priority for national Governments and the NHS. In order to understand what the term alcohol misuse means and what can be done, it is necessary to explore how populations use alcohol.

Table 18.1 Source of relative risk estimates and AAFs

Condition		Source
Wholly attributable conditions	Alcohol—induced pseudo-Cushing's syndrome	By definition these conditions are wholly attributable to alcohol consumption
	Mental and behavioural disorders due to use of alcohol	
	Degeneration of nervous system due to alcohol	
	Alcoholic polyneuropathy	
	Alcoholic myopathy	
	Alcoholic cardiomyopathy	
	Alcoholic gastritis	
	Alcoholic liver disease	
	Chronic pancreatitis (alcohol induced)	
	Ethanol poisoning	
	Methanol poisoning	
	Toxic effect of alcohol, unspecified	
	Accidental poisoning by and exposure to alcohol	
Partially attributable chronic conditions	Malignant neoplasm of lip, oral cavity and pharynx	Corrao et al. (2004)
	Malignant neoplasm of oesophagus	Corrao et al. (2004)
	Malignant neoplasm of colon	Corrao et al. (2004)
	Malignant neoplasm of rectum	Corrao et al. (2004)
	Malignant neoplasm of liver and intrahepatic bile ducts	Corrao et al. (2004)
	Malignant neoplasm of larynx	Corrao et al. (2004)
	Malignant neoplasm of breast	Hamajima et al. (2002)
	Diabetes mellitus (type II)	Gutjahr et al. (2001)
	Epilepsy and Status epilepticus	Rehm et al. (2004)
	Hypertensive diseases	Corrao et al. (2004)
	Ischaemic heart disease	Corrao et al. (2004)

Table 18.1 *(Contd.)*

Condition		Source
	Cardiac arrhythmias	Gutjahr *et al.* (2001)
	Heart failure	Single *et al.* (1996)
	Haemorrhagic stroke	Corrao *et al.* (2004)
	Ischaemic stroke	Corrao *et al.* (2004)
	Oesophageal varices	Corrao *et al.* (2004)
	Gastro-oesophageal laceration-haemorrhage syndrome	English *et al.* (1995)
	Unspecified liver disease	Corrao *et al.* (2004)
	Cholelithiasis	Gutjahr *et al.* (2001)
	Acute and chronic pancreatitis	Corrao *et al.* (2004)
	Psoriasis	Gutjahr *et al.* (2001)
	Spontaneous abortion	Gutjahr *et al.* (2001)
Partially attributable acute conditions	Road traffic accidents — non-pedestrian	Ridolfo and Stevenson (2001)
	Pedestrian traffic accidents	Ridolfo and Stevenson (2001)
	Water transport accidents	Ridolfo and Stevenson (2001)
	Air/space transport accidents	Ridolfo and Stevenson (2001)
	Fall injuries	Single *et al.* (1996)
	Work/machine injuries	Single *et al.* (1996)
	Firearm injuries	Ridolfo and Stevenson (2001)
	Drowning	Ridolfo and Stevenson (2001)
	Inhalation of gastric contents	English *et al.* (1995)
	Food causing obstruction of the respiratory tract	Single *et al.* (1996)
	Fire injuries	English *et al.* (1995)
	Accidental excessive cold	Single *et al.* (1996)
	Intentional self-harm/event of undetermined intent	Single *et al.* (1996)
	Assault	Corrao *et al.* (2004)

Effects of alcohol

Alcohol or Ethanol (C_2H_5OH) is a depressant drug which, when taken orally, diffuses from the stomach and small intestine to water containing parts of the body. Alcohol peaks in the blood within an hour of consumption. While in the system alcohol interacts with nerve cell membranes and has effects on neurotransmitter pathways resulting in a number of brain effects such as sedation, impaired judgement and reduced muscular control. Most alcohol is metabolized in the liver into acetaldehyde. The average healthy human liver will metabolize alcohol at roughly one unit per hour. There are numerous and multiple effects on body cells and organs and prolonged excessive use can result in dependence.

The effects of alcohol intoxication with which one would be familiar, through observation if not experience, are due to the effects on the areas of the brain controlling emotion, motor function, balance, problem solving, memory, judgement, impulse control, social and sexual control, vision and language. The perceived immediate positive effects of this are feelings of self-confidence and social relaxation. The potential short-term negative effects can manifest themselves as loss of control over violent anger, unprotected or unwanted sex, or becoming a victim of accidents or crime.

As indicated above, alcohol may be easily identifiable as a contributory factor among patients presenting with injuries from assaults or accidents, headaches and nausea. However it may also be a significant factor in numerous common conditions and symptoms which may not intuitively be associated with alcohol such as sleep disorders, sexual impotence, anxiety and depression, dehydration, stomach inflammation, hypertension and some cancers.

Most patients whose mental or physical ill health may be exacerbated or caused by their alcohol use are quite likely to be unaware that this is the case. Surveys show that most people are also unaware of the unit content of drinks and therefore, of how much alcohol they actually drink. All health practitioners can play a key role in helping people to make the links between alcohol and health.

A significant proportion of those with alcohol dependency are also receiving care for a mental health problem. The Adult Psychiatric Morbidity Survey (Singleton *et al.*, 2001) found that 14% of alcohol dependent adults were receiving treatment for a mental or emotional problem. Women were more likely to be receiving mental health treatment than men; 26% compared with 9% of men. Alcohol is also associated with up to 1,000 suicides per year (Cabinet Office, 2003).

Social effects of alcohol misuse

The Interim Analytical Report of the Cabinet Office Strategy Unit Alcohol Harm Reduction project reported that:

- In 1999, an estimated 1.2 million violent incidents (half of all violent crimes) were alcohol related.
- There are about 360,000 alcohol-related incidents of domestic violence.
- There are 85,000 cases of drink driving.
- Up to 17 million days are lost annually due to alcohol-related absence.
- Between 0.78–1.3 million children are affected by alcohol misuse in the family.
- Around a third of incidents of domestic violence are linked to alcohol misuse.
- There are up to 20,000 street drinkers in the UK.

Cabinet Office (2003)

Information and Analytical Directorate for the Department of Work and Pensions (DWP) has identified a number of recurring themes from research into the psycho-social effects of excessive alcohol consumption.

Family problems

- Increased family tension,
- Increased levels of quarrelling and violence,
- Destabilized relationships,
- Partners may become anxious, depressed, socially withdrawn and may drink excessively themselves,
- Detrimental effects on the children leading to behavioural problems and underperformance at school,
- Increased rates of divorce.

Work difficulties

There may be deterioration in performance, conflict with colleagues, an increase in workplace accidents and a worsening attendance record. This is likely to result in repeated dismissals ultimately leading to long-term unemployment.

Crime

Excessive drinking is associated with crimes that include petty theft, driving offences, fraud, sexual offences and crimes of violence.

Social

Social effects of alcohol misuse that may indicate moderate disability include:

- Unemployment,
- Social isolation,
- Contact with other people is confined to other drinkers,
- Debt,
- Divorce,
- Legal problems such as theft and crimes of violence.

Department of Work and Pensions (2010)

Units of alcohol

Alcohol used to be measured by 'standard drinks', however, this is unreliable due to variations in the alcohol by volume (ABV) content of drinks such as wine and beer and the tendency for drinks to be served in larger measures. In the UK alcohol is now measured in units. One alcohol unit is measured as 10ml or 8g of ethyl alcohol. This equals one 25ml single measure of spirit (ABV 40%), or about half a pint of beer (ABV 3.6 per cent) or roughly a third of a large (250ml) glass of wine (ABV 12 per cent).

The units in any drink can be calculated using the formula (Volume in ml/1000) x % abv.

Because regular consumption of alcohol is known to increase the risk of chronic ill health the Chief Medical Officers for the four UK nations have issued guidance on how to use alcohol but stay healthy. See **http://www.drinking.nhs.uk/questions/recommended-levels/**

- Men should not exceed three to four units per day on a regular basis.
- Women should not exceed two to three units per day on a regular basis.

The limits are the levels of regular drinking that present only a low risk of contributing to future health problems. Drinking above these levels on a regular basis is associated with an increasing risk of diseases and the more often drinker exceeds the limits, the higher the risk.

It's regularly exceeding these limits that poses the higher risks and the guidance recognizes that on certain occasions some people will exceed the limits. After such occasions the guidance recommends at least 48 hours with no alcohol in order to give the body a chance to recover.

These limits recognized that no amount of alcohol is completely safe and the guidance also recommends not drinking at all before strenuous exercise, operating machinery, driving or if on certain medicines.

The limits are given as ranges ('two to three' and 'three to four') because the same amount of alcohol can affect different people in different ways, depending on gender, weight, height, any current ill health and many other factors. The thresholds for individuals therefore are not 'gear changes' but more a continuum of risk that should be taken as a broad guide for the general population.

They're lower for women because women and men process and tolerate alcohol differently; for example, women's bodies have a higher ratio of fat to water, so that alcohol becomes more quickly concentrated in the body's fluids and can't be processed as easily as in men.

The limits are given as daily figures for regular consumption because it's important to recognize that regular daily levels add up. This is also intended to discourage the belief that a week's units can safely be saved up and drunk all at once — binge drinking is harder on the body and may put the drinker or others at immediate risk from accidents or crime.

Relative risks from alcohol

Drinkers are usually categorized in the scientific literature by the World Health Organization terms: hazardous, harmful or dependent. These terms were found to be not easily understood by the general public so it is more common for public-facing material and discussions with patients to use language that makes clear the continuum of health risk described above — such as lower, increasing or higher risk.

- 'Lower risk drinking' is drinking within the recommended limits.
- 'Increasing risk drinking' means regularly drinking more than 2–3 units a day if you're a woman or more than 3–4 units a day if you're a man.
- 'Higher risk drinking' means regularly drinking more than 6 units per day for women or more than 8 units per day for men or more than 35 units per week (women) and more than 50 units per week (men).

Some higher risk drinkers may also be dependent on alcohol. Dependency too is a continuum, ranging from mild to moderate and severe. Alcohol dependence is a particular form of higher risk drinking and has a particular set of characteristics. Rather than being defined by intake, dependency is essentially typified by an increased drive to use alcohol and difficulty controlling its use, despite negative consequences. For some severely dependent drinkers there is also a risk of alcohol withdrawal on stopping drinking. In such cases it can be dangerous to stop without medical supervision.

Pregnancy

Excessive alcohol consumption during pregnancy can damage the developing foetus, as the brain and central nervous system of the unborn child are highly susceptible to prenatal alcohol exposure (Streissguth, 1997). Foetal Alcohol Syndrome (FAS) refers to an amalgamation of physical and mental defects that may develop in infants whose mothers have consumed alcohol during pregnancy. FAS is an organic brain disorder which is commonly demonstrated by affects to the central nervous system, growth retardation, and characteristic facial features (Stratton, Howe, and Battaglia, 1996). It is estimated that around 10% of children of alcohol-dependent mothers suffer from foetal alcohol effects (Alcohol Concern, 1999).

Even moderate drinking can produce less severe but undesirable effects on the growing foetus. The National Institute for Health and Clinical Excellence (NICE) and the National Collaborating Centre for Women's and Children's Health updated advice in March 2008 on the care that should be offered to women during pregnancy. This advice is an update of the original document published in 2003.

The guideline includes recommendations for doctors and midwives on the advice they should give to pregnant women about drinking alcohol.

NICE recommendations are that:

- Pregnant women and women planning to become pregnant should be advised to avoid drinking alcohol in the first 3 months of pregnancy, because there may be an increased risk of miscarriage.
- Women should be advised that if they choose to drink alcohol while they are pregnant they should drink no more than 1–2 UK units once or twice a week.
- There is uncertainty about how much alcohol is safe to drink in pregnancy, but at this low level there is no evidence of any harm to their unborn baby.
- Women should be advised not get to drunk or binge drink (drinking more than 7.5 UK units of alcohol on a single occasion) while they are pregnant because this can harm their unborn baby.

Young people

Young people aged 16–24 are the heaviest drinkers they are more likely to drink above the recommended limits than older people. Alcohol use among younger children (11–15 years) has been rising and the proportions drinking have been increasing sharply with age. In 2003, 25% of 11–15 year olds in England had drunk alcohol in the week prior to interview; this figure had risen steadily from 21% in 1992 to 27% in 1996 and has since fluctuated within this range, showing no clear pattern over recent years (DH, 2004b).

A survey of drinking behaviour among young people in Northern Ireland in 2003 showed that 41% of young people aged between 11–16 years old had never taken an alcoholic drink. However, abstinence was shown to decrease with age and by the age of 16 only 19% have never had a drink. The greatest increase appeared to be between the ages of 11–13 (Health Promotion Agency for Northern Ireland and Irish Temperance League, 2005).

According to the National Institute for Health and Clinical Excellence (NICE, 2007) there are no national guidelines on what constitutes safe and sensible alcohol consumption for children and young people, so the recommendations focus on:

- encouraging children not to drink,
- delaying the age at which young people start drinking,
- reducing the harm it can cause among those who do drink.

NICE has produced a 'Quick Reference Guide for School-based interventions on alcohol', which includes the following recommendations:

What action should they take?

- Ensure alcohol education is an integral part of the national science, PSHE and PSHE education curricula, in line with Department for Children, Schools and Families (DCSF) guidance.
- Ensure alcohol education is tailored for different age groups and takes different learning needs into account (based, for example, on individual, social and environmental factors). It should aim to encourage children not to drink, delay the age at which young people start drinking and reduce the harm it can cause among those who do drink.
- Education programmes should:
  - Increase knowledge of the potential damage alcohol use can cause physically, mentally and socially;
  - Including the legal consequences;
  - Provide the opportunity to explore attitudes to and perceptions of alcohol use;
  - Help develop decision-making, assertiveness, coping and verbal/non-verbal skills;
  - Help develop self-esteem;
  - Increase awareness of how the media, advertisements, role models and the views of parents, peers and society can influence alcohol consumption.
- Introduce a 'whole school' approach to alcohol, in line with DCSF guidance. It should involve staff, parents and pupils and cover everything from policy development and the

school environment to the professional development of (and support for) staff.

- Where appropriate, offer parents or carers information about where they can get help to develop their parenting skills. (This includes problem-solving and communication skills, and advice on setting boundaries for their children and teaching them how to resist peer pressure.)

NICE, 2007

Binge drinking

Binge drinking is a term frequently used in the media, which can be unhelpful in health settings because its health impacts are difficult to predict. It's definition is not standardized and it can be defined as drinking more than 6 units for women and more than 8 units for men i.e. twice the daily limit on a single occasion or simply as drinking to get drunk. It is probably more meaningful to assess patients risk against the lower, increasing, higher risk categories. Those who binge drink only occasionally may not be incurring any significant longer-term health risk as a result whereas those who do so regularly are likely to fall into the higher risk category.

How the population drinks

Fig. 18.1 indicates how the adult population in England and Wales (90% of the UK population) drinks, based on the ONS General Household Survey (2006) and the Alcohol Needs Assessment Research Project (ANARP), DH (2005).

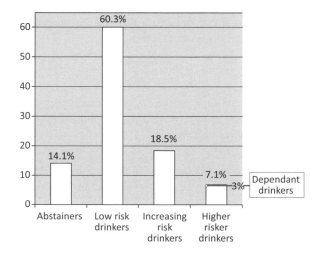

Fig. 18.1 Drinking patterns amongst the adult population in the UK. Adapted from DH (2009) Signs for Improvement.

Lower risk drinking

This group (estimated around 24.8 million people in England) drink alcohol in line with the recommended lower risk limits. There is good evidence to show that preventive activity such as provision of brief (5 minute) advice and information can encourage maintenance of lower risk drinking.

Increasing risk drinking

This group is the largest group of people misusing alcohol (estimated at around 7.6 million people in England). These are adults who regularly exceed the recommended limits for lower risk drinking but are not regularly drinking at the higher risk levels. These drinkers might not currently be experiencing harm from their drinking but are at increasing risk of long-term physical and mental ill health and of being victims of crime, contracting sexually transmitted infections and having unplanned pregnancies. There are also risks to others such as aggression towards family members, general disorder, accidents and assaults.

Higher risk drinking

This group (estimated around 2.9m people in England) regularly drink well over the recommended limits. Higher risk drinkers are those men who regularly drink more than 50 units a week or regularly drink more than 8 units a day and those women who regularly drink more than 35 units a week or regularly drink more than 6 units a day. This group is at a much greater risk than others of the wide range of alcohol-related health harms.

Increasing and higher risk drinkers account for most of the costs (estimated £2.2bn in England) caused by alcohol-related harm to the health economy. This equates to approximately £14.4 million per Primary Care Trust (PCT) in England. Brief (5 minute) information and advice is known to be effective in encouraging increasing and higher risk drinkers to reduce their drinking to lower risk.

Dependent drinking

This group is relatively small. The Alcohol Needs Assessment Research Project for England (DH 2005) found that 3.6% of adults are alcohol dependent; 6% of men and 2% of women. Dependent drinking is identified in some increasing risk drinkers but is more prevalent in higher risk drinkers. Dependent drinkers are more likely to need, and benefit from, access to specialist alcohol treatment interventions at a range of intensity – both for management of the dependence and to reduce risk or costs of other serious health harms. Although only a minority of drinkers become addicted to alcohol, dependent drinkers cost the health economy twice as much per person as other drinkers. In England this equates to £512m nationally or £3.4m per PCT.

Addressing alcohol harm

'Models of Care for Alcohol Misusers (MoCAM)' Department of Health and National Treatment Agency 2006**b**) provides best practice guidance which describes in detail a framework of stepped care for addressing alcohol-related harm.

MoCAM describes four tiers of increasingly intensive evidence-based interventions that should be in place to reduce the harm across the risk groups:

Tier 1 interventions: alcohol-related information and advice; screening; simple brief interventions; and referral

Definition

Tier 1 interventions include provision of: identification of increasing risk, higher risk and dependent drinkers; information on sensible drinking; simple brief interventions to reduce alcohol-related harm; and referral of those with alcohol dependence or harm for more intensive interventions.

Settings

Tier 1 interventions can be delivered by a very wide range of agencies and in a range of settings, the main focus of which is not alcohol treatment. For example: primary health care services; acute hospitals, e.g. A&E departments; psychiatric services; social services departments; homelessness services; antenatal clinics; general hospital wards; police settings, e.g. custody cells; probation services; the prison service; education and vocational services; and occupational health services.

Such interventions can also be provided in highly specialist non-alcohol-specific residential or inpatient services, which have service users with high levels of alcohol-related morbidity who may require care plans and support to facilitate their access to alcohol-specific provision. Examples include: specialist liver disease units, specialist psychiatric wards, forensic units, residential provision for the homeless, and domestic abuse services.

Tier 2 interventions: open access, non-care-planned, alcohol-specific interventions

Definition

Tier 2 interventions include provision of open access facilities and outreach that provide: alcohol-specific advice, information and support; extended brief interventions to help alcohol misusers reduce alcohol-related harm; and assessment and referral of those with more serious alcohol-related problems for care planned treatment.

Settings

Tier 2 provision may be delivered by the following agencies, if they have the necessary competence, and in the following settings: specialist alcohol services; primary health care services; acute hospitals, e.g. A&E and liver units; psychiatric services; social services; domestic abuse agencies; homelessness services; antenatal clinics; probation services; the prison service; and occupational health services.

Tier 3 interventions: community-based, structured, care-planned alcohol treatment

Definition

Tier 3 interventions include provision of community-based specialized alcohol misuse assessment, and alcohol treatment that is care coordinated and care planned .

Interventions

Tier 3 interventions include:

- Comprehensive substance misuse assessment;
- Care planning and review for all those in structured treatment, often with regular keyworker sessions as standard practice;
- Community care assessment and case management of alcohol misusers;
- A range of evidence-based prescribing interventions, in the context of a package of care, including community-based medically assisted alcohol withdrawal (detoxification) and prescribing interventions to reduce risk of relapse;
- A range of structured evidence-based psychosocial therapies and support within a care plan to address alcohol misuse and to address coexisting conditions, such as depression and anxiety, when appropriate;
- Structured day programmes and care planned day care (e.g. interventions targeting specific groups);
- Liaison services, e.g. for acute medical and psychiatric health services (such as pregnancy, mental health or hepatitis services) and social care services (such as child care and housing services and other generic services as appropriate).

Settings

Tier 3 interventions are normally delivered in specialized alcohol treatment services with their own premises in the community (or sometimes on hospital sites). Other delivery may be by outreach (peripatetic work in generic services or other agencies, or domiciliary or home visits). Tier 3 interventions may be delivered alongside Tier 2 interventions. Some of the Tier 3 work is based in primary care settings (shared care schemes and GP-led prescribing services), but alcohol specialist-led services are required within the local systems for the provision of care for severe or complex needs and to support primary care. The work in community settings can be delivered by statutory, voluntary or independent services providing care planned , structured alcohol treatment.

Tier 4 interventions: alcohol specialist inpatient treatment and residential rehabilitation

Definition

Tier 4 interventions include provision of residential, specialized alcohol treatments which are care planned and coordinated to ensure continuity of care and aftercare.

Interventions

Tier 4 interventions include:

- Comprehensive substance misuse assessment, including complex cases when appropriate;
- Care planning and review for all inpatient and residential structured treatment;
- A range of evidence-based prescribing interventions, in the context of a package of care, including medically assisted alcohol withdrawal (detoxification) in inpatient or residential care and prescribing interventions to reduce risk of relapse;
- A range of structured evidence-based psychosocial therapies and support to address alcohol misuse;
- Provision of information, advice and training and 'shared care' to others delivering Tier 1 and Tier 2 and support for Tier 3 services as appropriate.

Settings

Tier 4 settings include:

- Specialized statutory, independent or voluntary sector inpatient facilities for medically assisted alcohol withdrawal (detoxification), stabilization and assessment of complex cases.

- Residential rehabilitation units for alcohol misuse.

- Dedicated specialized inpatient alcohol units are ideal for inpatient alcohol assessment, medically assisted alcohol withdrawal (detoxification) and stabilization. Inpatient provision in the context of general psychiatric wards may only be ideal for some patients with co-morbid severe mental illness, but many such patients might benefit from a dedicated addiction specialist inpatient unit.

- Those with complex alcohol and other needs requiring inpatient interventions may require hospitalization for their other needs (e.g. pregnancy, liver problems) and this may be best provided for in the context of those hospital services (with specialized alcohol liaison support).

The role of nurses in addressing alcohol

Tiers 2 to 4 alcohol interventions are, by their nature, interventions involving increasing levels of specialism from the practitioner and many of those practitioners will be nurses with specialist expertise. However, Tier 1 interventions are necessarily delivered in non-alcohol-specialist settings, they rely on large scale implementation in order to have an epidemiological impact, improve public health and reduce long-term harm. All health practitioners in virtually any setting and those in a number of non-health professions have an important role to play in identifying those whose health is at risk from their alcohol misuse, delivering simple brief advice about alcohol use and referring those who need more intensive treatment.

The public health white paper **'Choosing Health' (DH, 2004) proposed that all health service staff should be in a position to give healthy lifestyle advice to patients.**

Identification and brief advice (IBA)

The primary Tier 1 activity is identification and brief advice (IBA) — sometimes also known as screening and brief intervention (SBI). There is very good evidence that, if implemented sufficiently widely, IBA will have an impact on the preventable health harm and associated costs caused by alcohol misuse. During the past 20 or so years, there have been numerous randomized clinical trials of Identification and Brief Advice in a variety of health care settings. Studies have been conducted in Australia, Bulgaria, Mexico, the United Kingdom, Norway, Sweden, the United States, and many other countries. Evidence for the effectiveness of brief interventions has been summarized in several review articles, including the following.

Bien, et al. (1993) In one of the earliest review articles, Bien, et al. considered 32 controlled studies involving over 6,000 patients, finding that brief interventions were often as effective as more extensive treatments. There is encouraging evidence that the course of harmful alcohol use can be effectively altered by well designed intervention strategies which are feasible within relatively brief contact contexts such as primary health care settings and employee assistance programs.

Kahan, et al. (1995) reviewed 11 trials of brief intervention and concluded that, while further research on specific issues is required, the public health impact of brief interventions is potentially enormous. 'Given the evidence for the effectiveness of brief interventions and the minimal amount of time and effort they require, physicians are advised to implement these strategies in their practice.'

Wilk, et al. (1997) Twelve randomized controlled trials were reviewed by Wilk, et al. who concluded that drinkers receiving a brief intervention were twice as likely to reduce their drinking over 6 to 12 months than those who received no intervention. 'Brief intervention is a low cost , effective preventive measure for heavy drinkers in outpatient settings.'

Moyer, et al. (2002) reviewed studies comparing brief intervention both to untreated control groups and to more extended treatments. They found 'further positive evidence' for the effectiveness of brief intervention, especially among patients with less severe problems. Cautioning that brief intervention should not substitute for specialist treatment, they suggested that they might well serve as an initial treatment for severely dependent patients seeking extended treatment.

The evidence shows that simple brief advice (5 minutes) delivered to increasing and higher risk drinkers will cause one in eight recipients to moderate their drinking. This is a high success rate for a public health preventive intervention. The reason for this level of success from such a simple and quick intervention is still a matter for speculation but it seems likely that a key factor is that most people want to make healthy lifestyle choices and are unaware of:

- a) The range of harm that alcohol can cause;
- b) The levels of alcohol that can cause those harms;
- c) How to calculate how much they actually drink.

With tools and training which are readily available, health practitioners can be in a position to help patients to an understanding of these three factors so that they can make the healthy choice.

To encourage more primary care practitioners to support patients to make healthier lifestyle choices a Directed Enhanced Service (DES) was introduced in England in April 2008 for alcohol-related risk reduction in order to:

- Encourage practices to review newly registered patients aged 16 or over;
- Where any patient is identified as possibly drinking alcohol at increasing or higher risk levels, to offer and deliver

a brief intervention aimed at reducing alcohol related risks.

This Directed Enhanced Service funds the activities undertaken by GP practices on their own registered practice population.

It was originally intended that the scheme run for a two year period however this was extended for a further year until March 2011.

IBA comprises two components, as its name suggests:

1. Identification of those whose drinking poses risk,

2. Brief advice/information.

Identification is achieved by means of a validated World Health Organization developed identification tool. The Alcohol Use Disorders Identification Test (AUDIT). The test consists of ten short questions which take less than a minute to complete and analyse and the resulting scores show a high degree of specificity and accuracy in identifying alcohol misuse and the degree of risk. Those identified as lower risk require no intervention, those identified as possibly dependent are offered referral to a local specialist alcohol service for full assessment and those identified as increasing or higher risk drinkers are offered brief advice.

Brief advice is based on motivational interviewing techniques which provide information, steer the recipient through a decision-making process and encourage positive affirmations. It is usually structured around a leaflet designed for the purpose. The advice session can be delivered in 5–10 minutes. An example of screening and advice tool is shown in Figure 18.3.

95% of adults have some relationship with alcohol and most will have views and perhaps preconceptions . It's important to bear in mind that the main target for health practitioners in terms of alcohol is not someone who has an obvious alcohol problem — though these should not be ignored. Those for whom IBA is most effective might consider themselves moderate drinkers and might even drink more moderately than many health practitioners. Some health care providers may have identified particular target groups as important for IBA — such as people on Quality and Outcomes Framework (QOF) registers for those with hypertension or diabetes. Alcohol, even at what may appear to some relatively moderate levels, does cause chronic disease and It's important that practitioners are non-judgemental in their approach to patients' alcohol use and that they deliver advice based on evidence rather than personal or anecdotal views.

Training in the delivery of alcohol IBA is available as e-learning http://www.alcohollearningcentre.org.uk/eLearning/

(see below for description of the Alcohol Learning Centre)

Case Study 18.1: Bradley

Bradley does not think his drinking is a problem as he states he has a high tolerance level. He and his wife drink a couple of bottles of red wine between them most nights. He believes that he is in generally good health, although he has recently been treated by his GP for hypertension.

He lives with his wife and two children but admits that his relationship with his wife is not good and they frequently argue quite violently. During the argument that led to his visit to the A&E Department, his wife threw an empty wine bottle at him, which struck him on the forehead. His wife is pregnant with their third child and he states that she is often stressed and anxious and he claims that her 'stressing' is often a trigger for their numerous arguments.

His older child aged 14 is having problems at school and has been sent home on a number of occasions for disruptive behaviour.

Discussion points

1. Why might Bradley's visit to A&E warrant screening for alcohol misuse?

2. From what he says, roughly how many units on average is Bradley is drinking each day?

3. How does this compare with recommended limit for males?

4. What are some of the physical health problems that Bradley may be susceptible to if he continues to drink at these levels?

5. What psycho/social problems might Bradley experience as a consequence of his misuse of alcohol?

6. What are the risk factors for Bradley's wife?

7. What are the risk factors for Bradley's children?

8. What action could you take?

As identified above, one of the common reasons for alcohol related attendance at A&E Departments is 'violent assault', along with incidents involving weapons, road traffic accidents, psychiatric emergencies, deliberate self-harm episodes. Screening for alcohol misuse in these instances therefore, is more likely to unearth problem drinking, which may lead to a behaviour changing intervention.

Bradley is drinking roughly a bottle of red wine a day so at least 9 units a day — see advice tool in the appendix for a bottle of wine at 12.5% abv—so he is regularly exceeding the lower risk recommendation of 3 to 4 units for men. He appears not to have alcohol free days.

Questions	Scoring system					Your score
	0	1	2	3	4	
How often do you have a drink containing alcohol?	Never	Monthly or less	2 - 4 times per month	2 - 3 times per week	4+ times per week	
How many units of alcohol do you drink on a typical day when you are drinking?	1 -2	3 - 4	5 - 6	7 - 9	10+	
How often have you had 6 or more units if female, or 8 or more if male, on a single occasion in the last year?	Never	Less than monthly	Monthly	Weekly	Daily or almost daily	
How often during the last year have you found that you were not able to stop drinking once you had started?	Never	Less than monthly	Monthly	Weekly	Daily or almost daily	
How often during the last year have you failed to do what was normally expected from you because of your drinking?	Never	Less than monthly	Monthly	Weekly	Daily or almost daily	
How often during the last year have you needed an alcoholic drink in the morning to get yourself going after a heavy drinking session?	Never	Less than monthly	Monthly	Weekly	Daily or almost daily	
How often during the last year have you had a feeling of guilt or remorse after drinking?	Never	Less than monthly	Monthly	Weekly	Daily or almost daily	
How often during the last year have you been unable to remember what happened the night before because you had been drinking?	Never	Less than monthly	Monthly	Weekly	Daily or almost daily	
Have you or somebody else been injured as a result of your drinking?	No		Yes, but not in the last year		Yes, during the last year	
Has a relative or friend, doctor or other health worker been concerned about your drinking or suggested that you cut down?	No		Yes, but not in the last year		Yes, during the last year	

Scoring: 0 – 7 Lower risk, 8 – 15 Increasing risk, 16 – 19 Higher risk, 20+ Possible dependence

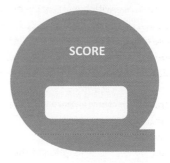

Fig. 18.2 To demonstrate the WHO's validated audit tool: The Alcohol Use Disorder Identification Test. Saunders, J. B. et al. (1993).

This is one unit...

For more detailed information on calculating unit see www.units.nhs.uk/unitCalculator.html

 Half pint of regular beer, lager or cider

 1 very small glass of wine(9%)

 1 single measure of spirits

 1 single glass of sherry

 1 single measure of aperitifs

 How many units did you drink today?

...and each of these is more than one unit

 2 A pint of "**regular**" beer, lager or cider

 3 A pint of "strong" / "premium" beer, lager or cider

 1.5 Alcopop or a 275ml bottle of regular lager

 2 440ml can of "regular" lager or cider

 4 440ml can of "super strength" lager

 3 250ml glass of wine (12%)

 9 Bottle of wine (12.5%)

Risk	Men	Women	Common Effects
Lower Risk	No more than 3-4 units per day on a regular basis	No more than 2-3 units per day on a regular basis	• Increased relaxation • Sociability • Reduced risk of heart disease(for men over 40 and post menopausal women)
Increasing Risk	More than 3-4 units per day on a regular basis	More than 2-3 units per day on a regular basis	*progressively increasing risk of:* • Low energy • Memory loss • Relationship problems
Higher Risk	More than 8 units per day on a regular basis or more than 50 units per week	More than 6 units per day on a regular basis or more than 35 units per week	• Depression • Insomnia • Impotence • Injury • Alcohol dependence • High blood pressure • Liver disease • Cancer

There are times when you will be at risk even after one or two units. For example, with strenuous exercise, operating heavy machinery, driving or if you are on certain medication.

If you are pregnant or trying to conceive, it is recommended that you avoid drinking alcohol. But if you do drink, it should be no more than 1-2 units once or twice a week and avoid getting drunk.

Your screeening score suggests you are drinking at a rate that increases your risk of harm and you might be at risk of problems in the future.

what do you think?

NHS

What's everyone else like?

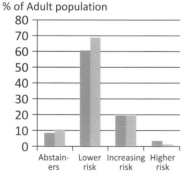

■ Male ■ Female

% of Adult population

The benefits of cutting down

Psychological/Social/Financial
• Improved mood
• Improved relationship
• Reduced risks of drink driving
• Save money

Physical
• Sleep better
• More energy
• Lose weight
• No hangovers
• Reduced risk of injury
• Improved memory
• Better physical shape
• Reduced risk of high blood pressure
• Reduced risks of cancer
• Reduced risks of liver disease
• Reduced risks of brain damage

What targets should you aim for?

Men
• Should not regularly drink more than 3-4 units of alcohol a day.

Women
• Should not regularly drink more than 2-3 units a day.

'Regularly' means drinking every day or most days of the week.
You should also take a break for 48 hours afetr a heavy session to let your body recover.

Making your plan

• When bored or stressed have a workout instead of drinking
• Avoid going to the pub after work
• Plan activities and tasks at those times you would usually drink
• When you do drink, set yourself a limit and stick to it
• Have your first drink afetr starting to eat
• Quench your thirst with non-alcoholic drinks before and in-between alcoholic drinks
• Avoid drinking in rounds or in large groups
• Switch to low alcohol beer/lager
• Avoid or limit the time spent with "heavy" drinking friends

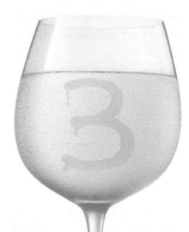

What is your personal target?

This brief advice is based on the **"How Much Is Too Much?"** Simple Structured Advice Intervention Tool, developed by Newcastle University and the Drink Less materials originally developed at the university of sydney as part of a W.H.O. collaborative study.

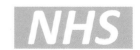 **NHS**

Fig. 18.3 Structured leaflet for giving brief advice.

From the information Bradley supplies it's likely that an AUDIT test would show that he is drinking at the higher risk level.

As well as a number of diseases which, by definition, are wholly attributable to alcohol consumption, such as alcohol poisoning and alcoholic liver disease, there are a number of conditions to which alcohol is a significant contributory factor (see Table 18.1 above) including diseases such as hypertension, stroke, ischaemic heart disease, malignant neoplasm, and diabetes. Compared to those drinking at lower risk levels, men drinking at the higher risk double their risk of stroke and quadruple their risk of hypertension.

As previously described, there a number of potential psycho/social consequences of his misuse of alcohol including **family problems,** work difficulties, crime, unemployment, social isolation, debt, mental and emotional problems.

His wife is pregnant and also under stress. She may also be drinking as a coping mechanism but be unaware of the potential risk to the foetus.

The effects of alcohol on Bradley's family environment may have a detrimental impact on his children leading to behavioural problems and underperformance at school. His children may also follow his example and begin to use alcohol themselves.

Bradley's mention of alcohol as a contributory factor in the injury with which he is presenting provides an opportunity to open a valuable dialogue about his drinking. An AUDIT test will only take a couple of minutes for him to complete and two or three minutes of brief advice using a structured leaflet, which guides both practitioner and patient, could make him aware of the potential harm his drinking may be doing and cause him to cut back.

If there isn't time or opportunity to undertake IBA there and then, it would be worth suggesting that he does talk to someone about his drinking as it could be affecting his health (e.g. the hypertension). An Alcohol Specialist Nurse employed in the hospital or his GP would be able to give him some advice. If an AUDIT shows that Bradley has developed some degree of alcohol dependency he should not be advised to stop, but should be referred to a local alcohol service for specialist assessment and you will need to make yourself familiar with points of contact specified in the local care pathway for alcohol specialist treatment.

> **Box 18.1** Key documents
>
> - **Safe. Sensible. Social. The next steps in the National Alcohol Strategy,** Department of Health, Home Office, Department for Education and Skills, Department for Culture, Media and Sport (DH, 2007).
> - **Models of Care**, MoCAM (DH, 2006b).
> - **Signs for Improvement: Commissioning interventions to reduce alcohol-related harm (DH, 2009a).**

- A summary of the **Review of the Effectiveness of Treatment for Alcohol Problems** (DH, 2006a).
- Local Routes — guidance on developing **Alcohol treatment pathways** (DH, 2009b).
- **Working Together to Reduce Harm, The substance misuse strategy for Wales 2008-2018** *(Welsh Assembly Government, 2008).*
- **Changing Scotland's Relationship with Alcohol: A Framework for Action** (Scottish Government, 2009).
- **New Strategic Direction for Alcohol and Drugs 2006-2011 Northern Ireland** (Department of Health, Social Services and Public Safety, 2006).

The Alcohol Learning Centre (ALC) was commissioned by the Department of Health (England) to develop, manage and disseminate a broad variety of online resources to assist commissioners, service mangers and practitioners nationally to increase their capacity to drive down the rates of alcohol-related hospital admissions.

The Alcohol Learning Centre is now established as an online 'one-stop-shop' providing online support and resources to commissioners, service managers and practitioners with a responsibility for, or an interest in, the prevention and treatment of alcohol misuse or alcohol-related ill health. The main features of the ALC include:

- Alcohol specific policy documents;
- Guidance and tools;
- Information from the Screening and Intervention Programme for Sensible Drinking (SIPS);
- The HubCAPP database of local implementation strategies and initiatives;
- E-learning modules to train health care professionals to deliver Identification and Brief Advice (IBA);
- Regional pages to support the work of Regional Alcohol Managers/Offices showcasing work with local delivery partners;
- Stakeholder area for the Department of Health's Alcohol Effects campaign.

Summary

Alcohol misuse is a major cause of disease and injury worldwide and is now recognized as one of the key challenges for public health in the UK. The predominant cause of chronic alcohol-related ill health and therefore, of the majority of the health harms and costs, is regular and frequent alcohol misuse

The number of people in the UK who drink at levels likely to present risk to their health has risen steadily over recent decades and rates of chronic alcohol-related illness are rising steadily year on year.

The harms caused by alcohol misuse extend beyond physical health and are associated with a range of psycho-social problems. These harms also extend to family members and wider society.

The majority of alcohol-related ill health is chronic and nursing staff have a crucial role to play in facilitating behavior change and promoting healthier lifestyles using 'Identification and Brief Advice' (IBA) — sometimes also known as screening and brief intervention (SBI). There is very good evidence that, if implemented sufficiently widely, IBA will have an impact on the preventable health harm and associated costs caused by alcohol misuse.

There is a growing variety of online resources to assist commissioners, service mangers and practitioners nationally to increase their capacity to drive down the rates of alcohol-related hospital admissions — including online training programmes. These can be accessed via the Department of Health's 'Alcohol Learning Centre'.

 Online Resource Centre

For more information on reducing problems caused by alcohol visit the Online Resource Centre —
http://www.oxfordtextbooks.co.uk/orc/linsley/

Further reading

http://www.drinking.nhs.uk/questions/recommended-levels/

http://www.alcohollearningcentre.org.uk/eLearning/

Alcohol Learning Centre http://www.alcohollearningcentre.org.uk/

Alcohol Concern (1999). *Proposals for a National Strategy for England.* London: Alcohol Concern.

Bien, T. H., Miller, W. R. & Tonigan, J. S. (1993). Brief interventions for alcohol problems: A review. *Psychotherapy: Theory, Research and Practice* 19: 276–288.

Cabinet Office (2003). *Interim Analytical Report.* Strategy Unit Alcohol Harm Reduction project. London: Cabinet Office.

Corrao, G., Bagnardi, V., Zambon, A. & La Vecchia, C., (2004). A meta-analysis of alcohol consumption and the risk of 15 diseases, *Preventive Medicine* 38(5):613–619.

Department of Health (2004) Choosing health: Making healthier choices easier. London: Her Majesty's Stationery Office.

Department of Health (2005). The Alcohol Needs Assessment Research Project (ANARP). London: Her Majesty's Stationery Office.

Department of Health (2006a). *A summary of the Review of the Effectiveness of Treatment for Alcohol Problems.* National Treatment Agency for Substance Misuse. London: Her Majesty's Stationery Office.

Department of Health (2006b). *Models of care for alcohol misusers (MoCAM),* London: Her Majesty's Stationery Office.

Department of Health (2007). *Safe. Sensible. Social. The next steps in the National Alcohol Strategy, The cost of alcohol-related harm to the NHS in England.* London: Her Majesty's Stationery Office.

Department of Health (2008). *Reducing Alcohol Harm: Health services in England for alcohol misuse* London: Her Majesty's Stationery Office.

Department of Health (2009a). *Signs for Improvement: Commissioning interventions to reduce alcohol-related harm.* London: Her Majesty's Stationery Office.

Department of Health (2009b). *Local Routes: Guidance for developing alcohol treatment pathways.* London: Her Majesty's Stationery Office.

Department of Health, Social Services and Public Safety (2006). *New Strategic Direction for Alcohol and Drugs 2006–2011.* Belfast: Department of Health, Social Services and Public Safety.

Department of Work and Pensions (2010). Social effects of alcohol misuse http://www.dwp.gov.uk/publications/specialist-guides/medical-conditions/a-z-of-medical-conditions/alcohol/social-effects-of-alcohol/, accessed 07.05.10.

English D.R., Holman C.D.J., Milne E., Winter M.J., & Hulse G.K. et al. (1995). *The quantification of drug-caused morbidity and mortality in Australia.*Canberra: Commonwealth Department of Human Services and Health.

Giovanni C., Vincenzo B., Antonella Z, & Carlo La V. (2004). A meta-analysis of alcohol consumption and the risk of 15 diseases, *Preventive Medicine* 38(5)613–619.

Gutjahr E., Gmel G., & Rehm J. (2001). Relation between average alcoholconsumption and disease. An overview. *European Addiction Research*, 7: 117–127.

Hamajima N., Hirose K., Tajima K., Rohan T., & Calle E.E., et al. (2002). Alcohol,tobacco and breast cancer — collaborative reanalysis of individual datafrom 53 epidemiological studies, including 58,515 women with breast cancer and 95,067 women without the disease. *British Journal of Cancer* 87:1234–1245.

Health Promotion Agency for Northern Ireland and Irish Temperance League (2005). *Drinking behaviour among young people in Northern Ireland: Secondary analysis of alcohol data from 1997 to 2003* Belfast: Health Promotion Agency for Northern Ireland.

Kahan, M., Wilson, L., & Becker, L. (1995). Effectiveness of physician-based interventions with problem drinkers: a review. *The Canadian Medical Association Journal* 152(6): 851–859.

Moyer, A., Finney, J. W., Swearingen, C. E & Vergun, P. (2002). Brief interventions for alcohol problems: a meta-analytic review of controlled investigations in treatment-seeking and non-treatment-seeking populations. *Addiction* 97: 279–292.

National Institute for Health and Clinical Excellence (2007). School-based interventions on alcohol, Quick reference guide, London: National Institute for Health and Clinical Excellence.

National Institute for Health and Clinical Excellence and National Collaborating Centre for Women's and Children's Health Antenatal Care (2008). *Routine care for the healthy pregnant woman, Clinical Guideline.* London: National Institute for Health and Clinical Excellence.

Rehm J., Room R., Monteiro M., Gmel G., & Graham K., *et al.* (2004). Alcohol use.In: Ezzati M., Lopez A.D., Rodgers A., & Murray C.J.L., (eds.) *Comparative quantification of health risks global and regional burden of disease attributable to selected major risk factors.* Geneva: WHO.

Ridolfo B., & Stevenson C. (2001). *The quantification of drug-caused mortality and morbidity in Australia 1998.* Canberra: Australian Institute of Health and Welfare.

Scottish Government (2008). Costs of Alcohol Use and Misuse http://www.scotland.gov.uk/Publications/2008/05/06091510/0.

Scottish Government (2009). Changing Scotland's Relationship with Alcohol: A Framework for Action http://www.scotland.gov.uk/Publications/2009/03/04144703/3 accessed 07.05.10.

Single E., Robson L., Xie X., & Rehm J. (1996). The cost of substance abuse in Canada. Ottawa: Canadian Centre on Substance Abuse.

Singleton, N., Bumpstead, R., O'Brien, M., Lee, A., & Meltzer, H. (2001). *Psychiatric morbidity among adults living in private households (2000).* London: The Stationery Office.

Stratton, K., Howe, C., & Battaglia, F. (1996). *Fetal Alcohol Syndrome: Diagnosis, Epidemiology,Prevention, and Treatment.* Washington: National Academy Press.

Streissguth, A. P. (1997). *Fetal Alcohol Syndrome: a Guide for Families and Communities.* Baltimore: Paul H. Brookes Publishing Co.

Welsh Assembly Government (2007). *Welsh Health Survey 2005–06.* Cardiff: Welsh Assembly Government.

Welsh Assembly Government (2008) *'Working Together to Reduce Harm',* the substance misuse strategy for Wales 2008–2018. Cardiff: Welsh Assembly Government.

Wilk, A. I., Jensen, N. M. & Havighurst, T. C. (1997). Meta-analysis of randomized control trials addressing brief interventions in heavy alcohol drinkers. *Journal of General Internal Medicine* 12 (5):274–83.

Chapter 19
Long-term conditions

Sian Maslin-Prothero and Andrew Finney

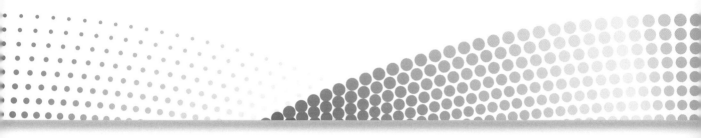

Introduction

The Department of Health estimates that about 78% of all health care spend relates to people with long-term conditions (LTCs), 80% of all General Practitioner (GP) consultations relate to long-term conditions and that patients with long-term conditions or complications utilize over 60% of hospital bed days, often as a result of an emergency admission (DH 2008a).

Understanding long-term conditions and their implications for us as public health practitioners is essential. By the end of this chapter you will be able to demonstrate an understanding of the following in relation to long-term conditions:

- Definitions of LTCs;
- Key figures and statistics relating to long-term conditions;
- Using a whole systems approach to deliver health and social care to people with long-term conditions;
- Self care and self management in long-term conditions, including how nurses can support this;
- Policy regarding long-term conditions across the United Kingdom (UK).

In 1998 a devolved form of government for Wales, Scotland and Northern Ireland was introduced and this has provided these political bodies with new freedoms to pursue and develop their own health policy. We have attempted to capture this in our chapter.

> **Box 19.1** Ten things about long-term conditions (DH, 2008a)
>
> 1. 15.4 million people, or almost one in three of the population, in England suffer from a long-termcondition.
> 2. Three out of every five people aged over 60 in England suffer from a long-termcondition.
> 3. Due to the aging population the number of people in England with a long-term condition is set to rise by 23% over the next 25 years.
> 4. 5% of the patients, the majority of whom have one or more long-term condition account for 49% of all in-patient hospital bed days.
> 5. Patients with long-term conditions are very intensive users of health care services. Those with long-term conditions account for 31% of the population, but use 52% of all GP appointments, and 65% of all outpatient appointments.
> 6. It is estimated that the treatment and care of those with long-term conditions accounts for 69% of the primary and acute care budget in England.
> 7. 6.4 million people have clinically identified hypertension. It is estimated that the same number again have unidentified hypertension, meaning that an estimated one in five of the population suffers from the condition.

8. Common mental health problems affect about one in seven of the adult population with severe mental health problems affecting one in a hundred.

9. The UK economy stands to lose £16 billion over the next 10 years through premature deaths due to heart disease, stroke and diabetes.

10. It is estimated that 85% of deaths in the UK are from chronic diseases. Within this, 36% of all deaths will be from cardiovascular disease and 7% from chronic respiratory disease.

Defining long-term conditions

Long-term conditions (sometimes referred to as chronic conditions) are defined by the World Health Organization (WHO, 2008) as health problems that require ongoing management over a period of years or decades. The Long-term conditions Alliance Scotland (LTCAS) say that long-term conditions are of prolonged duration that may affect any aspect of the person's life (LTCAS, 2008). The Department of Health (DH) states that long-term conditions are those conditions that cannot, at present, be cured but can be controlled by medication and other therapies, and that many people live with a condition that limits their ability to cope with day-to-day activities (DH 2007a). These long-term conditions can be life threatening, affecting people physically, mentally and emotionally and include a wide range of health conditions such as:

- **Non-communicable diseases** such as cancer and cardiovascular disease; **Communicable diseases** such as HIV/AIDS;

- Asthma; diabetes; epilepsy, psoriasis; arthritis; chronic pain;

- Other conditions to consider are certain mental health disorders like schizophrenia or depression;

- Ongoing impairments in structure, for example blindness or joint disorders.

This list is by no means exhaustive (London Health Observatory (LHO), 2008, LTCAS, 2008). In Northern Ireland heart disease, stroke, diabetes, asthma, cancer and chronic obstructive pulmonary disease are the most common long-term conditions (Chartered Society of Physiotherapists (CSP), 2008).

Many other conditions now fall into the category of chronic or long-term for example; changes in society require the recognition of childhood conditions such as **attention deficit hyperactivity disorder** (ADHD) which can also affect adults on a smaller scale. Childhood and adult obesity is also a condition that causes long-term problems and has been a media target of recent years.

'Chronic diseases are diseases of long duration and generally slow progression. Chronic diseases, such as heart disease, stroke, cancer, chronic respiratory diseases and diabetes, are by far the leading cause of mortality in the world, representing 60% of all deaths. Out of the 35 million people who died from chronic disease in 2005, half were under 70 and half were women'
WHO, 2008

Some people are born with long-term conditions whilst others will be affected at different ages and stages of life. Many people have more than one long-term condition; usually there is no cure but there are things that can be done to maintain and improve quality of life (LTCAS, 2008). There is evidence of inequalities; the prevalence of chronic conditions increases with age, social class and geographical location — for example in a study into social class inequalities in Britain, Wales had high rates of poor health in comparison with other regions across all seven social classes (Doran, Drever and Whitehead, 2004). Because the prevalence of chronic conditions is highest in older people and that there is an ageing of the population across all four countries of the UK, it is likely that most people aged 65 and over will have at least one chronic condition. This will have an impact on the provision of a public health service because long-term conditions have a direct impact on health and social care services (National Public Health Service for Wales, 2005).

Tackling the challenge

The **British Medical Association** (2006) has highlighted that one of the major challenges in improving the management of long-term conditions is in the redeployment of resources — human and financial — in health and social care. This can be illustrated by the fact that many older people are admitted to secondary care not because of a medical problem but because of a lack of social and domestic support. One way that this challenge can be addressed is through using a whole systems approach described as a structured, consistent approach that can be used in order that local health and social care partners can deliver integrated long-term care.

A **whole systems approach** is concerned with all agencies working together in their localities, in partnership. Using this approach recognizes that a wide range of demographic, social and economic factors and available services interact with agencies, for example clients and their families, professional health and social services —that is nothing works independently of the other. Therefore a problem or issue is not the responsibility of one factor, individual or team, but is addressed by working together with the relevant agencies to find solutions. A whole systems approach also acknowledges that systems can be complex and dynamic.

Working with a whole systems approach, recognizing the roles and responsibilities of the many professions within health and social care, and the important role of voluntary and charitable agencies — is a necessary requisite of nursing today and the future. It has been acknowledged that changes in the management of long-term conditions and earlier discharges from the acute sector have resulted in increasing pressure on the workload of community services (Baldwin, 2006; Department of Health (DH) 2005a; DH, 2008b).

The growing emphasis on improved management of long-termchronic conditions will further shift the emphasis from secondary care to primary care (DH, 2004). These developments, coupled with the **European Working Time Directive** (EWTD) reducing junior doctors' hours, are opening up a number of opportunities for nurses, midwives and health visitors to extend and expand their roles (Chief Nursing Officer (CNO), 2003) through, for example, the creation of community matron posts.

An evaluation of integrated health and social care working — referred to as whole system demonstrators programme — using assistive technologies, i.e. telecare and telehealth, is being undertaken at three sites in the UK: Kent, Cornwall and Newham. The focus is on people with chronic pulmonary disease (CPD), heart disease and diabetes, and adults with social care or health and social care needs who are at risk of hospital admission — that is long-term conditions. Using a randomized controlled trial, data are to be collected by the NHS on emergency admission rates and bed days, patient/carer experience and quality of life, and the impact on primary care; providing an evaluation of the impact of long-term conditions on health and social services (DH 2008c). The evaluation aims to see whether integrated care, using assistive technologies actually improves the care of older people with long-term conditions.

The aim of the document '**Supporting People with Long-term conditions : An NHS and Social Care Model** to support local innovation and integration' (Department of Health (DH) 2005a) was to set out a strategy for the management of people with long-term conditions. An important requirement for local health communities in England for example, is to recognize all patients with long-term conditions within their area, and the most appropriate treatment for each individual. This has been set into three levels based on need (London Health Observatory (LHO), 2008) (see Fig. 19.1) long-term conditions.

The NHS and social care long-term conditions model uses and builds on the Kaiser Permanente Triangle and aims to provide a system that matches care with need.

Level 1: Supported self care. This level would apply to 70–80% of the long-term condition population and involves helping individuals and their carers to care for their conditions effectively.

Level 2: Disease specific care management. This would apply to people who have a complex single need or multiple conditions.

Level 3: Case management. This level would apply to 3–4% of the long-term condition population, and requires the identification of the very high intensity users of unplanned secondary care.

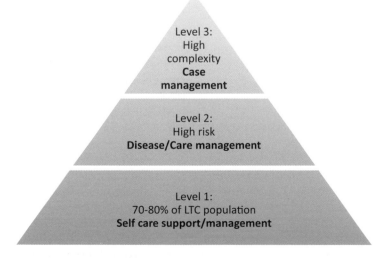

Fig. 19.1 The NHS and social care long-term conditions. Department of Health (2007b).

Case Study 19.1: George and Margaret

George is 63 year old retired farmer who lives with his 70 year old sister Margaret. George was diagnosed with rheumatoid arthritis when he was 40 and has experienced many years with extreme pain and joint inflammation. George has been a regular service user for over 20 years and spent long periods of time in hospital in his 40's and 50's with arthritic flares that required high usage of steroids to get George back to his regular lifestyle of heavy farm labour and long hours.

As a smoker since his teens George is finding breathing difficult. He was encouraged to give up smoking at the age of 59, when he was diagnosed with Type 2 diabetes. George is visited by a heath care support worker from the District Nurse team once a week who records his blood glucose levels due to poor concordance, and checks his compliance with his diet and insulin intake. The community nurse also guides Margaret (who is George's carer) on managing his insulin requirements.

George also has joint deformities of his toes and fingers, his breathing is now restricting his mobility and he is very conscious to the fact that he has osteoarthritis. George visits his local hospital once a month. He has blood tests to monitor the drugs he takes (Methotrexate and Sulphasalazine) and sees the diabetes nurse specialist for guidance and advice.

Margaret has developed venous leg ulcers and has to have a visit from the community nurse twice a week to monitor and redress her ulcers; the community nurse has suggested that despite the regular compression bandaging and the lack of infection in the wounds, they are not improving.

Questions:

What is the long-term outlook for George and his sister Margaret?

In terms of the DH social care model, at what level do George and Margaret find themselves?

Discussion points

What is the long-term outlook for George and his sister Margaret?

There is a lot of community nurse intervention taking place (primary care) but the outlook seems poor for the brother and sister. Margaret may ultimately need hospitalization if her leg ulceration worsens which leaves George without a carer. There is the potential for both George and Margaret to lose their mobility. The main goal is to keep them at home which requires keeping them healthy and mobile. Both Margaret and George are heavily reliant on the multidisciplinary team. Margaret will

benefit from a thorough review by the Tissue Viability Nurse in order to prevent a hospital admission. At present the community nursing intervention is helping. A social care assessment would assess the needs of both siblings. The involvement of an independent carer may take some pressure from both George and Margaret enabling them to relinquish some of their daily tasks and manage better at home.

In terms of the DH social care model, at what level do George and Margaret find themselves?

Level 2: Disease specific care management. This would apply to people who have a complex single need or multiple conditions. George and Margaret currently require a lot of attention for their complex needs. Without suitable intervention to keep them at their current health state they may become level 3.

Level 3: Case management. This level would apply to 3–4% of the long-term condition population, and requires the identification of the very high intensity users of unplanned secondary care.

The prevalence of long-term conditions

Evidence of the success of a National Health Service (NHS) in Britain can be seen historically through our ageing population and improved life expectancy. Life expectancy for those reaching the age of 65 in the United Kingdom (UK) has reached its highest level (National Statistics, 2006). In the last 25 years life expectancy has increased by 4 years for men and by 2.8 years for women; life expectancy from birth in 2006 was projected to be 88.1 years in males and 91 years in females in the UK (National Statistics, 2006). The ageing of society has been driven by the ageing of the 'baby boom' post world war two generation and the increase in life expectancy (DH, 2008d). This has been accompanied by a reduction in the birth rate such that the population has an increase in the numbers of older people compared to the young.

The DH (2008d) state that the probability of having a long-term condition increases with age; a survey for England suggests 60% of those aged 65 or over say they have a long-term condition compared to only 17% of those under 40 (DH 2008d). This begs the question, if long-term conditions are so prominent in an ageing population, and the ageing population is continuing to increase, what will the effect be on the demands of health and social care providers in the future? In the United States of America (USA) a 2004 survey suggested that 133 million individuals had at least one long-term condition and that by 2020 that figure could rise to 157 million which would equate to half of the population (Partnership for Solutions, 2004).

The DH (2008d) document **'Raising the Profile of Long-term Conditions Care'**, is a compendium of information aimed at raising awareness of the increasing demands of long-term conditions. Surveys have suggested that by 2025 the number of people over 65 will have increased by 42% in England alone. This equates to the number of people with one known long-term condition increasing from 3 million to 18 million. Those people with the long-term conditions will be the main users of both primary and secondary care services. Long-term conditions account for 52% of GP appointments, 65% of outpatient appointments and 72% of inpatient bed days (DH, 2008d).

This all adds up to a huge increase in cost of what equates to the most expensive services. A best estimate by DH (2008d) suggests that treatment and care for those with long-term conditions will account for 69% of the total heath and social care spend in England. Considering that people with long-term conditions are less likely to be able to work, we are looking at a huge burden on the economy if current trends and DOH predictions are not taken seriously.

The Quality and Outcomes Framework (QOF 2007 cited in DH 2008d) is a reward and incentive programme for General Practices that attempts to focus health care on priority areas. Its 2006/2007 figures for England presented prevalence counts for a number of long-term conditions, and the number of those affected by a long-term condition was:

- Hypertension: 6,706,000;
- Asthma: 3,100,000;
- Diabetes: 1,962,000;
- Coronary Heart Disease: 1,899,000;
- Stroke and Transient Ischemic Attack: 863,000;
- Chronic Obstructive Pulmonary Disease: 766,000;
- Cancer: 489,000.

If we also consider neurological disorders, such as multiple sclerosis, Parkinson's disease and motor neurone disease, as well as musculoskeletal conditions — such as, osteoarthritis and osteoporosis — it is easy to see how we reach figures of 15.4 million for people with a long-term condition in Britain.

world that long-term conditions are inevitable. Increasing life expectancy, along with many other factors related to health, means diseases and conditions that would once be expected to kill are now considered chronic and there for the long-term. Larsen (2006) considers advances in bacteriology, immunology and pharmacology as considerable developments in public health that have caused a drop in mortality rates. This along with advances in medicine and its procedures have ultimately led to a growth of long-term conditions.

Children with cystic fibrosis (CF) may now have the benefit of a lung transplant; adults with disabling osteoarthritis may get a new hip or knee. The people that may have once died of a myocardial infarction are now long-term patients with heart disease. The same can be said of neurological, respiratory and endocrine conditions. Larsen (2006) suggests that health care in USA was never intended for the treatment of long-term conditions and because of the system of 'component style care' where the patient pays individually for different types of care; no one is able to manage the whole illness or disease. This means higher costs may occur.

The British government along with the Department of Health (DH) have aimed to be responsive rather than reactive to these demands. A national health service that that is non-profit-making and free at the point of care has the opportunity to make sure that care for long-term conditions is not compartmentalized but has a structured systematic approach that delivers treatment and care for all patients with long-term condition when it is required.

For example, in Scotland the Long-Term Conditions Collaborative (LTCC) was launched in April 2008. This programme is being developed to support NHS Scotland in using tools and techniques for clinical systems improvement that will enable all staff to be involved in continuously improving the delivery of patient centred services. There are 3 work streams: self management; specialist care; and complex care. It also incorporates improvement work led by the Scottish Primary Long-term Care Collaborative (LTCC 2008).

Public health

Public health is seen as the need for each country to safeguard the health and well-being of their nation. In England the Department for Health (DH) considers health protection, health improvement and health inequalities as the key issues. Sir Donald Acheson, a former Chief Medical Officer described public health as:

'... the science and art of preventing disease, prolonging life, and promoting health through the organized efforts of society'
Acheson, 1988: 1

The success of a modern health service must not be understated; public health has improved so much in the developed

Self-care and self-management

Self-care

Self-care was highlighted in the **NHS Plan** (DH 1997) and is a key component of the model for supporting people with long-term conditions (DH 2005b). There are number of reasons for self care being promoted including current health and social policy in the United Kingdom (UK) which demonstrates a clear commitment by government to make patients and carers the focus of services (DH, 2005b); service redesign and delivery to take into account the changing demographic of the population and lessons learnt from overseas (Battersby *et al.*, 2002; Battersby, 2005).

Jones (2006) conducted a systematic review of the literature relating to self-care and identified a number of different terms and definitions. Self-care is seen as a multidimensional construct with definitions varying as to who is involved, why self care occurs, what is entailed, and how self-care is accomplished (Becker *et al.*, 2004). Essentially, self management indicates the active participation of patients in their treatment (Lorig and Holman, 2003), and self-management support involves:

'[the person with the chronic disease] engaging in activities that protect and promote health, monitoring and managing the symptoms and signs of illness, managing the impact of illness on functioning, emotions and interpersonal relationships and adhering to treatment regimes'
Center for the Advancement of Health 1996

Self-care is a part of daily living; it is the care taken by individuals and carers towards their own health and well-being and includes the care extended to their children, family, friends and others, whether in their homes, neighbourhoods, local communities, or elsewhere. Self-care also includes the actions individuals and carers take for themselves, their children, their families and others to stay fit and maintain good physical and mental health; meet social and psychological needs; prevent illness or accidents; care for minor ailments and long-term conditions; and maintain health and well-being after an acute illness or discharge from hospital.

The benefits of supporting self-care include Improvement to health outcomes, improvement to quality of life, increased patient satisfaction, a more appropriate use of NHS resources, and a reduced demand on services (DH, 2005c; Chodosh *et al.*, 2006; Coulter 2006). Since **'The New NHS'** (DH, 1997) self-care has been a growing theme in UK health and social care policy, with a recognition of the need to provide greater support for people with long-term and chronic health conditions, and helping them to take care of their conditions more effectively (DH, 2004, 2005c, 2005d, 2006).

Self-management

Self-management allows people to understand their health behaviours and develop strategies to live their lives as fully and productively as possible through: taking care of their illness (i.e. medical management), carrying out their normal activities (i.e. role management), and managing their emotional changes (Bodenheimer *et al*, 2002; Lorig and Holman, 2003). Key strategies for improving outcomes involve: assessment of patient-specific needs and barriers, goal setting, enhancing skills, problem-solving, follow-up and support, and

increasing access to resources. However, there is a need to recognize that patients need different interventions, and that they are not always ready to take on the responsibilities of self-management.

The core competencies for self-management support are:

- Relationship building,
- Assessing patients' needs,
- Expectations and values,
- Information sharing,
- Collaborative goalsetting,
- Action planning,
- Problem-solving,
- Follow-up on progress.

Success requires a commitment by health care organizations:

- A delivery system design that supports self-management support and care teams;
- Training for patients, carers and care givers about self-management support and what is expected from them;
- Information systems that prompt and remind staff and patients.

Bodenheimer *et al.* (2002) said that people with chronic conditions are the principal caregivers. They proposed that health care professionals should act as consultants, supporting them in this role. Everyday patients are making decisions about what they do —eating, drinking, going out, taking medication. The Flinders model of care (Battersby, 2005) incorporates:

- A patient-centred approach (holistic), behavioural change towards improved self-management,
- Evidence-based guidelines,
- Prospective care planning,
- Prevention focused, improved coordination of care,
- System change.

The Flinders team have identified six principles for self-management from the patient perspective and these are:

- Know your condition;
- Have active involvement in decision-making with your GP or health workers;
- Follow the care plan that is agreed with your GP and other health professionals;
- Monitor symptoms associated with the condition(s);
- Respond to, manage and cope with the symptoms, manage the physical, emotional and social impact of the condition(s) on your life;
- Live a healthy lifestyle.

The key to success is to integrate the self-management care plan with the health care plan, in a patient-centred way, and to systematically monitor and measure health outcomes. The Flinders model of care acknowledges that people do not always follow theoretical models, recognizes the characteristics of good self-managers and that good self-managers do not require as much input from practitioners. The Flinders model is a tool that can be used to coordinate care as well as a training programme, a system of assessment and support in South Australia, it has been integrated into the pre-registration medical programme, as well as an online postgraduate certificate at Flinders University (Battersby, 2005).

In the UK, Tomlins and Collins (2006) undertook a project aimed at promoting optimal self-care and supporting people in their own care by promoting awareness across health and social care communities of the fundamental importance of self-care, to dispel common myths about self-care. Through enabling conversations with people, by placing interventions into a context of planned rehabilitation, and understanding and incorporating change management skills training for people (through gathering and evaluating information, problem solving, pacing, cost-benefit analysis, planning, goal-setting) Tomlins and Collins (2006) believe that patients are going to demand self-care support from practitioners; we therefore need to be trained to cope with this new demand, and have an understanding of the theoretical models underpinning the promotion of self-care.

There is also a need to address issues of abandonment felt by the client/patient when discharged so that they see that their care is being transferred; the importance of participation, emotional support, respect, and continuity of care has been identified by Coulter (2006), and this fits with the self-care agenda. There is a difference between knowing and understanding your condition, and the practitioner's role in facilitating the move and filling any gaps in knowledge.

The Long Term Conditions Alliance Scotland (LTCAS) is a group that brings together different voluntary and community organizations across Scotland to give a national voice to ensure that the interests and needs of people living with long-term conditions are addressed. Their vision is where people with long-term conditions enjoy, not endure, full and positive lives, free from discrimination and supported by access to high quality services, information and support (LTCAS, 2008). This group have worked collaboratively with health providers and policymakers in order to influence health strategies for example the development of the 'Self Management Strategy for Long-term conditions in Scotland' (2008).

The patient journey

There is a need for practitioners to understand the patient journey and why self-help groups have developed — many of these groups were born out of desperation. For example, people with tinnitus were told to 'go away and live with it' but no one told these people how to live with tinnitus; so they created a self-help group as a means of support (see the British Tinnitus Association web site: http://www.tinnitus.org.uk/).

Some key issues to consider when talking to patients:

- The importance of language, that is patients are people therefore should be referred to as 'people with diabetes' (not 'diabetics'), and so on. If there is to be true partnership, then appropriate language is an important requisite of good clinical practice.

- The need to embrace opportunities; for example, being on a waiting list for an operation could be seen as a further delay for treatment, but it can be viewed is an opportunity to use this time to the benefit of the patient; such as losing weight or improving fitness prior to surgery.

- There are practitioners who erode peoples ability to self-care, because they do not encourage patients to take responsibility for their well-being This can be due to their personal approach, which can be 'disabling' rather than 'enabling'.

- The requirement to direct and signpost places for people to get information and support about their condition.

Case Study 19.2: Louise

Louise is a 15 year old girl with cystic fibrosis (CF). She was diagnosed with CF at a very early age and therefore has no memories of not being what she considers 'labelled' by the condition. Louise and her parents managed well with the condition throughout her childhood. Her parents were taught lots of nursing skills during her many hospital admissions as a child and also benefited from the guidance of physiotherapists. At home Louise's parents were guided by a community team and were able to administer intravenous antibiotics and provide an element of chest physiotherapy for their daughter. Louise has had reoccurring chest infections now for the last few years and has particularly struggled with **pseudomonas**. Her lungs have started to deteriorate so badly that her GP has suggested that she will require a transplant, and has put her on a waiting list. Louise has confided in the CF nurse specialist whilst she has been unwell and has stated that she has been secretly smoking for 2 years. She is fearful of the fact that she is now addicted to smoking and also concerned that she will not be well enough to take her GCSE exams.

Questions

What are the risks associated with Louise smoking?

What support can be put in place for Louise whilst she is awaiting a lung transplant?

Discussion points

What are the risks associated with Louise smoking?

The presence of copious mucous in those people suffering with cystic fibrosis means that Louise already has lungs that do not work to full capacity and is prone to infection. Smoking will only increase the speed of the deterioration of Louise's respiratory function.

What support can be put in place for Louise whilst she is awaiting a lung transplant?

The deterioration in Louise's condition means that she will need a network of support prior to surgery. The inability of the body to take on board required nutrition with cystic fibrosis means that Louise may have problems with diabetes and may have problems with eating in general. A diabetic link nurse would be beneficial to Louise as well as a dietician referral — to assess nutritional support. The long-term outlook may require her to use a Percutaneous Endoscopic Gastrostomy (PEG). The smoking addiction may benefit from the help of a smoking cessation nurse. Perhaps the most useful support for Louise would be psychological support. These problems will bare a huge mental weight to Louise as her condition is so multifaceted.

A multidisciplinary and interdisciplinary team approach

The terms **interdisciplinary** and **multidisciplinary** are often used as mutually exchangeable terms (Marriott, *et al.*, 2005). Multidisciplinary (MDT) refers to where the discipline focuses on their own particular contribution, role, and works in parallel with other disciplines. The interdisciplinary approach is more integrated and coordinated, where the team endeavours to overcome some of the professional and organizational boundaries and seeks to:

'...blur the professional boundaries and requires trust, tolerance, and a willingness to share responsibility'
Nolan, 1995

Characteristics of interdisciplinary working:

- Emphasizes the similarities across professional groups,
- Facilitates a single assessment approach and person centred goal setting,
- Acknowledges areas of shared skills,
- Promotes shared understanding and viewpoint,
- Relies on shared training, mutual trust and respect.

Marriott and Wright, 2002

A musculoskeletal example

Musculoskeletal disorders account for a high number of long-term conditions. The specialism of rheumatology has benefited

hugely from positive research into the many disorders and the management of them. The most common form of inflammatory arthritis is rheumatoid arthritis, affecting approximately 387,000 people in the UK (Arthritis Research Campaign (ARC), 2002); this autoimmune condition is characterized by joint inflammation, giving rise to, pain, swelling, heat and stiffness. Rheumatoid arthritis primarily affects the synovial joints such as the shoulders, wrists, fingers, knees, ankles and toes (ARC, 2002). Ryan and Oliver (2002) suggest that key factors in managing the condition include relieving pain whilst maintaining the patient's optimal function. Fig. 19.2 shows everyone in the multidisciplinary team (MDT) that will work with a patient who has rheumatoid arthritis.

Case Study 19.3: Philip

Philip has had rheumatoid arthritis for 14 years, first starting when he was 28, when the condition came on very quickly. Recently he noticed swelling and stiffness in his hands, which soon spread to most of his joints. At this stage Philip was in a lot of distress and discomfort; he was very stiff and felt like he had the 'flu. His GP realized it was rheumatoid arthritis straight away and because of Philip's clinical history and the obvious joint involvement, Philip was sent for a short spell of intensive treatment in hospital.

Shortly after diagnosis Philip struggled to do his job as an IT technician and became unemployed. He felt unable to apply for other roles due to the unpredictability of his condition as this may cause periods of sickness.

Philip's condition sometimes settles down. He has developed deformities of his hands and fingers, and has had an operation to replace his hip which was damaged by the rheumatoid arthritis. He uses night splints for his wrists and fingers and takes tablets every day.

Philip is now well. He has had to be careful and respect his arthritis. But he can do all the things he wants to and

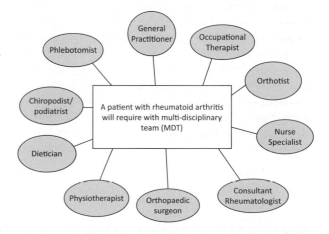

Fig. 19.2 The multidisciplinary team (MDT).

has no difficulty in getting out and about. He still gets pain and stiffness, but it is well controlled and he feels healthy.

Discussion points

Drawing on Fig. 19.2 Philip uses all members of the members of the MDT as follows:

General Practitioner (GP)

Philip makes regular visits to the GP because he relies heavily on **non-steroidal anti-inflammatory drugs (NSAID's)** for which he requires a prescription. His use of NSAID's also means he needs a proton pump inhibitor (PPI) as this will protect his stomach from ulceration sometimes caused by excessive use of NSAID's. Philip is prescribed Omeprazole. He also uses regular analgesia for migraines, a side effect of his treatment for arthritis.

Occupational Therapist (OT)

Philip relies heavily on splints that are cast for his fingers and wrists; these splints keep his fingers flexed and his wrists straight and comfortable in a neutral position through the night. The OT team have also raised the height of Philip's chairs and bed to make getting up from a sitting position easier. He has grab rails by his bath and doors; he also has a toilet raise and a converted shower. The OT also showed him a device to tip his kettle, without having to lift it which stops strain on his wrist joints and a device to put his socks on without reaching down.

Orthotist

Philip was seen by the orthotist who looked closely at what his condition might do to the joints in his feet and toes. He does not need specialist shoes but has been given advice on what footwear is best, and has purchased a pair of house slippers with a very wide and easy to use fastener.

Rheumatology nurse specialist

Philip has recently been started on a new drug for his condition called Infliximab. It is a biologic therapy and works alongside his other specialist drug — a cytotoxic drug called Methotrexate. Due to this treatment Philip sees the nurse specialist once a month, and his blood results are checked and monitored for assessment of disease activity. The medication used can have detrimental side-effects and show abnormal liver tests, therefore his dosage may be adjusted accordingly. Philip has found the nurse specialist helpful over the years; he has had periods of depression and she has helped him develop coping strategies and directed him to counselling groups.

Consultant Rheumatologist

Philip has developed a good, working relationship with the rheumatologists over the years. When his treatment has failed or faltered they have always helped him identify alternative solutions. The consultants working in collaboration with the nurse specialists are the people that recommended Philip for the biologic therapy, which to date, has been very successful.

Orthopaedic Surgeon

The rheumatology centre that Philip attends has strong links between the rheumatologists and the orthopaedic surgeons. Phillip was seen by the two consultants together at one of his scheduled appointments. They both decided upon the need for Philip to have a total hip replacement which made him feel very secure in his decision to have the surgery. He was helped by the opportunity to speak to both specialists about his fears of surgery and its benefits.

Physiotherapy

Initially, Philip thought that physiotherapy may be too intense for him — causing more pain and stiffness than he was already experiencing. However after persuasion Philip realized that gentle exercise was actually beneficial; for example he learned to adapt the way he walked, especially up and down stairs; then he commenced hydrotherapy, which helped to build strength through movement and build muscle tone through immersion in a warm water swimming pool. When an inpatient, Philip had always had hydrotherapy treatment; on discharge the physiotherapists recommended an exercise programme, and he now attends his local swimming pool once a week.

Dietician

In the first few years of his condition Philip became inactive and gained weight; this affected his rheumatoid arthritis, and his mobility was reduced because of his excessive weight. The dietician worked with Philip to educate him regarding his lifestyle, nutrition, and how a well balanced diet would help him keep his weight within a healthy range for his height and age.

Podiatrist/Chiropodist

Because of reduced hand dexterity, Philip was unable to grip or use scissors or nail clippers; regular visits to the podiatrist/chiropodists have ensure that his needs are met.

Phlebotomist

Philip visits the phlebotomist every time he sees the nurse specialist. That way he has blood results for her to evaluate when he visits the outpatients department. Blood monitoring is essential to identify any blood dyscrasias.

Over the last 14 years there have been times where Philip has also needed a carer and a community nurse.

Summary

This chapter has highlighted current health policy and practice with regards to long-term conditions, self-care and self-management. This reflects other policy drivers, including the drive to bring care closer to home with the aim of ensuring acute hospital beds are used appropriately with enhanced care provision being provided in the community setting. The management of long-term conditions using examples of rheumatoid arthritis, cystic fibrosis and older people have illustrated the importance of empowering people to change and adapt lifestyles to improve health and well being and the role of other members of the interdisciplinary team in meeting their needs. Using a whole system approach recognizes and embraces the roles and responsibilities of the different professionals within health and social care a necessary requisite of inter-professional care today and in the future.

 Online Resource Centre

For more information on long-term conditions visit the Online Resource Centre —
http://www.oxfordtextbooks.co.uk/orc/linsley/

Further reading

Evolving Practice
http://www.evolvingpractice.org/home
Accessed 04.01.10.

Evolving Practice is a website that allows practitioners to record, share and celebrate patient focus and public involvement. It is coordinated by the Scottish Health Council.

Long-term conditions Alliance (LTCA)
http://www.ltca.org.uk/pages/about_lmca.html
Accessed 24.09.08.

LTCA was a UK charity that was started in 1989 by a group of national voluntary organizations that wanted to campaign on areas of shared concern relating to long-term conditions. LTCA now has over 100 member organizations, from the largest health charities down to small unfunded support groups staffed by volunteers. In 2008 it became National Voices (see http://www.nationalvoices.org.uk/about-us).

Long-Term Conditions Collaborative (LTCC)
The Long-Term Conditions Collaborative gather, store and share information about self management and long-term conditions in Scotland.
http://ltcscotland.wik.is/
Accessed 04.01.10.

Long-Term Conditions Alliance Northern Ireland (LTCANI)
http://www.ltcani.org.uk/index.asp
Accessed 04.01.10.
The Long-Term Conditions Alliance Northern Ireland (LTCANI) is an umbrella body for voluntary and not for profit organizations working with and for people with long-term conditions in Northern Ireland. Collectively LTCANI member organizations represent approximately 500,000 people with long-term conditions in Northern Ireland.

Long-Term Conditions Alliance Scotland (LTCAS)
http://www.ltcas.org.uk/index.php?id=23
Accessed 04.01.10.

NHS Direct Wales
http://www.nhsdirect.wales.nhs.uk
Accessed 04.01.10.

National Library for Health
Managing long-term conditions
http://www.library.nhs.uk/HealthManagement/ViewResource.aspx?resID=32021&tabID=290&catID=4031
Accessed 04.01.10.

References

Acheson, D. (1988). *Committee of inquiry into the future development of the public health function*. Public Health in England. London: HER MAJESTY'S STATIONERY OFFICE.

Arthritis Research Campaign (ARC) (2002). *Arthritis: The Big Picture*. Chesterfield: ARC.

Baldwin, M. (2006). The Warrington workload tool: determining its use in one trust. *British Journal of Community Nursing*. 11 (9): 391–395.

Battersby, M. W. (2005). Health Reform through coordinated care: SA HealthPlus *British Medical Journal*. 330: 662–665.

Bodenheimer, T., Wagner, E.H., & Grumbach, E. (2002). Improving Primary Care for Patients With Chronic Illness. *JAMA*. 288:1775–1779.

British Medical Association (2006). Improving the management of long-term conditions in the face of system reform. **http://www.bma.org.uk/healthcare_policy/community_care/longterm-conditions.jsp** Accessed 04.01.10.

Chartered Society of Physiotherapists (CSP) (2008). New arrangements must deliver better care for people of Northern Ireland. **http://www.csp.org.uk/director/newsandevents/news.cfm?item_id=E5590AE89C44EB02725DE9D3D7B312B3**. Accessed 04.01.10.

Chief Nursing Officer (CNO) (2003). Rising to the challenge of the working time directive. The CNO Bulletin. **www.doh.gov.uk/cno/bulletindetail_nov.htm#topnews** Accessed 12.12.03. – no longer available

Chodosh, J., Morton, S.C., Suttorp, M.J. &Shekelle, P.G. (2006). Self-Management Education for Osteoarthritis. Annals of Internal Medicine. 18 April, 144 (8), 617–618.

Coulter, A. (2006). *Engaging Patients in their Healthcare*. Oxford: Picker Institute Europe.

Department of Health (2004). *Research Evidence on the Usefulness of self-care support networks for care of people with minor ailments, acute illness and long-term conditions and those taking initiatives to stay healthy*. London: DH.

Department of Health (2005a). *Supporting People with Long-term conditions, An NHS and Social Care Model to support local innovation and integration*. London: DH.

Department of Health (2005b). *The NHS Improvement Plan: Putting people at the heart of public services*. London: DH.

Department of Health (2005c). *The National Service Framework for long-term conditions*. London: DH.

Department of Health (2005d). *Self Care — A Real Choice, Self Care Support — A Real Option*. London: DH.

Department of Health (2005e). *Independence Well being and Choice*. London: THE STATIONERY OFFICE.

Department of Health (2006). *Our Health, Our Care, Our Say*. London: DH.

Department of Health (2007a). *Long-term conditions : Background* http://www.dh.gov.uk/en/Healthcare/Longtermconditions/DH_4128521 Accessed 04.01.10.

Department of Health (2007b). The NHS and Social care long-term conditions model. http://www.dh.gov.uk/en/Healthcare/Longtermconditions/DH_4130652.Accessed 04.01.10.

Department of Health (2008a). Ten things you need to know about long-term conditions http://www.dh.gov.uk/en/Healthcare/Longtermconditions/DH_084294. Accessed 04.01.10.

Department of Health (2008b). Long-term conditions model. http://www.dh.gov.uk/en/Healthcare/Longtermconditions/DH_084296 Accessed 04.01.10.

Department of Health (2008c). Whole system demonstrators http://www.dh.gov.uk/en/Healthcare/Longtermconditions/wholesystemdemonstrators/index.htm Accessed 04.01.10.

Department of Health (2008d). Raising the Profile of Long-term conditions Care: A Compendium of Information. London: DOH.

Doran T., Drever F., Whitehead M. (2004). Is there a north-south divide in social class inequalities in health in Great Britain? Cross sectional study using data from the 2001 census. *British Medical Journal* 328: 1043–1045.

King's Fund Report (2004). *Case Managing Long-term conditions.* London: King's Fund.

Larsen P.D. (2006). In: Lubkin I.M., Larsen P.D. (2006). *Chronic Illness, Impact and Interventions* (Sixth Edition). London: Jones and Bartlett publishers.

London Health Observatory (2008). Monitoring Health and Healthcare in the capital, supporting practitioners and informing decision makers. http://www.lho.org.uk/viewResource.aspx?id=9739.Accessed 04.01.10.

Long-term conditions Collaborative (LTCC) (2008). http://ltcscotland.wik.is/ Accessed 04.01.10.

Marriott A. & Wright H. (2002). All for one. Community Care. May:38–39.

National Assembly for Wales. *Welsh Health Survey October 2003-March 2004 provisional results* (unpublished). Cited in: National Public Health Service for Wales (2005) *A profile of long-termand chronic conditions in Wales*. Wales: National Public Health Service for Wales.

National Statistics (2006). National Statistics, Life expectancy continues to rise. http://www.statistics.gov.uk Accessed 08.09.08 – no longer available

Nolan M. (1995). Towards an ethos of interdisciplinary practice. British Medical Journal. 311:306.

Partnership for Solutions (2004). Chronic Conditions: Making a case for ongoing care. A Project of Johns Hopkins University and The Robert Wood Johnson Foundation. http://www.partnershipforsolutions.org/DMS/files/chronicbook2004.pdf Accessed 04.01.10.

Quality and Outcomes Framework (QOF) (2007). cited In: Department of Health (2008d) Raising the Profile of Long-term conditions Care: A Compendium of Information. London: DH.

Ryan, S., Oliver, S. (2002). Rheumatoid arthritis. *Nursing Standard*. 16 (20): 45–52.

Tomkins, S. &Collins, A. (2006). Promoting Optimal Self Care: Consultations techniques that improve quality of life for patients and clinicians. Dorset: Dorset and Somerset Strategic Health Authority. http://www.networks.nhs.uk/uploads/06/02/optminising_self_care.pdf Accessed 04.01.10.

Chapter 20

The future of nursing and public health: challenges and debates

Paul Linsley, Roslyn Kane and Sara Owen

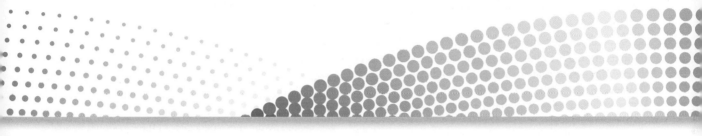

Introduction

The substantial changes in health care and service provision that have occurred over the last decade have been supported by the nation's renewed interest in the development of more relevant and flexible health care services. Clinical effectiveness, service quality and clinical governance along with a strong focus on preventative health care interventions, are major strands of the current drive to develop and modernize the National Health Service (DH, 2006a).

The recent reforms require that nurses posses the essential skills and knowledge to function in a continually evolving health care environment. This book has provided an analysis of what is needed to equip nurses for contemporary and future practice. A number of different perspectives on public health have been discussed and the different theoretical models relating these to practice have been examined; encouraging thought and debate through various activities and learning points.

The story so far

Section 1 of the book presented an overview of public health and the changing nature of health care delivery and service provision (Chapter 1). This was achieved by exploring the

context and direction of health care, highlighting important service developments and contemporary thinking. It looked at the influences on health and the causes of ill health across the lifespan (Chapter 2), emphasizing the need for a broad range of preventative activities, and strong partnership working with patients and their families. The case was made for nurses to become more actively involved in promoting health and well being as well as looking after those who are ill (Chapter 3).

Section 2 described the subsequent changing role of the nurse (Chapter 4) and the inter-professional dimensions of care (Chapter 5), recognizing that care is not delivered in a vacuum but best achieved through partnership working and shared education and learning. The importance of working with patients and their families was further reinforced (Chapter 6). Chapter 7 provided insight into the power and transformative potential that information technology can bring to health care delivery and management. The section ended by looking at the political and legal issues underpinning much of nursing practice today (Chapter 8).

Section 3 took a more practical approach, examining the core skills now required of the nurse in clinical practice. While the new opportunities for nurses that are emerging throughout the continuum of public health practice are exciting, they require that nurses be proactive in demonstrating their expertise in assessment (Chapter 9), planning and designing programmes of intervention (Chapter 10), delivering care (Chapter 11) and evaluating interventions (Chapter 12).

Section 4 explored various key topic areas of public health nursing and practice; including smoking cessation (Chapter 13); tackling health inequalities (Chapter 14); tackling obesity (Chapter 15); improving sexual health (Chapter 16); improving mental health (Chapter 17); tackling alcohol misuse (Chapter 18) and caring for people with long-term conditions (Chapter 19). These chapters above all, provide insight into what it is to work within the public health arena and the skills required of the nurse in promoting health and well-being amongst individuals and populations.

It is important that nurses develop and are able to articulate both the general and specific aspects of their practice with patients, families, other professionals and the general public. In doing so, they ensure that the roles they undertake are appropriate and meet the needs of those they care for. It is crucial that nurses remain focused on what they do whilst being mindful of the changing health care environment and their contribution to this. Throughout the book there is an acknowledgement that there will be professional, political, financial and organizational challenges to face in developing the nursing profession in alignment with the new direction of health and health care.

Key policy documents

There has been for some time a formal commitment to increasing the contribution nurses make to public health and tackling inequalities (Linsley *et al.,* 2008). Several key policy documents have been introduced throughout the book. In brief, key recent reports all point to the same policy and practice direction. Health care staff are now expected to play an active role in developing their own understanding of the determinants of health and in helping people to achieve healthy lifestyles (Hardsley *et al.*, 2007).

Since the publication of the Acheson report in 1998, the need for a radical approach to improving the health of the population has been recognized. In 1998 an official statement of intent to examine the role of nurses within the public health arena was published by the European and UK Chief Nursing Officers.

This was later further enforced in the Munich Declaration, when ministers pledged to 'enhance the roles of nurses and midwives in public health, health promotion and community development'. It was recognized, however, that this would not be possible without an accompanying shift in the focus of the workforce (DH, 2002). In 2004, the White paper **Choosing Health: Making Healthy Choices Easier** (DH, 2004a) made direct reference to the need to 'develop training and support for all NHS staff to develop their understanding and skills in promoting health and to foster and expand a comprehensive range of community health improvement services'. It also highlighted how new skills needed to be developed and

old-fashioned professional boundaries broken down to pave the way forward towards the sharing of existing skills between a range of public health practitioners (DH, 2004a).

This focus on prevention was further reiterated in a number of key policy documents including, **The Future Nurse: the RCN vision** (RCN, 2004), **The Future Nurse: the future for nurse education** (DH, 2007), and **Modernizing Nursing Careers: setting the direction** (DH, 2006b). Health professional are now being asked to work together in partnerships with other agencies to make inroads into helping people achieve and maintain good health, particularly the most disadvantaged (Dion, 2008, DH, 1999, DH, 2003, DH, 2004a).

The Wanless reports: a key turning point

So change is already happening and a shift in the direction of the nursing role is gaining momentum (Linsley *et al.* , 2008). A key turning point was the publication of the two reports by Derek Wanless in 2002 and 2004. Wanless (a former banker) was invited by the then chancellor of the Exchequer to advise on future health trends and on the ability of a health service funded by central taxation to meet future health care demands (Hunter, 2007). Wanless recognized that the UK could no longer afford to fund the health care of a population that is living longer and has increasing long-term demands on its health service (Wanless, 2002, 2004). He highlighted what has been described as 'one of the most protracted and impassioned debates in health policy' (Hunter, 2008:146): the imbalance between the resources devoted to health care as distinct to health. Hunter (2007) summarizes one of his key observations:

'From a financial point of view Wanless argued that health and wealth were inextricably linked: good health relies on good economics and better public health measures could significantly effect the demand for health care'
Hunter, 2007

Health in the Community

Wanless was critical of the prevailing bias in favour of acute hospital care, recognizing that investment in public health would bring wider benefits by increasing productivity and reducing inactivity in the working age groups (Hunter, 2007). The Wanless reports gave prominence to the importance of public health and are seen as a key development in the thinking around public health issues.

The reports recommended more primary and community based care with public involvement in health improvement. This change in focus was echoed in the NHS Improvement Plan (DH, 2004b), which further signaled the need for major cultural change to address this move from sickness to health.

Acute clinical care has been provided traditionally in hospitals, by staff specifically trained to care for ill people in that setting. However there is growing recognition that simply pouring resources into health care services, especially acute hospital care, cannot be equated with good health (Hunter, 2008). Consequently there is now much more focus on community based care. Non-emergency, every day public health practice that reduces health inequality and improves health and well-being — the landscape for practice in multidisciplinary public health in the twenty-first century is now just as likely to be in a community centre as a hospital setting (Hardsley *et al.*, 2007).

A holistic vision of care

There has also been a shift away from a biomedical, disease focussed approach to a more holistic vision of care (DH, 2005). Nurses are now far more mindful of the need to see beyond specific signs and symptoms and to be aware of and addressing the social, environmental and psychological determinants of health. Nurses must understand that health care is not just about the delivery of care to the sick. It is also about recognizing that health enhancing activities should be available to all regardless of income, geography, gender, ethnicity, ability or level of education. Furthermore, it is necessary to have a firm understanding of the ways in which the socio-economic environment in which a person lives, can in turn influence their behaviour and ultimately their health status.

Inevitably the shift in focus from policy at governmental level has necessitated an accompanying shift in clinical practice and this has resulted in the need for a shift in focus of 'frontline' staff (Hardsley *et al.*, 2007), with the nursing profession now having to revisit its core skills. Where roles and responsibilities change so to do the skills and educational preparation needed to underpin this new direction. The nursing profession must change to meet the changing needs of the population. The education curriculum needs to examine the public health aspects and roles nurses play in the twenty-first century and ensure that qualified nurses are fit for purpose.

Nursing knowledge and skills for the future

This is reflected in a recent move by the Nursing and Midwifery Council (NMC). The NMC has recently undertaken a thorough review of pre-registration nursing education and has consulted widely with professionals, service users and carers on the development of new standards for nurse education (Mitchell, 2008). From September 2011, these new standards will be used by all educational institutions in the UK to design and develop nurse education programmes. The standards have a strong emphasis on the preparation of student nurses to be competent to deliver holistic care in a variety of settings.

Also recently published is the report of the Prime Minister's Commission on the future of nursing and midwifery in England. The Commission was established in March 2009 to explore and make recommendations on how the nursing and midwifery professions could implement and accelerate the agenda of the Darzi report (DH, 2008), which itself was commissioned to set out a vision for a quality NHS.

The Commission held an extensive engagement programme and considered the views of the public, service users and front line staff. Its report (published on 2 March 2010) sets out a vision for the future of nursing and midwifery. Twenty recommendations on seven key themes were made:

- high quality,
- compassionate care,
- the political economy of nursing and midwifery,
- health and well-being,
- caring for people with long-term conditions,
- promoting innovation in nursing and midwifery,
- nurses and midwives leading services,
- careers in nursing (and midwifery),
- PM's Commission 2010.

Specifically, in relation to health and well being it recommends that:

'Nurses and midwives must recognize and scale up their important role in the design, monitoring and delivery of services to improve health and wellbeing and reduce health inequalities'.

Further emphasizing the increasing importance of nurses to the prevention of ill health. Interestingly it also recommends that:

'Nurses and midwives must acknowledge that they are seen as role models for healthy living, and take personal responsibility for their own health. Their employers must value and support staff health and wellbeing' (PM's Commission, 2010).

Contemporary nursing practice requires that the nurse looks beyond the individual to the health needs of the community. Nurses must broaden the context of their care and the responsibility and understanding they bring to the care-giving situation. Opportunities exist for nurses and other health care professionals to actively participate in the shaping of services and the construction of new and innovative ways of working. The current practice of nursing requires greater sensitivity to the social environment and the advocacy needs of patients and their families and communities. It also mandates thoughtful consideration of complex legal and ethical dilemmas that arise from a delivery system that is focused on the efficiencies of managed care, which can disadvantage and discriminate against those with an illness or disability. New ways of working also require greater skill in interdisciplinary collaboration that is built on the nurse's clinical competence and professional self-assertion and balanced by a clear understanding of what it is they do and can deliver. Each of these elements must influence the education, research, and clinical components of contemporary nursing practice.

Interdisciplinary working

An essential part of contemporary nursing practice is working in partnership with other health care professionals and providers (McKimm and Philips, 2009). However, interdisciplinary working does not always run smoothly. There are many barriers to interdisciplinary collaboration including inappropriate education and training of team members, traditional organizational structures, goal and role conflict, competitive and accommodating interpersonal interactions, power and status inequities, and the personal qualities of individuals that do not promote shared problem solving (Mullins, 2007). If roles, functions, and channels of communication among the various team members are not clarified and agreed on, confusion, resentment, crossing of boundaries, and inappropriate use of team members are likely to result. It is important that nurses take charge and set their own practice agenda and that they communicate this to other team members; whilst at the same time promoting compromise and consideration of other health professional groups' ways of working. Without this understanding and respect, health teams will not function at an optimum level and the autonomy of the nurse will be compromised (Girvin, 1998).

As roles become blurred between the health care professions and in particular between nursing and medical professions, it is important that nurses recognize the value and legitimacy of their own voices and what it is they do. Nursing contains political, academic, managerial and clinical domains each containing varied priorities and languages (Antrobus and Kitson, 1999). This is of particular significance as nurses seek to become part of strategic planning and development rather than simply responding to imperatives from government and other agencies (Crossan, 2003). They need to understand the many connections between their work and that of society. This will allow nurses to mobilize their workplaces and effect community and legislative action. Nurses need to involve themselves in the community in which they work and in the wider political arena. Passive acceptance of decisions made by other professionals and legislators and government should be replaced by proactive strategies and political engagement (Kitson, 2001).

Leadership and management

This highlights the importance of the nurse as a leader and manager. Increasingly, nurses are being encouraged to take a more active part in the management of services and staff. What is required is a nurse manger, not a manager who used to be a nurse with management training. Clinical leaders, acting and thinking as clinicians rather than managers have the potential to provide a more value orientated approach to both leadership and health management (Callaly and Minas, 2005). Such leadership has an effect on the care that patients receive; it also strengthens and expands the contribution of nursing to the larger health care system. Conversely, poor nurse leadership can be argued as leading to poor care.

It is important to recognize here that whilst nurses cannot affect all the factors that make up the context of nursing, they can now, attain enough influence over their immediate practice to govern the direction, rate and expression of change in nursing. Within this wider context, the leadership approach is to translate the varied priorities into the clinical domain to enhance staff awareness of how and why organizational changes impact upon their practice (Hurley and Linsley, 2008).

Nurses must use their leadership skills and clinical knowledge to work as agents of change to a greater degree than they do currently. To this end nurses can initiate change; assist by supporting, participating, or implementing change; and evaluate completed change (Hyde and Cook, 2004). To do this, nurses need to take risks. The nurse must develop the ability to calculate potential risks surrounding the implementation of change and then decide whether these risks are worth taking.

Nursing research and evidence

If the quality of health and social care is to be improved, existing knowledge about effective clinical and organizational practice must be applied and new information to monitor and evaluate care must be generated and interpreted. Increasingly, nurses are involved in the commissioning and shaping of services, and taking responsibility for the effective use of resources and delivery of contracts. The relationship between practice, theory and research is highlighted in the development of the nursing role. For theory to be useful, it must have implications for practice, and for practice to be tested and validated, it must be based on theory. Theory that arises out of practice is validated by research, which returns to direct practice and has implications for clinical care and service development.

This progression of observing from practice, theorizing, testing in research and subsequently modifying practice must continue to be an essential part of nursing.

Research and evidence-based practice are central to the developing role of the nurse such that a nurse becomes what has been described as a 'knowledgeable doer'. In order to advance this agenda there is a need to benchmark infrastructure and standardize the education and development of nurse education and nurses undertaking advanced practice roles. There is also a need for continued debate on the future of the health care workforce, informed by research, to facilitate correct and cost effective decision-making. The importance of modernizing education and training to ensure that the workforce is properly equipped to deliver the new health agenda is acknowledged as part of the process of reform. *Modernising Nursing Careers: Setting the Direction* (DH, 2006b) highlighted the changing context of health care and set out a series of priorities for all nurses across the UK. Education was a key theme of the document, which advocated a review of the content and level of educational preparation for nursing, the development of new postgraduate career pathways and a review of nurse educator roles designed for future needs. Formal accredited awards will need to be explicitly linked to individuals' development (UK Clinical Research Council, 2008) (for example the development of Masters degrees in Research, in Clinical Research and post doctoral programmes). Educators will need to be expert in areas of practice with the associated skills and knowledge.

Professional development and new ways of working

Following the above, as an individual's career progresses, the focus on development needs become more specific. Professional education must be responsive to the rapidly changing demands and needs of the service. Nurses need to be appropriately skilled, adaptable responsive and flexible if they are to effectively anticipate and respond to the new roles and competencies that are expected of them. The challenges that are most salient to the nurse are to differentiate their roles among other health professionals while creating a support environment for advanced nursing practice; creating a climate whereby the integrity of the education system is maintained and to provide a service with clear authoritative guidelines about the clinical and cost effectiveness of their interventions.

In part these changes reflect developments in science and technology, which enable new forms of diagnosis, treatment and delivery of health care. Greater emphasis on improving the health of the population and this will require the collection and aggregation of information across practices to assess health needs and health impacts, reduce inequalities, and monitor the quality of care in comparison to agreed standards, best achieved through these advances in technology (Thede, 2003). As with any innovation, technology also presents many challenges, some involved in adapting the innovation to our needs, others due to the to new issues that such technology brings. Any introduction of a new system changes ways of working, and in itself can be a source of conflict within teams, for example, who gets what information?

As we have seen in Chapter 7 there is the danger that nurses have become data inputters and not users of data. If nursing practice and consequently patient care is to improve then nurses not only need to have a say in developing technological systems of support but ensure that such systems meet the requirements of nurse practice. Nurses, along with other health care professionals, need to explore approaches to effectively manage public health knowledge so that it can be appropriately used according to need and audience and aid and assist in decision-making.

Finally, any health alliance approach to promoting health involves recognition by the nurse, of the need to consider the views and experiences of the general public and those that use their services. True consultation and community participation are key elements of a health alliance approach and ones which the nurse can be positively engaged with. Despite this, there are areas of contention. The issue of management legitimizing and creating the right conditions for health and social care providers to engage in community participation processes is key. This is where organizational development work on the part of the statutory agencies is so vital in order to facilitate a climate in which staff as individuals and teams, can fully pursue participation and the principles that underlie it. Participation and partnership working is a pragmatic element of health care and is a route to promoting and maintaining health within an individual and community. Nurses need to be supported in this by their leaders and managers.

References

Antrobus, S. & Kitson, A. (1999). Nursing leadership: influencing and shaping health policy and nursing practice. *Journal of Advanced Nursing* 29:746–753.

Callaly, T. & Minas, H. (2005). Reflections on clinician leadership and management in mental health. *Australasian Psychiatry* 13, 1: 27–32.

Cook, M. & Leathard, H. (2004). Learning for clinical leadership. *Journal of Nursing Management* 12 (6): 436–444.

Crossan, F. (2003). Research philosophy: Towards an understanding. *Nurse Researcher*, 11 (1): 46–55.

Department of Health (1999c). *Making a difference: strenghthening the nursing, midwifery and health visiting contribution to health and healthcare.* London: DH.

Department of Health (2000). *NHS Plan.* London: The Stationery Office.

Department of Health (2001). *Shifting the Balance of Power*. London: The Stationery Office.

Department of Health (2002). NHS Reform. London: The Stationery Office.

Department of Health (2003). *Tackling health inequalities: A programme for action*. London: The Stationery Office.

Department of Health (2004a). *Choosing Health: Making Healthy Choices Easier*. London: The Stationery Office.

Department of Health (2004b). *NHS Improvement Plan*. London: The Stationery Office.

Department of Health (2005). *Commissioning a Patient-led NHS*. London: The Stationery Office.

Department of Health (2006a). *Our Health, Our Care, Our Say*. London: The Stationery Office.

Department of Health (2006b). *Modernizing Nursing Careers—Setting the Direction*. London: Her Majesty's Stationery Office.

Department of Health (2007). *World Class Commissioning*. London: Her Majesty's Stationery Office.

Department of Health (2008). *High Quality Care For All NHS Next Stage Review Final Report*. London: DH.

Dion, X. (2008). Developing Programmes, Services and Reducing Inequalities. In: L. Coles & E. Porter (eds.) *Public Health Skills: A practical guide for nurses and public health practitioners*. Oxford: Blackwell Publishing.

Girvin, (1998). *Leadership and Nursing*. New York: Palgrave.

Hunter, D. (2007). Public health: historical context and current agenda. In: A. Scriven & S. Garman. *Public health: social context and action* Milton Keynes: Open University Press.

Hunter, D. (2008). *The Health Debate*. Bristol: The Policy Press.

Handsley S. & Moira, S. (2007). Working with communities to promote public health. In: C.E. Lloyd, S. Handsley, J. Douglas, S. Earle, & S. Spurr.: *Policy and practice in promoting public health*. London: Sage/Open University Press.

Hurley, J. & Linsley, P. (2007). Leadership challenges to move nurses toward collaborative individualism within a neo-corporate bureaucratic environment. *Journal of Nursing Management*, 15: 749–755.

Hyde, J. & Cook, M. J. (2004). *Managing and Supporting People in Health Care*. London: Bailliere Tindall in association with the RCN.

Kitson, L. (2001). Nursing leadership: bringing caring back to the future. *Quality Health Care*, 10(2): 79–84.

Linsley, P., Kane, R., McKinnon, J., Spencer, R. & Simpson, T. (2008). Preparing for the future: nurse education and workforce development. *Quality in Primary Care*. 16 (3):171–176.

Mitchell, D. (2008). *A Review of pre-registration nursing education — Report of consultation findings*. Prepared by Alpha Research Ltd for Nursing & Midwifery Council http://www.nmc-uk.org/aDisplayDocument.aspx?documentID=4917

Mullins, L. J. (2007). *Management and Organizational Behaviour* (8th edn.) London: Prentice Hall.

Phillips, K. (eds.) (2009). *Leadership and Management in Integrated Services* (2nd edn.). Poole: Learning Matters.

Prime Minister's Commission on the Future of Nursing and Midwifery in England (32010) Front Line Care: the future of nursing and midwifery in England. Report of the Prime Minister's Commission on the Future of Nursing and Midwifery in England 2010. http://webarchive.nationalarchives.gov.uk/20100331110400/http://cnm.independent.gov.uk/wp-content/uploads/2010/03/front_line_care.pdf

Royal College of Nursing, (2004). *The Future Nurse: the RCN vision*. London: Royal College of Nursing.

Royal College of Nursing (2007). *The Future Nurse: the future for nurse education. A discussion paper*. London: Royal College of Nursing.

Thede, L. (2003). Informatics and Nursing Opportunities and Challenges (2nd edn.). London: Lippincott Williams and Wilkins.

United Kingdom Clinical Research Collaboration (UKCRC) (2008). *Developing the best research professionals. Qualified graduate nurses: recommendations for preparing and supporting clinical academic nurses of the future*. London: UKCRC.

Wanless D. (2002). *Securing our Future Health: taking a long-term view*. London: Her Majesty's Stationery Office.

Wanless, D. (2004). *Securing Good Health for the Whole Population*. London: Her Majesty's Stationery Office.

Glossary

Chapter 1 Definition

Allied health professionals A health care professional with expert knowledge and experience in certain fields but with no medical degree.

Association of Public Health Observatories (APHO) The Association of Public Health Observatories represents a network of twelve public health observatories (PHOs) working across the five nations of England, Scotland, Wales, Northern Ireland and the Republic of Ireland.

Communicable diseases Any disease that can be transmitted from one person to another.

Community care The provision of help and treatment for people in their home environment.

Health gain Health gain is a way to express improved health outcomes. It can be used to reflect the relative advantage of one form of health intervention over another in producing the greatest health gain.

Health trainers Health trainers offer practical advice and good connections into the services and support available locally. They are an essential common-sense resource in the community to help out on health choices. A guide for those who want help, not an instructor for those who do not, they will provide valuable support for people to make informed lifestyle choices.

Integrated care pathways A multidisciplinary plan for delivering health and social care to patients with a specific condition or set of symptoms.

Intermediate care The care of people who do not need acute tertiary care in hospitals but are not sufficiently independent to be self-caring in their own homes at specific outcomes for rehabilitation or recuperation, and is provided for a time limited period of up to six weeks.

Primary care Comprehensive health care for individuals and families in the community provided through an integrated network of services covering the treatment of common illnesses and injuries.

Secondary care Health care provided by hospital clinicians for a patient whose primary care was provided by the general practitioner or other health professional who first diagnosed or treated the patient.

Chapter 2 Definition

Disability-free life expectancy A modification of conventional life expectancy to account for time lived with disability. It is the number of years (free from disability) of life that can be expected on average in a given population. It is generally calculated at birth, but estimates can also be prepared at other ages. It adjusts the expectation of years of life for the loss on account of disability, using explicit weights for different health states.

Healthy life expectancy A modification of conventional life expectancy to account for time lived free from ill health. It is the number of healthy years of life that can be expected on average in a given population. It is generally calculated at birth, but estimates can also be prepared at other ages. It adjusts the expectation of years of life for the loss on account of ill health, using explicit weights for different health states.

Life expectancy A number of years a person can expect to live based on statistical averages.

Local health profiles (LHP) A description of indicators of health status in a given population or geographical area. Health profiles provide a snapshot of health using key health indicators, which enables comparison locally, regionally and over time. They are designed to help with decisions about key health priorities and where to target resources locally.

National Service Frameworks (NSFs) A series of guidelines for the future of public health care.

Office for National Statistics (ONS) The organization responsible for producing official UK statistics in relation to the economy, population and society and local and national level.

Public Health Observatories

Self-agency

Chapter 3 Definition

Community capacity The capacity and skills of members of a community to identify and meet their needs to participate more fully in society

Critical consciousness Focuses on achieving an indepth understanding of the world, allowing for the perception and exposure of social and political contradictions. Critical consciousness also includes taking action against the oppressive elements in one's life that are illuminated by that understanding.

Empowerment Refers to increasing the spiritual, political, social, or economic strength of individuals and communities. It often involves the empowered developing confidence in their own capacities.

Models A representation or description of something that aids in understanding or studying a set of assumptions about relationships used to study interactions. Models help guide thinking about an event or activity in a theoretical way; they do not attempt to explain the processes underlying the activity, but only to represent them.

Rate of adoption The speed and rate by which an individual or community adopts a health innovation.

Theories A set of ideas, based on evidence and careful reasoning, which offers an explanation of how something works or why something happens, but has not been completely proved.

Chapter 4 Definition

Acute settings In an acute care setting, patients receive short-term medical treatment for acute illnesses or injury, or to recover from surgery.

Advanced nurse practitioner The RCN (2010, Advanced nurse practitioners an RCN guide to the advanced nurse practitioner role, competences and programme accreditation) defines an advanced nurse practitioner as a registered nurse who has undertaken a specific course of study of at least first degree (Honours) level and who:

- **Makes** professionally autonomous decisions, for which he or she is accountable.
- **Receives** patients with undifferentiated and undiagnosed problems and makes an assessment of their health care needs, based on highly developed nursing knowledge and skills, including skills not usually exercised by nurses, such as physical examination.
- **Screens** patients for disease risk factors and early signs of illness.
- **Makes** differential diagnosis using decision-making and problem-solving skills.
- **Develops** with the patient an ongoing nursing care plan for health, with an emphasis on preventative measures.
- **Orders** necessary investigations, and provides treatment and care both individually, as part of a team, and through referral to other agencies.
- **Has** a supportive role in helping people to manage and live with illness.
- **Provides** counselling and health education.
- **Has** the authority to admit or discharge patients from their caseload, and refer patients to other health care providers as appropriate.
- **Works** collaboratively with other health care professionals and disciplines.
- **Provides** a leadership and consultancy function as required.

Chronic diseases Chronic diseases are diseases of long duration and generally slow progression. Chronic diseases are diseases such as heart disease, stroke, cancer, chronic respiratory diseases and diabetes, and are the leading cause of mortality in the world.

Congestive cardiac failure Inability of the heart to maintain an adequate output of blood of one or both ventricles, resulting in manifest congestion and over distension of certain veins and organs with blood, and inadequate blood supply to the body tissues, and excessive retention of water and salt.

Flexible sigmoidoscopy Enables the physician to look at the inside of the large intestine from the rectum through the last part of the colon, called the sigmoid.

Knowledgeable doer The knowledgeable doer was a term that arose from the education move in the 1980s to Project 2000, which acknowledged the gap between theory and clinical practice. The new nurse education system aimed to produce nurses who could base their clinical practice on a sound body of knowledge that was itself research and science-based.

New public health agenda Public health concerns such as obesity, smoking and poverty are a key driver for government action, in recognition that inequalities in health experience are increasing. Public health activity is wide-ranging including health protection, education and prevention as well as healthy public policy and community empowerment.

Patient self-management Refers to a care model in which patients on a particular medication measure the relevant physiological parameters, interpret the results, and adjust their medication accordingly, for example patients on anticoagulation therapy in this model of care will measure their own International Normalised Ratio (INR), interpret the result themselves, and adjust their dosage according to the value obtained and within the range recommended for treatment

Chapter 6 Definition

Attachment theory The psychological framework which describes human beings as preprogrammed as prosocial at birth with the need to 'attach' themselves to trusted others particularly in times of vulnerability and trauma being positively related to health.

Concordance A partnership of equals between nurse and patient on which care planning is negotiated.

Consumerism The ideology in which health care is treated as market place and patients as consumers in that market place.

Empathy The ability to understand the experience of another in the way that they experience it.

Engagement The demonstration of willingness to become involved; the evidence of a desire to pursue an understanding of another's situation.

Nurse-patient relationship A mutual trust and respect which exists between patient and nurse which informs health care practice and facilitates patient-centred care.

Paternalism The ideology in which one knows what is best for another by virtue of one's authority or expertise.

Patient-centredness The mindset in which the interpretations and concerns of the patient have primacy in care and fuel care planing.

Personhood The condition of being an individual.

Chapter 7 Definition

Business intelligence Business intelligence is a broad concept encompassing the processes, software and technologies for gathering, storing, analysing, and providing access to data to help users make better decisions. In essence, it is 'the art of sieving through large amounts of data, extracting information and turning that information into actionable knowledge'.

Caldicott Guardian A senior person responsible for protecting the confidentiality of patient and service-user information and enabling appropriate information-sharing. The Guardian ensures that organizations satisfy the highest practicable standards for handling patient identifiable information.

Clinical decision support software are interactive computer programs which are designed to assist health professionals with decision making tasks.

Clinical informatics The use of health care data, information and knowledge for supporting patient care, research and education (Deleany, 2001).

Clinical information systems A CIS is a comprehensive, integrated information system designed to manage the administrative, financial and clinical aspects of a health care organization.

Data Facts, readings, measurements items that are essentially 'value free'.

Data Protection Act 1998 sets out rules for the processing of personal information held in paper form or/and in computer files. It establishes eight principles of good information handling.

Data quality relates to the building blocks of information, i.e. data items. Until data are assembled and interpreted they are not information.

Data standards A set of rules that impose structure on information so that its meaning and format are the same regardless of who views it or what kind or information technology system they use to access it

e-Health A term used to refer to the whole scope of IT usage in health and healthcare. This includes, Patient Internet Usage, SMS text messaging, Healthcare Professional Internet Usage, NHS Direct/NHS 24 Services, Electronic Patient Record, Telemedicine, Telecare and Telehealth.

European Computer Driving License is the European wide qualification demonstrating competence in computer skills.

Hard copy The paper record.

Information Data that has been interpreted or to which commentary has been added by a user for a purpose, making it 'value laden'.

Information & Communications Technology Information & Communications Technology is the technology or set of tools that enables information to be managed—to be collected, recorded, stored, processed, and transmitted. It includes hardware and software.

Information governance (IG) ensures necessary safeguards for, and appropriate use of patient and personal information. Key areas are information policy for health and social care, IG standards for NPfIT systems and development of guidance for NHS and partner organizations.

Information management Improving the quality, availability and effective use of information in an organization.

Information technology A means of capturing, storing and distributing information towards a more productive way of working.

Legitimate relationship An LR is an electronic record stored on the Spine. It details the care relationship between a patient and a health care professional (or group of health care professionals)

Local service provider (LSP) The organization responsible for making sure the new systems and services delivered through the NPfIT meet local requirements and are implemented efficiently.

National Programme for Information Technology (NPfIT) Responsible for procurement and delivery of the investment in new information and technology systems to improve the NHS.

NHS Clinical Knowledge Summaries A reliable source or evidence-based information and practical 'know how' about the common conditions managed in primary care.

Nursing indicators Nursing sensitive indicators reflect the structure, process and outcomes of nursing care.

Nursing intelligence Information gathered from nurses in their nursing work (managing knowledge in health care)

Personal digital assistant A PDA is a handheld computer also know as palmtop computer.

Public health is 'the science and art of preventing disease, prolonging life and promoting health through the organized efforts and informed choices of society, organizations, public and private, communities and individuals.

Role-based access is an approach to restricting system access to authorised users.

Short message service A communication protocol allowing the interchange of short text messages between mobile telephone devices. Most SMS messages are mobile to mobile text messages, though the standard supports other types of broadcast messaging.

Telecare The passive monitoring of patients with mechanisms such as fall sensors, panic buttons and flood detectors connected to an emergency call and response service

Telehealth Involves the patient taking responsibility for measuring vital signs of their state of health, such as blood pressure or glucose levels. The information is monitored remotely by clinicians who can send instructions to the patient on medication, diet or behaviour or call them in for a consultation.

®Telemedicine Involves the intervention of a clinician at both ends, for example, a nurse practitioner sending information to a consultant for remote diagnosis.

Chapter 8 Definition

Capitalism Capitalism is an economic system characterized by private or corporate ownership of capital goods

Ethical recruitment A system of moral principles applied to the recruitment of staff. Recruitment ethics provide guidelines for acceptable behaviour by organizations in recruiting staff ensuring that all those that apply for a job have a fair and equal chance of getting it.

Preceptorship The aim of preceptorship is to provide a structured, supportive programme of learning and development during the transition from student nurse to practitioner.

Statute A statute is a formal written enactment of a legislative authority that governs a state, city, or county. Typically, statutes command or prohibit something, or declare policy.

Glossary

Chapter 9 Definition

Bristol Stool Form Scale Developed by Dr K. W. Heaton, Reader in Medicine at the University of Bristol. It provides a pictorial representation of seven general types of stool consistency or form, ranging from Type 1 (hard and difficult to pass) to Type 7 (entirely liquid). It can be used as a general guide to aid in the objective reporting of symptoms and to inform comprehensive patient assessment.

Glasgow coma scale The Glasgow Coma Scale was initially developed as a research tool to study the level of consciousness **(LOC)** in patients following severe head injury. It is now recognised as a widely used and reliable tool to objectively measure and assess **LOC** in a range of clinical settings.

Gold Standards Frameworks (GSF) A systematic evidence-based approach to optimising the care for patients nearing the end of life delivered by generalist providers. It is concerned with helping people to live well until the end of life and includes care in the final years of life for people with any end stage illness in any care setting.

Makaton An internationally recognized communication programme. Makaton was developed using the words most frequently used in everyday conversation. Signs from the British Sign Language, used by the deaf community were then matched to these words, allowing simultaneous sign and speak. Makaton also uses symbols, in the same way that signs support speech.

Malnutrition Universal Screen Tool 'MUST' is a five-step screening tool to identify adults, who are malnourished, at risk of malnutrition (undernutrition), or obese. It also includes management guidelines which can be used to develop a care plan. It is designed for use in hospitals, community and other care settings and can be used by all care workers.

Task-orientated approach A reductive way of conceptualising nursing, in which the delivery of care is perceived merely as a series of jobs to complete, rather than each aspect of care being viewed as having intrinsic value in contributing to the holistic well-being of the patient.

Waterloo Score The Waterlow Score pressure ulcer risk assessment and prevention tool was developed by Judy Waterlow, in 1985. It comprises a risk assessment scoring system and guidance on nursing care, types of preventative aids associated with three identified levels of risk status, wound assessment and suggested dressing types. It is intended for use by nurses, health care professionals and carers working in the hospital, community and within care homes. It is necessarily simplistic and therefore requires the exercise of professional judgement in determining the risk assessment for each individual patient.

Chapter 10 Definition

Activity The basic unit in health promotion planning. A health promotion programme is made up of a series of activities.

Advocacy A combination of individual and social actions to gain political support for a particular health goal or intervention. Action may be taken on behalf of individuals or groups to create conditions that promote healthy living (WHO, 1998).

Aim A broad statement of what is to be achieved.

Collaboration Working together for the achievement of common goals.

Empowerment 'Empowerment may be a social, cultural, psychological or political process through which individuals and social groups are able to express their needs, present their concerns, devise strategies for involvement in decision-making, and achieve political, social and cultural action to achieve those needs'.

Epidemiology The study of how often disease occurs in different groups of people and why.

Evidence-based Evidence-based practice is an approach to health care that draws upon and integrates best available research evidence, professional expertise and client characteristics to guide decision-making.

Intervention An activity or course of treatment that seeks to modify outcomes. An intervention is usually implemented to treat ill health or promote good health.

LogFrame Matrix The Logical Framework Approach (LOGFrame) is an analytical, presentational and management tool which can help planners and managers to:

1. analyse the existing situation during project preparation;
2. establish a logical hierarchy of means by which objectives will be reached;
3. identify some of the potential risks;
4. establish how outputs and outcomes might best be monitored and evaluated; and
5. present a summary of the project in a standard format.

Mass population strategy An intervention or activity that seeks to address risk factors in the population as a whole not simply people identified as 'high-risk'.

Methods Techniques and approaches used.

Objectives Precise measurable statements of what is to be achieved by an activity.

Personal, Social and Health Education Provides young people with the knowledge and skills needed to lead healthy and responsible lives as confident individuals and members of society (Qualifications and Curriculum Authority, 2000).

Plan A systematic arrangement of activities required to achieve a set of given aims and objectives.

Planning Refers to the organization of a series of actions to achieve a specified outcome.

Policy A plan or course of action developed by government, organizations, groups and individuals, intended to determine decisions and actions.

Risk factors Something which can increase the chances of disease developing. For example, age, sex, ethnicity, family history.

Setting A location or context that may be used to carry out a health promotion activity such as a school, hospital, or workplace.

Stakeholders A stakeholder is a person, group or organization that has an interest in, or might be affected by, the actions and outcomes of a particular project or intervention.

Strategy A plan of action designed to achieve a particular aim or goal.

Targeting The selection of particular groups at which health promotion messages and activities should be directed.

Thinking shower The generation of ideas and thoughts on a given task or scenario.

Chapter 11 Definition

Case Manager Care management and assessment constitute one integrated process for identifying and addressing the needs of individuals within available resources, recognising that those needs are unique to the individuals concerned. For this reason, care management and assessment emphasise adapting services to needs rather than fitting people into existing services, and dealing with the needs of individuals as a whole rather than assessing needs separately for different services.

Chapter 12 Definition

Action research A research methodology that pursues action (or change) and research (or understanding) at the same time, achieved by using a cyclic or spiral process that alternates between action and critical reflection, and in later cycles continuously refines methods, data, and interpretation in the light of understanding developed in the earlier cycles.

Analysis The separation of substances into their components for examination and determination of their properties.

Generalizable The extent to which information about a program, project, or instructional material collected in one setting can be used to reach a valid judgment about how it will perform in other settings.

Impact The effect or impression made by something.

Qualitative data collection Data collection which is concerned with describing meaning, rather than with drawing statistical inferences. They provide in depth and rich descriptions.

Quantitative data collection Methods which focus on numbers and frequencies rather than on meaning and experience. Quantitative methods (e.g. experiments, questionnaires and psychometric tests) provide information which is easy to analyse statistically.

Quasi-experimental designs Experimental designs distinguished by the researcher randomly assigning test units to experimental groups and randomly assigning treatments to experimental groups. Quasi-experimental designs were developed to provide alternate means for examining causality in situations, which were not conducive to experimental control. Designs that apply part of the procedures of true experimentation yet lack full experimental control.

Chapter 13 Definition

Airway hyper-responsiveness Airway hyper-responsiveness is a characteristic feature of asthma and consists of an increased sensitivity of the airways to an inhaled constrictor agonist for example sudden exposure to changes of temperature can cause bronchospasm leading to shortness of breath, cough, wheeze.

A medical test for airways hyper-responsiveness is methylcholene challenge.

Bronchodilator therapy The use of drugs that relax the airways smooth muscle tissue. This is usually as inhaled medication either as hand held devices or nebulised but can also be given intravenously when a person is severely ill.

Carcinogens Any substance that, when exposed to living tissue, may cause the production of cancer.

Chronic obstructive pulmonary disease A disease of adults, especially those over the age of 45 with a history of smoking or inhalation of airborne pollution.

Cilia Microscopic hair-like projections from certain epithelial cells.

FEV1 Forced expiratory volume in 1 second. This is the amount of air that a person can force out in 1 second from their deepest breath in and using their maximum effort. It is one of the most basic of lung function measurements.

Fixed obstructive airway disease Fixed airway disease is often a result of asthma which has not been well controlled but can have other underlying causes. This condition of 'fixed airways' indicate that there is little of no response to bronchodilators or steroids due to long-term inflammation which has led to collagen strands being deposited within the airways thereby 'hardening' or 'fixing' them.

FVC Forced vital capacity

Forced vital capacity The amount of air which can be forcibly exhaled from the lungs after taking the deepest breath possible. Because chronic obstructive pulmonary disease causes the air in the lungs to be exhaled at a slower rate and in a smaller amounts compared to that in a healthy person, measuring how well air cab forcibly be exhaled can help determine the presence of the disease.

Mucociliary escalator The cilia of the respiratory epithelium beat in concert cranially, effectively moving secreted mucus containing trapped foreign particles toward the oropharynx, for either expectoration or swallowing to the stomach where the acidic pH helps to neutralize foreign material and micro-organisms. This system is collectively known as the *mucociliary escalator* and serves two functions: to keep the lower respiratory tract sterile, and to prevent mucus accumulation in the lungs.

Mucolytics A mucolytic agent or expectorant is any agent which dissolves thick mucus and is usually used to help relieve respiratory difficulties.

Mutagenic An agent Capable of causing genetic mutations.

Peak expiratory flow rate A patient's maximum speed of expiration

Reversible condition

Self-efficiency The belief that one is able to behave in a certain way to achieve certain goals and that control over your beliefs and therefore your ability one has to achieve these goals.

Chapter 14 Definition

Beveridge Report The Beveridge Report was the Report of the Inter-Departmental Committee on Social Insurance and Allied Services chaired by William Beveridge, an economist. The report identified five 'Giant Evils' in society: squalor, ignorance, want, idleness and disease, and went on to propose widespread reform to the system of social welfare in the United Kingdom to address these. Highly popular with the public, the report formed the basis for the post-war reforms known as the Welfare State, which include the expansion of National Insurance and the creation of the National Health Service.

Health disparities Also called health care inequality in some countries. Refers to gaps in the quality of health and health care across racial, ethnic, sexual orientation and socio-economic groups.

Health inequities Health inequalities can be defined as differences in health status or in the distribution of health determinants between different population groups. For example, differences in mobility between elderly people and younger populations or differences in mortality rates between people from different social classes. It is important to distinguish between inequality in health and inequity. Some health inequalities are attributable to biological variations or free choice and others are attributable to the external environment and conditions mainly outside the control of the individuals concerned. In the first case it may be impossible or ethically or ideologically unacceptable to change the health determinants and so the health inequalities are unavoidable. In the second, the uneven distribution may be unnecessary and avoidable as well as unjust and unfair, so that the resulting health inequalities also lead to inequity in health.

Health variations During the 1980s and early 1990s health inequalities were not very high on the political agenda in the UK. However with the ever-increasing evidence of the impact of socio-economic status on health, the then conservative government conceded that there were variations in health across the population. The term health variations was used in political rhetoric during this period. However it has now fallen out of use in academic circles, with the recognition that there are actually inequalities, rather than simply variations, to be addressed.

Ottawa Charter for Health Promotion A document produced by the World Health Organization. It was launched at the first international conference for health in 1986 promotion that was held in Ottawa, Canada.

Social capital A sociological concept, which refers to connections within and between social networks.

Social exclusion A multi-dimensional process of progressive social rupture, detaching groups and individuals from social relations and institutions and preventing them from full participation in the normal, activities of the society in which they live

Victim blaming Holding the victims of a crime, an accident, or any type of abusive maltreatment to be entirely or partially responsible for the unfortunate incident that has occurred in their life.

White Paper A government report containing statements of policy intentions.

Chapter 15 Definition

Adrenal disorders Conditions that interfere with the normal functioning of the adrenal glands. They are characterized by adrenal insufficiencies, where there are deficiencies in the availability of steroids that are produced by the adrenal glands. They may cause hyperfunction or hypofunction, and it may be congenital or acquired.

Anovulatory Cessation or absence of ovulation.

Atypical antipsychotic drugs Atypical antipsychotic drugs — a group of recently developed (compared to the typical antipsychotics) drugs used to treat conditions such as schizophrenia, drugs in this class include clozapine and risperidone.

Bariatrics The branch of medicine that deals with the causes, prevention, and treatment of obesity.

Central adiposity Adipose tissue (fat) which is located around the trunk.

Duodenal switch A procedure, also known as Biliopancreatic Diversion with Duodenal Switch (BPD-DS) or Gastric Reduction Duodenal Switch (GRDS), is a weight loss surgery procedure that is composed of a restrictive and a malabsorptive aspect.

Evidence-based Evidence-based refers to practice which utilises the best available evidence i.e. demonstrating statistically significant effectiveness of treatments for specific problems.

High density lipoprotein One of the five major groups of lipoproteins that enable lipids like cholesterol and triglycerides to be transported within the water-based bloodstream. In healthy individuals, about thirty percent of blood cholesterol is carried by HDL.

Hypothyroidism The disease state in caused by insufficient production of thyroid hormones by the thyroid gland.

Laparoscopic adjustable gastric banding Also known as a Lap-Band, is an inflatable silicone device that is placed around the top portion of the stomach, via laparoscopic surgery, in order to treat obesity.

Laparoscopic gastric bypass One of four types of operations for morbid obesity.

Leptin A protein, produced by adipose tissue that has a role in regulating eating: an increase in adipose tissue results in higher concentrations of leptin, which reduce food intake.

Low density lipoprotein One of the five major groups of lipoproteins (chylomicrons, VLDL, IDL, LDL, HDL) that enable lipids like cholesterol and triglycerides to be transported within the water-based bloodstream. It is used medically as part of a cholesterol blood test, and since high levels of LDL cholesterol can signal medical problems like cardiovascular disease, it is often called bad cholesterol.

Mono and dizygotic twins Mono-zygotic twins are identical, arising from one zygote which splits early in development. Dizygotic are non-identical arising from the fertilisation of 2 ova released during the same ovarian cycle.

Morbid obesity An individual with a BMI over 40 is classified as morbidly obese. Weight is a real and imminent threat to health in individuals who are morbidly obese.

Oestrogen signalling

Open gastric bypass Gastric bypass carried out as open surgery, i.e. not keyhole.

Plasma triglycerides Plasma concentrations of triglycerides.

Prader-Willi Syndrome An inherited (autosomal dominant) condition due to an abnormality of paternal chromosome 15.

Relative risk A mathematical value used to compare the risk in two different groups of people.

Sleeve gastrectomy A surgical weight-loss procedure in which the stomach is reduced to about 15% of its original size, by surgical removal of a large portion of the stomach, following the major curve. The open edges are then attached together (often with surgical staples) to form a sleeve or tube with a banana shape. The procedure permanently reduces the size of the stomach. The procedure is performed laparoscopically and is not reversible.

The Cochrane Collaboration A group of over 27,000 volunteers in more than 90 countries who review the effects of health care interventions tested in biomedical randomized controlled trials.

Thermogenesis The process of heat production in organisms.

Z score A statistical value which indicates how far and in what direction, that item deviates from its distribution's mean, expressed in units of its distribution's standard deviation. Also called a standard score.

Chapter 16 Definition

Vertical transmission also known as **mother-to-child transmission**, is the transmission of an infection or other disease from mother to child immediately before and after birth during the perinatal period.

Social marketing is the systematic application of marketing, along with other concepts and techniques, to achieve specific behavioral goals for a social good

Genotypes The genetic makeup, as distinguished from the physical appearance, of an organism or a group of organisms.

Chapter 17 Definition

Control and choice The power to determine action without restraint; to follow personal preference or choice without interference.

Mental functioning Functions or processes such as perception, introspection, memory, creativity, imagination, conception, belief, reasoning, volition, and emotion—in other words, all the different things that we can do with our mind.

Pre-morbid functioning The persons level of functioning preceding the occurrence of disease or illness.

Reactive depression Reactive or situational depression is a usually transient depression that is precipitated by a stressful life event or other environmental factor.

Resilience The ability to recover quickly from illness, change, or misfortune.

Self-determination The power or ability to make a decision for oneself without influence from outside.

Helping relationships Face-to-face interactions in which the nurse applies effective human relations skills to assist a client attain a goal or goals.

Chapter 19 Definition

Attention deficit hyperactivity disorder A mental disorder, usually of children, characterised by a grossly excessive level of activity and a marked impairment of the ability to attend, resulting in aggressive disruptive behaviour.

British Medical Association An independent trade union representing all doctors from all branches of medicine throughout the UK, for negotiation on pay and conditions.

Chronic diseases Chronic diseases are diseases of long duration and generally slow progression. Chronic diseases are diseases such as heart disease, stroke, cancer, chronic respiratory disease and diabetes, and are the leading cause of mortality in the world.

Communicable diseases An infectious disease that is transmitted from one person to another, directly or by an animal or insect vector or a carrier.

European Working Time Directive A collection of regulations concerning hours of work, designed to protect the health and safety of workers. Key features are the limiting of the maximum length of a working week to 48 hours in 7 days, a minimum rest period of 11 hours in each 24 hours and a minimum number of paid leave days per annum.

Interdisciplinary Denoting the overlapping interests of different fields of health and social care.

Kaiser Permanente Triangle The Kaiser permanente triangle represents the overall framework for case management proposed by the Department of Health, adapted from Kaiser Permanente (DH, 'Chronic Disease Management'. A compendium of Information', 2004).

Long-term conditions (LTCs) Long-term conditions (also called chronic conditions) are health problems that require on-going management over a period of years or decades. This includes a wide range of health conditions including non-communicable diseases (e.g. cancer and cardiovascular disease), communicable disease (e.g. HIV/AIDS), certain mental disorders (e.g. Schizaphreni depression), and ongoing impairments in structure (e.g. blindness, joint disorders).

Long-term conditions collaborative The Long-Term Conditions Collaborative (LTCC) is a programme developed to support NHS Scotland in using tools and techniques for clinical systems improvement. The collaborative helps people to deliver improvements in patient centred services and change the way care is provided for people with long-term conditions.

Multidisciplinary Combining or involving several separate academic disciplines.

NHS Plan A framework, published in July 2000, outlining radical changes to the way the NHS is organised and managed.

Non-communicable diseases A disease which is not contagious.

non-steroidal anti-inflammatory drugs Medications that acts as painkillers and reduce inflammation.

Glossary

Primary care

Pseudomonas A genus of gram-negative, rod-shaped and polar-flagella bacteria. Most live in soil and decomposing matter.

Secondary care Secondary care can be defined as a service provided by health professionals who generally do not have first contact with patients. Secondary care is usually delivered in hospitals or clinics and patients have usually been referred to secondary care by their primary care provider (usually their GP)

Whole systems approach The process of involving key stakeholders working together in partnership for example clients and their families, professional health and social services. A problem or issue is not the responsibility of one individual or team, but is addressed by working together with the relevant agencies to find solutions. All parties are encouraged to think about the way the whole service delivery system works, rather than focusing only upon their own service.

Index

Note: page references to tables, figures, and diagrams are given in italics